Helping Couples
Get Past the Affair

Helping Couples Get Past the Affair

A Clinician's Guide

Donald H. Baucom
Douglas K. Snyder
Kristina Coop Gordon

THE GUILFORD PRESS
New York   London

© 2009 The Guilford Press
A Division of Guilford Publications, Inc.
72 Spring Street, New York, NY 10012
www.guilford.com

Printed in the United States of America

This book is printed on acid-free paper.

Last digit is print number: 9   8   7   6   5   4   3   2

Library of Congress Cataloging-in-Publication Data
Baucom, Donald H.
    Helping couples get past the affair : a clinician's guide / Donald H. Baucom,
Douglas K. Snyder, and Kristina Coop Gordon.
        p. ; cm.
    Companion to: Getting past the affair / Douglas K. Snyder, Donald H. Baucom,
Kristina Coop Gordon. c2007.
    Includes bibliographical references and index.
    ISBN 978-1-60623-067-1 (alk. paper)
    1. Marital psychotherapy.   2. Adultery.   I. Snyder, Douglas K.   II. Gordon,
Kristina Coop.   III. Snyder, Douglas K. Getting past the affair.   IV. Title.
    [DNLM: 1. Marital Therapy—methods.   2. Extramarital Relations—
psychology.   WM 430.5.M3 B337h 2009]
    RC488.5.B373 2009
    616.89'1562—dc22

                                                                    2008048491

With love and appreciation to our spouses:
Linda, Linda, and Andrew

You have taught us much about commitment
and staying true to our values.

D. H. B.
D. K. S.
K. C. G.

About the Authors

Donald H. Baucom, PhD, is Richard Lee Simpson Distinguished Professor of Psychology at the University of North Carolina at Chapel Hill. His research focuses on couples and marriage, with an emphasis on the integration of basic research and applied treatment outcome investigations and has been funded through grants from the National Institutes of Health and various foundations. Through his approximately 175 publications, Dr. Baucom has helped to shape an understanding of the role of cognitions in intimate relationships, which has contributed to the development of cognitive-behavioral couple therapy. He also helped develop and evaluate the efficacy of couple-based interventions for the treatment of marital distress, recovery from infidelity, prevention of marital discord, enhancement of satisfied relationships, treatment of psychopathology within a couple context, and the application of couple-based interventions to a variety of health problems.

In addition to his empirical investigations, Dr. Baucom has written and edited several books on couple treatment and observational coding of couple interaction, which are fundamental readings for the field. He has served as Associate Editor for *Behavior Therapy* and is on the editorial boards of numerous journals. Dr. Baucom also is a noted teacher, speaker, and mentor. He is the recipient of several awards for excellence in undergraduate teaching and mentoring graduate students as well as the Mary Clarke Award for lifetime contributions to psychology in North Carolina. Dr. Baucom gives workshops throughout the world training professionals in couple therapy, serves as an advocate for individuals with mental health problems, and maintains an active clinical practice working with couples and individuals around relationship difficulties.

Douglas K. Snyder, PhD, is Professor of Psychology and Director of Clinical Training at Texas A&M University in College Station. Nationally recognized for his research on marital assessment and for his outcome research on marital therapy, Dr. Snyder is the author of the widely used Marital Satisfaction Inventory. He has published one of the few controlled studies comparing behavioral with nonbehavioral approaches to couple therapy. A 4-year follow-up study of his couple treatment research funded by the National Institute of Mental Health was recognized by the American Association for Marriage and Family Therapy as the Outstanding Research Contribution in 1991.

Dr. Snyder is coeditor of the books *Treating Difficult Couples* and *Emotion Regulation in Couples and Families*. In 2005, he received an award from the American Psychological Association for Distinguished Contributions to Family Psychology. He is a Fellow in the Divisions of Family Psychology, Clinical Psychology, Psychotherapy, and Evaluation and Measurement of the American Psychological Association; of the Society for Personality Assessment; and of the American Association for Applied and Preventive Psychology. Dr. Snyder has served as Editor of the *Clinician's Research Digest* and as Associate Editor of the *Journal of Consulting and Clinical Psychology* and *Journal of Family Psychology*. He also serves on the editorial boards of numerous clinical psychology and family therapy journals. In addition to his research and teaching, Dr. Snyder maintains a clinical practice emphasizing couple therapy.

Kristina Coop Gordon, PhD, is Associate Professor and Associate Director of Clinical Training in the clinical psychology program at the University of Tennessee–Knoxville. She has served as Vice-President for Science of Division 43 (Family Psychology) of the American Psychological Association and is currently chair of its task force on empirically validated couple and family therapies. Dr. Gordon also has served as copresident of the Association for Behavioral and Cognitive Therapies Couples Research and Therapy Special Interest Group. She has authored numerous articles and book chapters on forgiveness, couple therapy, and dyadic processes in journals such as the *Journal of Family Psychology, Journal of Marriage and the Family, Journal of Marital and Family Therapy*, and *Family Process*. Dr. Gordon conducts research on forgiveness and family processes and also maintains a clinical practice specializing in couple therapy.

Acknowledgments

This book evolved from, and is the culmination of, our clinical experiences, empirical research, discussions with couples, and interactions with numerous colleagues over many years that reflect on how to help couples address significant interpersonal traumas such as infidelity. In all of these contexts, a consensus arose: Healing from infidelity is extremely difficult for couples and presents a significant challenge for couple therapists.

In this book, we recommend that couples take advantage of all possible resources at their disposal to complete the challenging journey before them, and we followed the same advice. At our respective universities and elsewhere, we have extraordinary colleagues and students who stimulate and challenge us, and we thank those individuals who have helped us grow individually and have supported our efforts. Collectively, we have been part of a larger group of colleagues who conduct research on infidelity, and we are especially appreciative to Beth Allen, Dave Atkins, and the late Shirley Glass, who helped us develop the book's overall conceptual framework. This collaboration and other collaborative research have greatly influenced the book.

Once the idea for a book takes shape in the minds of the authors, a strong publishing company becomes an essential partner in the process of turning ideas into a finished product. In our experience, there is no better publisher than The Guilford Press in helping authors to shape the content and presentation of ideas for an intended audience. Our sincere thanks to Kitty Moore, who not only encouraged us to write this book, but also encouraged us to write the 2007 self-help book for couples *Getting Past the Affair: A Program to Help You Cope, Heal, and Move On—Together or Apart.* Jim Nageotte was a superb editor for this book, shepherding it through every step in the process, with the very able assistance of Jane Keislar and developmental editor Barbara Watkins. Three anonymous reviewers provided insightful feedback on the manuscript, which contributed significantly to the quality of the book.

Over the life of a relationship, many things change yet many things remain constant. Fortunately for all three of us, what is important in our home lives remained unchanged. We began formally thanking and acknowledging our spouses in our doctoral dissertations many years ago, and our appreciation continues today. Linda, Linda, and Andrew, you did it again, which allowed us to do it again! We especially thank Linda Baucom, who not only kept Don on course personally but, by using her professional editorial skills in revising the entire book, brought it to a higher level of literacy and readability. Wonderful partners are hard to find; we are blessed to have them in our lives.

Preface

This book is about healing. For individuals in a committed relationship such as marriage, few statements carry more pain than "My partner is involved with someone else." For many injured individuals, this statement reflects a recognition that a lifelong dream of love and commitment has been shattered. For others, it brings to the forefront a sense of being taken advantage of, deceived, or duped. Yet for some individuals, there is a sense of self-blame: "Where did I fail? What did I do wrong? How did I fall short as a partner?" For many injured partners, these and other ideas race through their minds as they struggle to understand what happened, at times forming a cacophony of confused thoughts that leave them feeling overwhelmed and shaken to the core. A multitude of emotions accompany these beliefs, including anger, sadness, fear, anxiety, guilt, and shame, at times alternating with a sense of numbness. Everyday life is disrupted as the injured person is preoccupied with his or her partner's infidelity. Routine interactions with the partner that previously formed the fabric of daily life have ceased to function as familiar patterns of sleeping, eating, and exercising have been disrupted. Similarly, the partner who has had the affair is frequently in turmoil and must deal with what he or she has done. For some individuals, facing this reality arouses a strong sense of guilt and remorse. For others, it raises fears of losing a long-term partner, of having to endure the embarrassment of public disclosure, or of becoming entangled in legal battles. For still others, on an immediate basis, there may be a sense of relief that the affair is finally out in the open and no longer a secret. For the couple, intense arguments often ensue, as well as threats, withdrawal, disengagement, or countless discussions of "Why did you do it? What were you thinking?" When such couples seek assistance from a therapist, not only do the couples often feel lost, overwhelmed, and out of control, but many therapists do as well. Treating couples who have experienced infidelity is an extremely complex and demanding clinical task, and couple therapists agree that it is one of the hardest clinical problems they face. Therapists themselves frequently are unsure of what to do when a couple arrives feeling shattered and alienated at a time that is often one of the most difficult and confusing the couple has ever experienced.

This book is intended for clinicians who work with these couples. It presents a road map to guide the clinician through this difficult terrain, providing broad principles to consider over the course of treatment, along with specific interventions to use when addressing various aspects of treatment. The treatment unfolds in three stages from (1) helping couples deal with the immediate crisis when the affair is acknowledged or first becomes known, to (2) helping them understand the major factors that contributed to the partner's decision to have an affair and that likely need to be addressed, to (3) helping them move ahead with their lives, either together as a couple or as separate individuals. In some instances, they will decide to move forward together as a couple. Other couples will decide to end the relationship, sometimes because the affair itself has taken too large a toll on the relationship and sometimes because the process of exploring the reasons for the affair has led one or both partners to recognize that the relationship is not healthy. Our task as clinicians is to help couples make wise decisions about how to proceed in life, whether it is together or apart, to help them implement the specific behaviors needed to achieve their goals, and ultimately to help them heal.

We hope that this book will assist clinicians who espouse a range of theoretical orientations. By emphasizing broad principles of treatment and goals that need to be established to help couples heal, the treatment can be adapted to different theoretical approaches, as long as these broad goals are addressed. For example, the major goal of Stage 2 of treatment is to help couples understand the variety of factors that contributed to the partner's decision to have an affair. To help couples achieve this goal, we often teach them a variety of communication skills and guide them through conversations. Other therapists might choose to help couples explore these same factors without the use of a skills-based approach. Throughout the book, we describe a wide range of specific interventions and strategies that clinicians might use to achieve these broader goals. Consistent with our own approach to clinical work, we also suggest exercises, assignments, or alternative ways in which couples might put into effect in their daily lives what is being discussed during treatment sessions.

We believe that the best clinical work typically is performed by a thoughtful, insightful clinician who is well informed generally about the clinical phenomenon being addressed, who understands the nuances of a particular couple's relationship, and who has access to a treatment model that is realistic for clinical settings and is grounded in sound research. This book is designed to equip the clinician in all three domains. Hence Part I presents an overview of infidelity and brings the clinician up to date on recent research, thus providing a thorough understanding of the clinical phenomenon. Here we also explain how to assess a couple who is presenting with an affair and how to create a therapeutic atmosphere in which to work with the couple successfully during this difficult phase in their relationship, thus individualizing treatment planning. Parts II, III, and IV correspond to the three stages involved in the treatment, which is informed by basic research on infidelity, trauma, and forgiveness. We have integrated findings from basic research with findings from two bodies of treatment-outcome research: (1) studies examining cognitive-behavioral and insight-oriented approaches to couple therapy in general, and (2) outcome research based on the infidelity treatment described in the book. The product of this integration is a model for understanding infidelity, a well-defined set of treatment goals and therapeutic principles, and a set of specific clinical interventions to help achieve these goals.

As authors, we view ourselves as "couple specialists" who have developed a theoretical model of infidelity derived from many years of basic and treatment research on infidelity, and who are practicing clinicians working with couples who have experienced affairs. We also have a passion for teaching, presenting, and learning from other professionals; this book is born from that passion.

Our self-help book *Getting Past the Affair: A Program to Help You Cope, Heal, and Move On—Together or Apart* (Guilford Press, 2007) is intended for couples to read and use on their own in addressing an affair. Likewise, this book can be used on its own by a clinician to guide a couple through treatment and does not require the use of the self-help book. Yet, since both books are based on the same treatment model, they can be used effectively in tandem. For this purpose we cross-reference, at the end of each chapter, supplemental reading material and exercises from the self-help book that can be assigned to the couple to be completed between sessions.

We began the model building, research, and development of our clinical treatment for infidelity many years ago, because we felt that our own knowledge was lacking and the state of the field was insufficient to equip us to deal with this vitally important yet complex clinical phenomenon. As we say to couples who have experienced infidelity, "This is a process; it takes time to

work through such a difficult, complex set of experiences." We remind ourselves of this same notion while we, as clinicians, strive to understand how
best to assist couples who are urgently asking for help when they are in crisis
following an affair. Writing this book has helped us to clarify for ourselves
what that clinical path looks like. We hope that after reading this book, your
path too will be straighter, shorter, and better illuminated as you help couples
heal from this most difficult experience of infidelity.

DONALD H. BAUCOM
DOUGLAS K. SNYDER
KRISTINA COOP GORDON

Contents

PART FOUR. STAGE 3 OF TREATMENT

PART ONE

PREPARING FOR TREATMENT

CHAPTER 1

Conceptualizing an Integrative Treatment for Affair Couples

Infidelity is one of the most destructive and common crises that couples face. Previous surveys indicate that 21% of men and 11% of women will engage in sexual infidelity during their lifetime, and evidence suggests that these rates are rising and the gender gap is narrowing (Lauman, Gagnon, Michael, & Michaels, 1994). Considering the profound betrayal of trust and the relationship trauma that infidelity typically produces, it is no wonder that couple therapists report infidelity as one of the most difficult relationship problems to treat (Whisman, Dixon, & Johnson, 1997).

Portraits of Infidelity

Patterns of infidelity are as diverse as the individuals participating in an affair, their injured partners, and the relationships in which infidelity occurs. Consider these snapshots:

- Gary and Heather both report a happy marriage of 15 years. Heather recently learned that Gary has been having an affair for the past year with a business associate in another town. Neither partner wants a divorce, but Gary doesn't want to end his other relationship.
- For several years, Miriam has asked Noah to go to couple therapy to pursue a more intimate marriage. After years of frustration, she

recently pursued a sexual relationship with a divorced father she met at her daughter's school.

- Keisha learned 2 months ago that her husband, Marcus, had a one-night sexual encounter with an old girlfriend after a wild bachelor party with friends at work. Marcus has expressed profound regret, but Keisha finds it difficult even to be around him.
- Colin has had three affairs in the past 5 years, each lasting a few months and each ending with a promise never to be unfaithful again. Maggie doesn't want to end their marriage but has lost confidence in Colin's commitment or ability to change.
- Laura has been married for 35 years and enjoys excellent health and a vibrant attitude toward life. Her husband, Ben, 7 years older than Laura, has been depressed for 5 years but refuses treatment. Recently, Laura pursued an affair with a kind, passionate widower who has no desire to establish a committed relationship or to intrude into Laura's marriage.
- Five years ago, Randy discovered Amy's affair, which she quickly ended. They both pledged to put her affair behind them and never discuss it again. Since then, their marriage has become progressively less intimate, with periodic conflicts erupting for no apparent cause. They report staying together primarily for their children's sake.
- Kayla recently pursued individual therapy after discovering that her husband, Finlay, has been leading a double life with another woman for the past 10 years. She is in shock and feels so profoundly depressed that she can barely get out of bed in the morning.
- Mark recently discovered that his wife, Tanya, had developed an Internet relationship with a man she had never met, who lives 2 hours away. Their recent e-mails revealed plans to meet in 2 weeks at an out-of-town hotel. When confronted, Tanya told Mark that she hadn't yet decided whether to carry out the plan.

Although the contexts within which infidelity occurs vary widely, both clinical observations and empirical investigations confirm that the discovery or disclosure of an affair typically has devastating consequences and can disrupt the emotional and behavioral functioning of both partners. Even experienced couple therapists frequently feel at a loss and have no clear or effective treatment plan for such couples. Standard couple interventions typically used with distressed couples might be insufficient, and no single set of interventions is likely to be effective for all couples, in part because the dynamics of affair couples can vary so dramatically, as the previous vignettes demonstrate. Some couples, particularly those in the very early stages after an affair is discovered, can be behaviorally and emotionally out of control; these couples require extensive containment and problem solving to control the damage and to avoid making the situation worse. On the other hand, some couples present as emotionally distant and disengaged, in which case strategies to uncover emotions and explore underlying conflicts might be necessary. Given the complexity of this presenting problem, many clinicians find themselves feeling as overwhelmed and frustrated as the couples they are treating.

Difficulties in Treating Affair Couples

What makes treating affair couples so difficult? There are many possible reasons. First, in the initial stage after discovery of an affair, couples are likely to be extremely dysregulated. Clinicians report that, for the injured partners, intense emotions often vacillate between rage directed toward the participating partner and inner feelings of shame, depression, powerlessness, victimization, and abandonment (Abrams-Spring & Spring, 1996; Brown, 1991). Moreover, the emotional upheaval that these couples often experience may impair their ability to think clearly, making it difficult for them to process and integrate new information and insights offered in treatment.

The dynamics of partners also can be confusing as they fluctuate between positions of victimization and vindication. Although infidelity seems to lend itself to the identification of a clear "victim" and "perpetrator," partners who participate in an affair may harbor their own resentments, hurts, or experiences of betrayal at the hands of the injured partner. Consequently, the participating partner may not be as contrite as the "victim" or therapist might expect, and this apparent lack of remorse may complicate therapy. Alternatively, the participating partner may have tolerated the injured partner's anger or abuse for so long that he or she finally refuses to offer further apology or restitution, potentially altering the power balance as the injured partner now struggles to bring about reconciliation to maintain the relationship.

Partners struggling after an affair can be uncooperative and verbally aggressive with each other and with the therapist. It is not surprising that such couples often display little collaboration, particularly early in treatment; their identity as a couple has been severely damaged, with little remaining trust or willingness to make themselves vulnerable. Although understandable, such behavior renders the therapist's task far more difficult.

Therapists also experience an added sense of urgency with affair couples. When partners are highly dysregulated, there is an acute sense that at any moment their relationship may spin out of control and self-destruct. In response, clinicians feel they need to intervene quickly and effectively to establish some control of the situation, but they often are unsure about where to start or how to proceed. Not uncommonly, people outside the couple's relationship also are intervening in ways that make matters worse. The outside-affair person may be continuing to pursue the affair or harass the couple, and well-meaning family members or friends may be urging the injured partner to leave the relationship, informing others in ways that erode the couple's fragile support network, promoting retaliation rather than efforts toward thoughtful decisions, or informing children in ways that disrupt the broader family's stability.

All the emotional upheaval, distorted thoughts, chaotic behaviors, and social pressures combine to heighten the couple's ambivalence about their relationship, and this ambivalence can make the clinician's job seem impossible. Partners frequently do not know what to expect of each other and themselves during this time, and this lack of predictability becomes even more anxiety provoking. They often are unsure whether to embrace or withdraw, to sleep together or in separate rooms, to pretend everything is okay, or to pretend that their partners do not exist. They lack a basic "map" of how to navigate this uncharted territory, and often the therapist does as well. Thus, it is not surprising that affairs are considered one of the most difficult relationship problems to treat.

Couples who have experienced an affair initially present with myriad questions. How did the affair develop? How could this happen? How can they come to trust each other again or move beyond their profound hurt? How can they ever feel safe again in their relationship? Will their lives ever return to normal? Helping couples address and resolve such critical questions requires that, as a therapist, you have a thorough understanding of what is known about affairs—their prevalence, their various patterns and trajectories—and ways of intervening effectively to guide couples through the difficult process of recovery. You need to help couples understand and cope with what they are experiencing in the moment. You also need to help them develop a clear and complete understanding of how they reached this crisis and then offer them an explicit strategy for how to work through the crisis and move on. This book presents the collective wisdom we have gained in working with affair couples over a combined 60 years of clinical experience and research on this topic. Although it cannot provide all the answers, we are confident this book does offer basic knowledge and a working conceptualization that will guide you in working with couples in these very difficult circumstances.

Current Knowledge: What Is Known about Infidelity?

Affairs Occur with a High Frequency

As we noted earlier, representative community surveys indicate a lifetime prevalence of sexual infidelity of approximately 21% among men and 11% among women (Lauman et al., 1994). Broadening infidelity to encompass emotional as well as sexual affairs increases these rates to 44% and 25%, respectively (Glass & Wright, 1997). Nationally representative samples indicate that, in any given year, between 0.6% and 1.5% of married individuals will engage in extramarital sexual activity (e.g., Lauman et al., 1994; Prins, Buunk, & Van Yperen, 1993; Whisman, Gordon, & Chatav, 2007; Whisman & Snyder, 2007). Infidelity is the most frequently cited cause of divorce (Amato & Rogers, 1997), with approximately 40% of divorced individuals reporting at least one extramarital sexual contact during their marriage (Janus & Janus, 1993). Clearly, extramarital sexual activity is a prevalent problem for couples and one that both individual and couple therapists are likely to encounter.

Affairs Occur for Many Different Reasons

To understand how and why affairs occur, we and our colleagues have developed a conceptual framework that systematically examines multiple domains of potential contributing factors across different time periods in the development, maintenance, and resolution of an affair (Allen et al., 2005). This framework is presented in Table 1.1, along with examples of the diverse factors that can influence the likelihood of an affair as well as partners' subsequent recovery.

Various characteristics in the couple's relationship can increase the likelihood that an affair might develop or that recovery might be more difficult. Most obvious are high levels of conflict and low levels of emotional or sexual intimacy (Atkins, 2003). More subtle influences include imbalances of power, discrepant expectancies regarding partners' roles, or lack of a common long-term vision for the marriage (e.g., Edwards & Booth, 1976; Prins et al., 1993; Treas & Giesen, 2000). In addition to serving as initial risk factors, chronic relationship conflict or emotional distance can also interfere with efforts to end the affair or with the partners' efforts toward recovery. Restoring trust and security in a marriage after infidelity is difficult enough, but it becomes even more challenging when the requisite skills of exchanging intimate feelings and negotiating the resolution of relationship conflicts are deficient. Although frequently contributing to the risk of infidelity, marital distress is far from being a necessary precursor to an affair; at least 56% of men and 34%

TABLE 1.1. Organizational Framework and Exemplars for Exploring Factors Related to Development of and Response to an Affair

Variable	Predisposing factors ("setting the stage")	Approach factors ("slippery slope")	Precipitating factors ("crossing the line")	Maintenance of extramarital relationship	Disclosure or discovery	Response: short and long term
Marriage or primary relationship	High conflict; low emotional warmth; neglect of pleasure	Anger and retreat	Increases in conflict or emotional distance	Increases in distress or conflict	Change in distress or in anticipated outcome	Conflict containment; gains in emotional expressiveness
Outside context	Role models; job demands	Increasing reinforcement from flirtations	Advances from outsider; "ideal" opportunity	Supportive peer environment; pleasure isolated to other	Threats of disclosure by other	Appropriate boundaries with other; social support
Person participating in affair	Insecurities about sexual self; pursuit of excitement	Denial of risks	Ambivalence about marriage; disinhibition; rationalizations	Increases in self-esteem; excitement; low guilt	Guilt; fear of discovery; pursuit of change	Reduced investment in the marriage; intolerance of partner's distress
Injured partner	Discomfort with closeness	Avoidance of relationship difficulties	Refusal to engage in couple therapy; threats to end marriage	Reluctance to confront partner or demand change	Increased vigilance or decreased avoidance	Emotional regulation; beliefs about forgiveness

of women who have participated in an affair report having been happily married at the time (Glass & Wright, 1997).

Couples with strong, healthy relationships also can experience increased vulnerability to an affair when their relationship is subjected to prolonged or overwhelming stress. Common stressors, such as demands from work or family responsibilities, financial strains, or physical health concerns, can erode the foundations of a relationship when they combine or persist over an extended time period. Individuals can become more susceptible to having an affair when they spend too little time with persons who encourage and support faithful and committed relationships or too much time with persons who undermine such values. Of particular risk is a partner's frequent exposure to situations or persons who provide opportunities for or actively encourage emotional or sexual involvement outside the marriage, including but not restricted to the outside-affair person (e.g., Atwood & Seifer, 1997; Buunk & Bakker, 1995; Lusterman, 1997; Vaughn, 1998). Healthy social support, or its absence, can also exert a powerful influence on partners' recovery, either buffering or exacerbating the emotional turmoil that follows discovery of an affair.

Either partner may bring individual characteristics into the relationship that place it at greater vulnerability to an affair or make recovery from infidelity more difficult. For the participating partner who has the affair, such characteristics can include enduring insecurities about him- or herself, high levels of sensation seeking or need for novelty, poor judgment or impulse control, lack of commitment or strong relationship values, and conflict avoidance leading to a denial of a relationship or outside factors threatening fidelity (e.g., Atwood & Seifer, 1997; Ellis, 1969; Glass & Wright, 1992; Greene, Lee, & Lustig, 1974). Similar factors can influence the participating partner's decision to disclose the affair or to end it once it becomes known. Also essential to recovery are participating partners' readiness to reinvest in their marriage and their capacity to tolerate their injured partner's emotional distress after discovery of the affair (Allen et al., 2005).

Various characteristics of injured partners also may influence either the vulnerability of their relationship to an affair or its subsequent recovery. We are careful to emphasize repeatedly to the couples with whom we work that no one is ever responsible for a partner's decision to have an affair. We strive diligently to ensure that the injured partner does not receive blame for the participating partner's choices. However, it is equally important to recognize and address the various ways in which injured partners have contributed to their relationship that potentially rendered it more vulnerable to an affair. For example, injured partners may exhibit enduring self-doubts that interfere with emotional or physical intimacy. They may lack emotion regulation or communication skills essential to working through difficult relationship conflicts. They may fear conflict and retreat from relationship problems in ways that cause the problems to linger and fester. Such characteristics potentially place a relationship at greater risk for an affair and can also compromise the couple's ability to work through the profound challenges of recovery. Unfortunately, perhaps because of the fear of "blaming the victim," very little research has been conducted on this topic; hence, much of what is understood about the contributions of injured partners stems primarily from clinical observations.

In struggling to recover from infidelity, couples need to develop a shared understanding of how the affair came about. Injured partners need such an understanding to regain a sense of security in their relationship. Participating partners need to work toward this understanding for their partners' sake but also to understand their own decisions to become involved in an affair. Developing a shared formulation of the affair is essential to addressing and resolving factors that initially increased the vulnerability of the couple's relationship. Couples often feel lost during this process, and sometimes they accept an oversimplified or inaccurate explanation of the affair as a way of ending their confusion. The framework outlined previously, and described in greater detail throughout this book, promotes a richer understanding for the couple and offers a conceptualization that more effectively guides clinical interventions targeting essential components of the partners' relationship and individual well-being.

Affairs Frequently Have Devastating Consequences

The effects of infidelity can be devastating for the person having the affair and for the partner, their relationship, and others in the immediate or extended family. The partner of the person engaging in an affair often experiences strong negative emotional reactions, including shame, rage, depression, anxiety, a sense of victimization, and symptoms consistent with those seen in posttraumatic stress disorder (PTSD; Beach, Jouriles, & O'Leary, 1985; Cano & O'Leary, 2000; Charny & Parnass, 1995; Glass & Wright, 1997; Gordon & Baucom, 1999; Gordon, Baucom, & Snyder, 2004). The partner participating in the affair also may experience guilt, depression, and negative feelings about him- or herself (Beach et al., 1985; Glass, 2003; Gordon et al., 2004; Spanier & Margolis, 1983; Wiggins & Lederer, 1984).

Affairs are the most commonly reported cause of divorce and are a common precipitant of domestic violence (Amato & Previti, 2003; Daly & Wilson, 1988). Couples entering therapy with issues of infidelity are more likely to separate and divorce relative to other distressed couples presenting for treatment (Glass, 2003), particularly if the husband was the participating partner (Betzig, 1989; Lawson, 1988; Veroff, Douvan, & Hatchett, 1995) . Combined sexual and emotional affairs pose an especially potent threat to the stability of a marriage; in one study, men in couple therapy who engaged in primarily sexual but not emotional affairs rarely left their marriage (Glass, 2003). In a separate study, women who experienced other marital stressors in addition to a major relationship betrayal were significantly more likely to separate or divorce (Cano, Christian-Herman, O'Leary, & Avery-Leaf, 2002).

In summary, although some couples may emerge with stronger marriages after an affair if they use the event as a precipitant to address long-standing relationship issues (e.g., Charny & Parnass, 1995), the more typical consequences of infidelity involve individual and relationship upheaval and distress.

Research also suggests that these adverse effects frequently persist over a long or indefinite period unless partners directly engage in a process focused on understanding and addressing the various factors contributing to the affair as well as its adverse consequences. Our own research indicates that after a relationship injury, persons who fail to demonstrate behaviors, thoughts, and emotional experiences consistent with forgiveness or "moving on" score lower on measures of marital adjustment, closeness, and trust than couples who have worked through and resolved these events (Gordon, Baucom, & Floyd, 2008). Additional findings from a large treatment–outcome project indicate that couple therapy is less likely to be successful when an affair has occurred and this affair remains unknown to the therapist or unaddressed in therapy (Atkins, Yi, Baucom, & Christensen, 2005). Hence, both our clinical experience and research findings suggest that failing to resolve the betrayal of an affair can lead to lasting adverse consequences, and it is important to confront and work through these issues when treating couples.

Treating Affairs and Promoting Recovery: A Three-Stage Approach

Based on theory, research, and clinical observations, we have developed a three-stage model for treating couples struggling with issues of infidelity. Our approach draws on the theoretical and empirical literature regarding responses to trauma (e.g., Janoff-Bulman, 1989; Resick & Calhoun, 2001) as well as interpersonal forgiveness (e.g., Gordon & Baucom, 1998, 2003; Gordon, Baucom, & Snyder, 2000). A brief overview of this model is given here, and a more comprehensive version and the accompanying research are available in our other publications (Baucom, Gordon, Snyder, Atkins, & Christensen, 2006; Gordon & Baucom, 1998, 2003; Gordon et al., 2004) .

We define major betrayals as negative, *traumatic* events that significantly disrupt spouses' basic beliefs about their relationships, their partners, or themselves. The literature on traumatic responses suggests that people are most likely to become emotionally traumatized when an event violates basic assumptions about how the world and people in general operate (Janoff-Bulman, 1989; McCann, Sakheim, & Abrahamson, 1988; Resick & Calhoun, 2001). The cognitive disequilibrium and emotional dysregulation resulting from an interpersonal trauma such as an affair may be more clearly understood when this trauma model is applied. Several vital marital assumptions may be violated by an affair, including the assumptions that partners can be trusted, that the relationship is safe and secure, and that partners can trust their judgments about each other. The trauma literature also suggests that when such basic assumptions are violated, the traumatized person often considers the future to be less predictable and consequently experiences a loss of control, leading to increased feelings of anxiety and depression (e.g., Joseph, Yule, & Williams, 1993; McCann et al., 1988).

These observations from the trauma literature map well onto the confusion, anger, loss, and anxiety expressed by couples who are struggling in the aftermath of an affair. For example, consider the case of Vicki and Bill, one of three couples we follow throughout this book (along with Pam–Tom and Gail–Brad). Vicki and Bill met through their former place of business, where they sold real estate. Vicki was lively, smart, and energetic, and Bill was more than her match. They enjoyed talking with each other and never seemed to run out of topics to discuss. Each could make the other laugh easily, and they shared a similar vision of what they wanted in life. Both were divorced with young children, all the kids got along well, and little conflict occurred when Bill and Vicki decided to marry and blend their families. Vicki, who had been ignored and emotionally abused in previous relationships, felt cherished by Bill. Bill felt that Vicki was the woman he was meant to be with and agreed with her that their early days were remarkably easy and warm. Even the birth of their son a year after their marriage was smooth, causing little disruption.

Bill and Vicki eventually decided to establish a real estate agency together. In the initial rush of the venture, their excitement carried them through a few minor arguments about business decisions. However, as the arguments became more frequent, each of them began to have trouble leaving these experiences at work. When they added a third partner to help manage the business's growth, the arguments intensified; Bill often felt that Vicki took the new partner's side over his. To complicate matters, Vicki's remaining parent, her alcoholic father, died under suspicious circumstances. Vicki became depressed, and Bill tried to support her but did not know what to do. During this time, he began to confide in a sympathetic mutual friend in their Sunday school class. Initially, Bill's intention was to gain a female point of view regarding his problems with Vicki, but the relationship eventually became emotionally intimate, and sexual intimacy soon followed.

Vicki attributed Bill's increasing distance to their arguments at work and stress regarding the business. However, late one night when Bill was asleep and Vicki was working on the business records using Bill's computer, she received a flirtatious instant message addressed to Bill. With her heart pounding, she replied, posing as Bill, and was horrified as the message became more sexually explicit in a manner suggesting that the writer knew her husband intimately. After a sleepless night, Vicki confronted Bill, who initially denied the relationship. Vicki then hired a private investigator, who discovered evidence of a relationship with a woman from their church. When faced with this evidence, Bill confessed the relationship and vowed to end it. Vicki and Bill decided to seek marital counseling to try to reestablish their relationship of 10 years, which was now shattered.

Upon entering treatment, Vicki expressed the feeling that she no longer felt that she knew Bill. Did he still love her? Did he ever love her? Could she trust him with the children? Could she believe anything he said? Long-held beliefs about the dependability and safety of the relationship were destroyed. Consequently, she alternated between shock and rage toward Bill and the other woman. She refused to sleep with Bill, questioned him endlessly about the affair and his motives, and stayed up many nights worrying about the future of their relationship and her family, even though he repeatedly expressed a desire to remain with her. She even questioned the happiness that they had initially experienced in their relationship. As Bill tearfully confessed in the first therapy session, Vicki said that she felt as if "the whole book of our marriage has been rewritten." She felt that she could no longer count on anything in their relationship.

The general conceptualization of affairs as traumatic, including the violation of important relationship assumptions, also means that not all affairs will be experienced as traumatic or will fit the model being proposed. The model that we introduce predicts that only those affairs resulting in major disruptions in couples' belief systems about themselves, their relationships, and their partners are likely to create a level of distress that could be termed traumatic. Preliminary findings provide some support regarding the association between trauma and violated assumptions: As the partners' assumptions about each other and themselves become more negative after the discovery of an affair, they become more likely to endorse trauma symptoms on a well-established measure of PTSD (Gordon, Dixon, Baucom, & Snyder, 2007). Furthermore, a similar implication of this model is that couples for whom affairs are expected or part of the cultural model of marriage would not be as likely to find affairs as traumatic and would be less likely to present in a therapist's office with trauma symptoms after the discovery of an affair. In the case of Vicki and Bill, although Vicki had experienced emotional abuse in previous relationships, Bill had seemed to be the exception, a man with whom she could feel safe and secure. She expected a great deal from him and their relationship and believed he would behave in a manner consistent with her best interests; therefore, the discovery of his deceit was extremely distressing and unexpected, which made it even more painful for her. Vicki heartily agreed that the discovery of the affair had been traumatic for her. Bill even felt it had been traumatic for him because it had disrupted his view of himself. He repeatedly asked himself how he could have inflicted so much pain on someone he cared about so deeply; he questioned why he would choose to act in a manner so inconsistent with his own values.

Conceptualizing affairs as potentially interpersonally traumatic events provides useful implications for planning effective therapy with these couples (Gordon, Baucom, & Snyder, 2005; Snyder, Baucom, & Gordon, 2007). For example, many of the responses observed in injured partners during the aftermath of an affair can be seen as resulting from disruption of their basic beliefs and their strong need to reconstruct a shattered worldview, all the while protecting themselves from further interpersonal harm. Thus, Vicki's excessive questioning of Bill can be seen as an attempt to understand what happened and make sense of the traumatic event. If recovery from an affair is conceptualized as a response to an interpersonal trauma, then the recovery process can be understood as unfolding in three major stages that parallel the stages involved in the traumatic response (Horowitz, 1985): (1) absorbing and addressing the traumatic impact of the affair; (2) constructing meaning for why the affair occurred; and (3) moving forward with life within the context of this new understanding. The following descriptions summarize couples' typical experiences during each stage of response to infidelity. This conceptualization forms the basis for the interventions that are described in detail throughout the rest of this book. More specifically, our treatment discusses how to assist couples in addressing problems and challenges at each of these stages. The following section outlines the conceptual model, provides a brief description of the kinds of interventions used, and indicates the types of therapies from which these interventions are drawn (e.g., cognitive–behavioral, developmental/affective–reconstructive, and forgiveness therapies).

Stage 1

In the first stage of the recovery process, the *impact stage*, the partners are attempting to comprehend what has happened. However, given that betrayals are unexpected and often have major implications for the injured person's well-being, this process usually is accompanied by an overwhelming array of emotions, such as fear, hurt, and anger, which can alternate with a sense of numbness or disbelief. As injured partners experience strong emotions or become emotionally dysregulated, they may find themselves acting in ways that are erratic or uncharacteristic. As described previously, all persons have assumptions about how their world and relationships function, and they expect themselves and their partners to behave accordingly. An affair disrupts these basic beliefs because the injured partners can no longer predict what will happen in the relationship or how the participating partner will behave. Their bonds of trust and emotional security have been shattered. As a result, their understandings of who their partners are and how to understand their partners are greatly disrupted, and well-established daily patterns of behavior become questioned or reinterpreted. For example, after thinking nothing of it for many years, an injured partner might now ask, "Why does she really get up early to check her e-mail?" Similarly, even the persons who engaged in the affair experience disruptions in their own beliefs about themselves and their relationships; many people who have affairs generally report that affairs are wrong (Greeley, 1994). Therefore, many people are acting outside of their own value system when they have an affair and experience a similar upheaval and loss of predictability; they begin to question themselves at times. As a result, the interactions between the partners are often chaotic, intensely negative, and likely to lead to further frustration and anger rather than feelings of resolution.

Given that the injured partner's sense of safety and trust typically has been violated, injured partners often retreat or establish barriers and boundaries to protect themselves. This strategy might involve responses such as sleeping in a different room, no longer sharing events of the day, and having little physical contact. Further, in an attempt to reconstruct their understanding of their partners and their relationships and thus reestablish some sense of safety, injured partners often obsessively question participating partners about the affair. However, because of the deleterious effects of negative emotion on information processing (e.g., Howell & Conway, 1992; Karney, Bradbury, Fincham, & Sullivan, 1994; Singer & Salovey, 1988; Sullivan & Conway, 1991), the strong emotions that dominate this stage often make it more difficult for the injured partners to process the information and work toward a better understanding of why the affair occurred.

Furthermore, the injured person may perceive that the balance of power in the relationship has shifted. The participating or offending partner may now appear to have more power, particularly if the injured partner feels victimized or if the outside third person is still seen as a potential threat to the relationship. In an attempt to correct this imbalance, the injured partner may lash out in destructive ways. For example, an injured partner may send demeaning letters about the participating spouse to colleagues at work or demand that the partner perform extraordinary tasks to "even the score," such as quit his or her job as a way of terminating contact with the outside-affair person. On the other hand, participating partners might experience a loss of power in their relationships as well. Given their major transgressions, they often feel that they now have no negotiating power in the relationship in any domain and must go along with whatever the injured partner wants or demands. They clearly are in the "doghouse" with little basis to complain about anything. As a result, interactions between the partners are particularly difficult to negotiate.

The emotional, cognitive, and behavioral upheavals that often characterize Stage 1 call for specific interventions targeting difficulties commonly experienced by partners during this initial phase of response to trauma, all of which are addressed in the following chapters. These include (1) setting clear and strong boundaries on how partners interact with each other and with persons outside their relationship; (2) promoting essential self-care by attending to physical well-being as well as both social and spiritual support; (3) teaching time-out and venting techniques as a way of regulating difficult negative emotions; (4) facilitating emotional expressiveness and empathic listening regarding the impact of the affair, along with offering a rationale for the importance of this process; (5) problem solving on immediate crises that demand a solution; and (6) helping both partners to recognize and cope with reexperiencing or "flashback" phenomena, including intense feelings, images, or recollections of the affair. Chapters 4–6 describe in detail the treatment strategies designed to help the couple contain the turmoil that frequently follows discovery of an affair and prepare to explore factors contributing to the affair. The techniques used in this stage tend to be more directive in order to help couples deal with their strong emotions and related behavior. Although some uncovering and exploratory techniques are used in helping the partners express their emotions and reactions surrounding the discovery of the affair, we have drawn largely from enhanced cognitive–behavioral couple therapy (Epstein & Baucom, 2002) to assist couples during this stage of recovery, although therapists from other orientations can achieve important goals of this stage using other techniques.

Stage 2

In the second phase of recovery, the *meaning stage*, the couple's primary task is to explore more thoroughly why the event occurred and place it in a more understandable context. Gaining new understanding about the affair and developing new assumptions about the relationship are critical for the couple to restore severed emotional bonds and move forward. Giving a traumatic experience some kind of "meaning," or coming to some understanding of "why" it happened, helps persons to move on from the event (Horowitz, Stinson, & Field, 1991; Resick & Calhoun, 2001). Therefore, the second stage of recovery involves seeking richer and more coherent narratives about why the traumatic event occurred; these are needed to replace the more negative, malicious, and often simplistic explanations often generated in Stage 1, such as "You did this just to destroy me" or "I now realize you are a total liar and always have been." This new, more thorough narrative and conceptualization help injured partners reevaluate and reconstruct their disrupted beliefs about their relationships, and in that process they begin to restore a capacity for attachment and regain some sense of predictability in their lives. Knowing why the affair happened gives both partners the ability to try to prevent it from happening again, eventually deciding either to stay together and make needed changes or to terminate an unhealthy relationship that cannot be repaired. Thus, a more thorough understanding of the affair can prepare the couple to "move on." Additionally, the search for a new understanding of the causes of the betrayal might allow the injured partner to experience more empathy and compassion for the participating partner, particularly if it becomes clear that the partner was acting out of his or her own past developmental needs or injuries.

This second stage comprises the heart of our treatment and demands the greatest amount of time. Couples need a road map for recovering trust and intimacy. Injured partners in particular need ways to restore emotional security and reduce their fear of further betrayal to the degree that these outcomes are realistic. Both partners often crave mechanisms for restoring trust: injured partners for regaining it and participating partners for instilling it. Reestablishing security is an essential precursor to letting go, forgiving, or moving on emotionally, either together or apart. Following an affair, couples who fail to restore security either remain chronically distant and emotionally aloof, craft a fragile working alliance marked by episodic intrusions of mistrust or resentment, or eventually end their relationship in despair.

The specific components comprising Stage 2 interventions are described in detail in Chapters 7–12. The conceptual model for examining potential contributing factors to affairs described earlier provides an organizational framework for interventions in this stage of recovery. As the therapist, you will guide partners in examining aspects of their relationship, stresses from outside the relationship, and issues specific to each of the partners for their potential role as predisposing or precipitating influences leading up to the affair, factors impacting maintenance of the affair and eventual discovery or disclosure, and influences bearing on partners' subsequent responses or recovery. The techniques we have used in this stage of treatment are largely cognitive or insight oriented and are drawn from cognitive–behavioral couple therapy, insight oriented couple therapy, or affective–reconstructive therapy (Snyder, 1999). Again, a variety of theoretical orientations and therapeutic interventions can be called upon as long as they help couples derive a clearer, more balanced perspective on why the affair occurred – the major goal of Stage 2. For example, emotionally focused couple therapy (e.g., Johnson & Denton, 2002) and integrative behavioral couple therapy (Jacobson & Christensen, 1996b) offer couples a variety of strategies to explore their understanding for why various events have occurred in their relationship.

After potential contributing factors have been examined across various domains, the therapist assists the couple in integrating the disparate pieces of information they have gleaned into a coherent narrative that explains how the affair came about. Developing a shared understanding of why the affair occurred is central to partners' gaining a new set of assumptions about themselves, each other, and their relationship. After constructing a shared narrative of the affair, you and the couple will examine what changes might be needed in several domains—each partner as an individual, their relationship, and how they relate to their environment—to allow them to move forward into the future, either together or separately. In this respect, the therapy begins to move from a focus on the past to a focus on the present and future of the relationship.

Stage 3

In the third, or *moving-on, stage*, partners must learn to move beyond the event and no longer allow it to control their lives. After developing a realistic narrative for why an event occurred, couples may feel more capable of putting the event behind them because they now have a better understanding of what needs to happen to allow them to move forward. However, for many couples, moving on from an affair means wrestling with the idea of forgiveness. In the current conceptualization, forgiveness of an affair involves moving forward by giving up the right to punish the partner and by committing to move beyond the negative emotions and thoughts about the event that have dominated one's own life. Furthermore, the understanding gained in Stage 2 often leads to a reevaluation of the partners' lives. At times, this reevaluation may mean altering the relationship or some other aspect of life in significant ways. In some instances, the couple must make decisions regarding whether they can make these alterations and whether they wish to continue with the relationship.

From a psychological perspective, forgiveness does not require reconciliation. One may forgive one's partner and yet still decide that the relationship is unhealthy and that the best outcome is to end the relationship. Furthermore, forgiveness does not require that anger disappear completely. In fact, it is expected that the emotions and thoughts associated with the event will recur, in a form similar to that of PTSD flashbacks or lesser forms of reexperiencing. However, concurrent with forgiveness or moving on, these thoughts and feelings will no longer be as severe or as disruptive as they once were, and the individual is able to move beyond them more quickly. Couples often have beliefs about forgiveness that impede their ability to grant or receive it; part of the therapist's work of this stage is to help couples to examine these beliefs. For example, during Stage 3 of therapy, one husband expressed fear that forgiving his wife, who had the affair, was "weak," a viewpoint that also was held by his family. After an exploration of various definitions of forgiveness, described in Chapter 13, the husband decided that he could choose to forgive his wife from a position of strength and that his choice to forgive did not mean that he condoned her action or gave her permission to "walk all over him." Therapeutic strategies used during this stage of treatment draw on the developing body of literature surrounding interventions promoting forgiveness (e.g., Worthington, 2005).

To move forward, the couple needs to achieve three goals by the end of Stage 3: (1) Develop a realistic and balanced view of their relationship; (2) experience a release from being dominated by negative emotion about the event, with the injured partner voluntarily relinquishing the right to punish the participating partner; and (3) evaluate the relationship carefully and make healthy decisions about its continuation.

Interventions in this stage of treatment, found in Chapters 13 and 14, are designed to help the couple address individual or relationship barriers to moving on. For example, partners may report difficulty related to beliefs that forgiving their partner is equivalent to declaring that what happened is acceptable or excusable. Or partners may equate forgiving with literal forgetting or with rendering oneself vulnerable to being injured in a similar way in the future. Sometimes one individual is still dominated by anger about his or her partner (e.g., because of perceived power imbalances after the affair or failure to regain an adequate sense of safety in the relationship). In each of these situations, it is important that as therapist you help both partners explore and work through barriers to achieving emotional resolution so that they can move forward in a healthy manner.

Additional strategies outlined in Chapter 14 help facilitate partners' integration of what they have learned about themselves and their relationship, well beyond the affair, to reach an informed decision about whether to continue in their relationship or move on separately. For couples deciding to move forward together, interventions emphasize additional changes partners will need to undertake either individually or conjointly to strengthen their relationship and reduce influences that potentially make it vulnerable to another affair or other destructive behaviors in the future. If one partner or the other reaches an informed decision to end the relationship, the couple will need help implementing that decision in order to move forward separately in ways that are least hurtful to themselves and others they love, including children, family members, and friends.

Research Support for This Treatment Model

Our model of recovery from an interpersonal trauma such as infidelity described previously has been evaluated in a community sample and appears to be consistent with couples' experiences with forgiveness of major betrayals in their marriages (Gordon & Baucom, 2003). This model of recovery also served as the basis for the treatment described in this book, which we have begun to evaluate empirically. More specifically, our treatment was assessed in an open trial using a series of replicated case studies. Findings from that open trial suggested that two thirds of the couples improved and maintained their gains after treatment (Gordon et al., 2004). In that treatment study, the injured partners demonstrated a level of trauma symptoms in the clinical range at the beginning of the study and significantly decreased their trauma symptoms to below clinical thresholds by the end of the study. Injured partners experienced benefits in other domains as well; that is, their levels of forgiveness, positive assumptions about their partners and themselves, and their empathy for their partners significantly increased, and their levels of anger and marital and psychological distress significantly decreased over the course of treatment. Participating partners also benefited from the intervention. They were distressed personally when treatment began, and their depression decreased notably by the end of treatment. Participating partners also reported that they learned much about themselves and their partners and felt the treatment was valuable in moving on from the affair.

Overall, the study just discussed provided preliminary evidence for the efficacy of this treatment in helping most couples recover and move on from an affair. This treatment incorporates empirically supported interventions from two approaches to treating couple distress: cognitive–behavioral (e.g., cognitive restructuring techniques and communication skills training; Epstein & Baucom, 2002) and insight-oriented (e.g., affective and developmental explorations of unmet needs and relational themes; Snyder, 1999). The American Psychological Association's (APA's) Division 12 task force on empirically supported treatments has determined both approaches to be promising efficacious treatments. For both of these treatments, approximately 70% of couples improve after treatment and 50% are considered to be no longer distressed. Along these lines, new therapies that combine elements of treatments that already have empirical support can be considered to have achieved Level 1 status: evidence-informed intervention/treatment based on recommendations by APA's Division 43 (Family Psychology) task force on identifying evidence-based couple and family treatments (Sexton et al., 2008). Furthermore, many of the techniques used in this intervention have been promoted elsewhere in the clinical literature on the treatment of couples recovering from infidelity. In addition, this approach is the *only* couple-based intervention designed specifically to address both individual and relationship consequences of infidelity that has been empirically examined and supported in clinical research (Gordon et al., 2004).

Thus, although the empirical evidence for this treatment is preliminary at present, it is positive. Further work is needed to evaluate the intervention in a large randomized controlled clinical trial and to compare its effectiveness directly with alternative treatments targeting affairs specifically or relationship distress more generally. Although treatment effect sizes were larger for injured compared with participating partners, this finding is not unexpected given the nature of the traumatic experience for persons learning of their partner's infidelity. Moreover, in narratives regarding the impact of treatment, even participating partners emphasized the positive effects of this intervention in promoting a fuller understanding of themselves and their partners.

Tailoring Treatment: Making This Work for You and Your Clients

To make this treatment manual more user-friendly, rather than presenting a step-by-step, session-by-session treatment manual, we elected to offer a theoretically based, coherent series of principle-driven interventions. This book is designed to describe the rationale underlying our clinical strategies and their timing so that you can understand the theory and the reasoning behind our sequencing of interventions. A clear understanding of the principles underlying this treatment should facilitate your ability to approach the split-second clinical judgments you are often called upon to make in treatment. Additionally, with a good understanding of the basic principles underlying each stage of therapy, you will be able to integrate your own clinical perspectives and skills to achieve goals focal to a given couple.

Therapists will likely approach this book from widely differing backgrounds, theoretical orientations, and training. Despite this variability, we believe that this integrative treatment approach will resonate with most therapists who work with affair couples. This treatment provides enough flexibility that you should be able to tailor the approach to your own style. For example, therapists will likely vary in their use of structure within sessions or homework assignments to achieve the major goals for each stage. They also will likely differ in the relative balance of behavioral- versus insight-oriented strategies used to accomplish various tasks. However, we believe that as long as you are able to accomplish the critical goals for each stage in the treatment model, this treatment approach can be successful across a range of therapeutic styles and theoretical orientations.

This treatment is best followed from beginning to end, because each phase of treatment builds on the previous phase. A clear rationale underlies the content and sequencing of these interventions, as you will discern as you read through this book. However, we are not suggesting that every intervention described here must be implemented with every couple. Chapter 3 describes how you can assess the unique characteristics of partners, their relationship, and their environment in order to focus your treatment efforts effectively. Some couples may be immersed in Stage 1 and require most or all of the interventions listed there, whereas others may need only a few Stage 1 interventions and may be ready to move quickly to Stage 2. The overriding goal is that your interventions with these couples be thoughtfully tailored to the partners' specific needs and that you not omit essential components of the treatment.

We have also written a book entitled *Getting Past the Affair: A Program to Help You Cope, Heal, and Move On—Together or Apart* (Snyder et al., 2007), which is designed for affair couples themselves and can serve as a companion to this treatment manual. This complementary resource for couples adopts a conceptual approach and process for recovery parallel to the one outlined here and includes specific exercises designed to promote partners' understanding and recovery at a deeper level. At the end of each chapter in the current treatment guide, we indicate how to incorporate features from *Getting Past the*

Affair to enhance your treatment with your couple, if you so elect. Although it is not essential to your use of clinical interventions described here, we believe that incorporating this complementary book for affair couples facilitates their work outside of the sessions and provides them with an additional resource as they struggle with difficult challenges between appointments. As such, it can strengthen and enhance your work with them during the sessions.

Finally, it is important to note that this treatment guide presumes that you have already acquired at least a general level of competence in conducting couple therapy. It is beyond the scope of this book to provide more specific training in how to treat general relationship distress or specific couple issues other than affairs. Toward that end, we refer you to a number of excellent texts on couple therapy, including some of our own. Please see the reference list at the end of the book for the titles.

We have written this book based on our clinical experience and research with couples struggling to recover from infidelity. Working with these couples is immensely difficult and yet enormously rewarding when the treatment proceeds in a thoughtful, well-reasoned manner. We anticipate that the treatment approach we describe here will increase your effectiveness, providing both you and your couples with a clear vision and specific steps for recovering from an affair.

CHAPTER 2

Initial Assessment
and Formulation

E ffective treatment of couples struggling with infidelity requires an initial assessment to determine the current status of the partners' own relationship, the extent and nature of interactions with the outside-affair person, the partners' individual strengths and vulnerabilities potentially influencing the recovery process, as well as outside stressors and resources. As we noted in Chapter 1, patterns of infidelity are as diverse as the participants and relationships in which affairs occur. Intervening effectively with affair couples requires that both the therapist and the couple understand where partners currently are in the trauma and healing processes and what factors are likely to influence the course of recovery. The assessment process should answer several critical questions. What do partners need most in order to function during the next few weeks? Based on the couple's history before the affair, as well as characteristics of the outside-affair relationship, what special challenges lie ahead? What unique resources can partners draw upon in themselves, in each other, or outside their relationship to minimize further damage, regain equilibrium, and work toward healthy decisions about moving forward?

In this chapter, we discuss strategies for assessing couples after an affair, aiming toward an initial formulation that provides both you and the couple with a tentative road map for working toward recovery. We emphasize clinical processes and domains of inquiry specific to affair couples, building on more general guidelines for assessing couples. For readers less familiar with basic strategies and techniques for assessing couples, several excellent resources are available (cf. Epstein & Baucom, 2002; Snyder & Abbott, 2002; Snyder, Heyman, & Haynes, 2005).

Obtaining Relevant Information

Initial Considerations

Couples struggling with a recent affair typically enter treatment in crisis. Recognizing this crisis early helps the therapist to gather information essential to promoting stabilization. Sometimes you will know of the affair even before the initial interview because of information provided at the time of scheduling the first session or because of prior contact with one partner. At other times the affair does not become known until the first session. To ensure identifying an affair in the initial session as early as possible, it is useful to ask as a part of introductory comments, "What do you want to make sure that we get to today before we end our session?"

Couples identify affairs as a relationship issue in various contexts. Often, the affair is recent or ongoing and constitutes the overriding concern demanding immediate and primary attention. In this book, treatment of infidelity is presented from this perspective so that the clinician can know what to do from the very beginning when an affair is first discovered or disclosed. However, the affair might have occurred in the remote past, as many as 5 or 10 years earlier. In such instances, it may still be presented as the primary issue, or it may be viewed as only one of many factors related to ongoing conflicts or emotional distance. When the affair was in the more distant past, its effects might still be very strong, yet the immediate turmoil of Stage 1 has long passed. In this instance, much of the work with the couple might begin with what is described in Stage 2 of treatment, which focuses on understanding the various factors that contributed to the context for the affair.

Sometimes a recent or current affair is embedded in a highly conflictual relationship with multiple problems. In this case, the treatment outlined in this book may need to be complemented by more general couple therapy to address relationship issues separate from the affair, and discussion of the infidelity must be integrated with more general interventions for ongoing relationship distress. Focusing only on the affair for several months in an ongoing destructive relationship would be extremely difficult because of the ongoing negative exchanges and therapeutically counterproductive because the couple's relationship would likely continue to deteriorate.

Once you learn of the affair and decide to address it as a focus of treatment, you will need to determine whether you intend to include individual sessions as part of the assessment process and, if so, communicate explicitly your policies for handling issues of confidentiality (see Chapter 3). Cogent arguments can be made for either including or excluding individual interviews. The material that follows does not presume that you follow one format or another. You may work toward completing the assessment in an extended session of 1½–2 hours, or you might separate the initial session from a subsequent formulation/feedback session by brief individual interviews. What is essential is that the assessment process (1) be sufficiently broad to gain an overview of the psychosocial context in which the couple is struggling, (2) target specific issues unique to affairs, and (3) be completed within a short time frame to address immediate needs for crisis containment.

Table 2.1 summarizes important domains to assess and their implications for treatment. By and large, assessment relies heavily on the clinical interview; exceptions involving questionnaires or structured behavioral observations are noted in the table and discussed further in the following sections.

Assessing the Couple's Relationship

As a therapist, you will need to ascertain quickly who the key players are in the couple's lives, how they are interacting currently, and how they have interacted in the past, beginning with the partners themselves. A brief marital history should include information about

- Length of the couple's relationship (before and since marrying).
- Previous marriages, how they ended, and ongoing contact with former spouse(s).
- Children by this or previous marriages and their current living arrangements.
- Previous affairs, separations, or experiences in couple counseling and the circumstances surrounding each of these.

Next, it is important to assess the extent of disruption in partners' basic patterns of interacting, in part to identify issues or crises requiring immediate attention. For example, are the partners still sharing meals or sleeping together? Have their basic ways of connecting either emotionally or physically been disrupted? If they have children, have both partners been able to maintain essential parenting roles, either separately or collaboratively? The couple may need guidelines for engaging on a limited basis or assistance in restoring basic routines such as arranging transportation for their children, ensuring

TABLE 2.1. Initial Assessment Domains, Strategies, and Treatment Implications

Domains	Strategies	Treatment implications
Couple's relationship		
Brief marital history	Clinical interview	Potential need to address (1) parenting arrangements concerning children by this or previous marriages, (2) couple's vulnerability as reflected in premorbid relationship functioning, and (3) anticipated issues related to previous affairs or couple therapy.
• Length of couple's relationship.		
• Previous marriages and how they ended.		
• Children by this or previous marriages.		
• Previous separations or affairs.		
• Previous couple therapy.		
Basic routines	Clinical interview	Restoring basic routines is a prerequisite to building predictability and reducing emotional turmoil. Clarifying intermediate arrangements (e.g., sleeping in separate bedrooms) may promote stability.
• Living and sleeping arrangements.		
• Sharing of meals or family routines.		
• Coparenting of children.		
• Managing routine household tasks.		
Communication patterns	Clinical interview; questionnaires; behavioral observations	Disrupting physical aggression and reducing verbal escalations are essential for constructive dialogue about the affair. Structured behavioral observations may be useful later in Stage 1.
• Decision-making discussions.		
• Sharing of thoughts and feelings.		
• Verbal or physical aggression.		
Relationship sentiment	Clinical interview; questionnaires	Premorbid relationship quality may influence (1) partners' motivation to restore the relationship and (2) the extent to which treatment will need to integrate more general couple therapy.
• Current versus previous relationship quality.		
• Specific areas of conflict.		
• Disclosure of affair to others (e.g., children, extended family, friends).	Clinical interview	Couple may need immediate assistance in decisions about what to disclose to whom and how best to do this
Outside-affair relationship		
Information regarding affair	Clinical interview	Therapy may need to focus initially on facilitating disclosure of basic information regarding status of affair. Partners may need specific direction regarding (1) evaluation of physical health risks and (2) dealing with outsiders who already know about the affair.
• Extent of undisclosed information.		
• When it began, whether it has ended.		
• Whether emotional, sexual, or both.		
• If sexual, whether any instance of unprotected intercourse.		
• Others' knowledge about the affair.		

(continued)

TABLE 2.1. *(continued)*

Domains	Strategies	Treatment implications
Outside-affair relationship *(continued)*		
Information regarding outside person • Nature of ongoing contact. • Marital status or expectations. • Potential adverse reactions of outside person.	Clinical interview	Couple may need assistance in (1) reaching agreement about further contact with the outside person or (2) dealing with outside person's efforts to retain affair or retaliate if it has ended.
Partners' strengths and vulnerabilities		
• Content, intensity, and regulation of negative emotion. • Suicidality. • Alcohol or other substance misuse. • Basic self-care, including nutrition, sleep, exercise, friendships. • Separate physical or emotional health problems.	Clinical interview; questionnaires; behavioral observations	Therapist needs to distinguish between "normative" turmoil after an affair versus frequency or intensity of emotional or behavioral responses that warrant additional interventions. Structured assessment of individual functioning may be useful, depending on partners' reactivity.
Environmental resources and stressors		
• Work-related stresses, particularly those related to affair. • Reactions of family, friends, coworkers. • Social or spiritual support.	Clinical interview	Initial interventions may be needed to constrain external stressors and to identify and draw upon external sources of both individual and relationship support.
Additional considerations		
• Children's emotional/social functioning. • Individual treatment(s). • Couple treatment receptiveness, goals.	Clinical interview	Couple may need assistance in understanding and managing children's responses to the affair. One or both partners may benefit from individual treatment, including psychotropic medications. Depending on partners' respective goals for treatment, additional interventions may be needed to promote collaborative alliance.

that bills are paid, or managing other everyday family and household responsibilities; Chapter 5 addresses how to promote these goals.

What assistance do the partners require immediately for containing turmoil related to the affair, preventing further damage, and reaching decisions
for managing the logistics of their household operations? For example, the
couple may need help in defining boundaries of interacting with one another
as a way of reducing intense negative escalations; Chapter 4 provides guidance on how to work with the couple to contain potential crises and problem-solve difficult interactions. Couples sometimes have enduring conflicts
in areas separate from the affair that may interact with turmoil related to the
affair itself; additional domains of conflict can be assessed in interview or by
questionnaires following the initial interview (see Snyder et al., 2005, for a
review and recommendations regarding such measures).

In eliciting information regarding basic interactions, it is also important
to assess what emotions each partner is experiencing and how well each person is able to regulate those emotions. To what extent does either partner
struggle to manage overwhelming feelings of hurt, anger, fear, loss, guilt, or
shame? Does either partner exhibit undercontrol of emotions in ways that
contribute to spiraling negative exchanges? For example, the participating
partner might be so sensitive to feelings of shame about his or her behavior
that he or she stonewalls the injured partner's efforts to discuss the affair,
which in turn leads the injured partner to escalate attempts to engage the
participating partner in discussions. Conversely, one or both partners may
be unable to access their feelings or may avoid uncomfortable interactions in
ways that prevent the couple from discussing what has happened or how to
begin recovery. Strategies for handling both of these circumstances are provided in Chapter 6.

Couples' capacity to engage constructively in discussions about the affair
or other relationship issues can be observed to some extent during the interview. However, because partners' interactions at home may differ from those
during the session, inquiry should be made about typical or problematic interactions at home as well. Structured observations in which partners are asked
to discuss problem issues on their own for 5–10 minutes without the therapist's
intervention can be useful to elicit more typical patterns of interaction (cf,
Heyman, 2001).

When inquiring about regulating strong feelings, it is critical to assess the
level of partners' verbal and physical aggression and the potential for violence.
The clinical literature reflects considerable divergence on how best to elicit
reliable information about physical violence while promoting partners' safety.

For example, research indicates that some persons experiencing a partner's physical aggression do not disclose this behavior in early interviews because of embarrassment, minimization, or fear of retribution (Ehrensaft & Vivian, 1996). Conversely, arguments against individual interviews for assessing partner violence emphasize potential difficulties in conjoint therapy if one partner has disclosed information to the therapist about which the other partner remains uninformed. We introduce the issue of verbal and physical aggression after initial background information has been obtained, some therapeutic rapport established and the couple has been invited to disclose about conflict-resolution patterns more generally. We then inquire, "During the times when your disagreements or arguments become most heated, does it ever become physical between the two of you—for example, grabbing, shoving, or anything more than that?" We ask each partner in turn and look for nonverbal indications of disagreement or distress as a cue for following up at a later time or using an alternative strategy.

For example, an additional method of assessing for verbal or physical aggression is to include measures of conflict tactics in a standard assessment battery for all couples, for example, the Conflict Tactics Scale (Straus, Hamby, Boney-McCoy, & Sugarman, 1996) or the Aggression Scale of the Marital Satisfaction Inventory—Revised (Snyder, 1997). However, if you choose this questionnaire method, you will still need to decide whether to follow up in a conjoint or an individual interview. Whether assessing for partner violence in either individual or conjoint sessions, it is critical to obtain information about both the frequency and the severity of aggression, to inquire in a tone that conveys concern for both the partners and their relationship, and to be explicit regarding your policies about containing physical aggression as a precondition for conjoint therapy. We refer readers to extended discussions of the complex issues involved in assessing and treating partner violence available elsewhere (e.g., Rathus & Feindler, 2004).

Couples often struggle upon disclosure or discovery of an affair with decisions about whom else to inform of their situation (e.g., children, extended family, friends, coworkers). Ill-advised decisions made early in the midst of chaos can wreak further havoc for months or even years to come. For example, partners' relationships with their children or with their own or each other's extended family can be irrevocably damaged by disclosing information about the affair. Punitive actions aimed at involving the participating partner's employer can produce adverse impact and enduring financial hardship. It is important to assess partners' struggles with such decisions early on and to provide explicit guidelines as needed to help them navigate these issues when present. These guidelines are addressed in Chapter 4.

To demonstrate how we obtain and formulate initial information about the couple's relationship, we use the example of Brad and Gail, another couple we follow throughout the book. This couple sought therapy after Gail's discovery of Brad's affair with a graduate student. Brad and Gail, 35 and 30 years old, respectively, had been married 6 years and had no children. Brad was an anthropology professor and Gail a recently hired instructor in the same department. Brad's affair was with Jill, a 25-year-old doctoral student. After recurrent rumors about Brad and Jill's relationship started to stir among the other students, Gail confronted Brad, but he denied that anything inappropriate was happening. Chaos ensued 2 weeks later when Brad's department head informed him that Jill had filed a formal grievance charging Brad with sexual harassment.

By the time Brad and Gail began couple therapy—a month after Brad's affair with Jill became public—considerable damage had already been done. Brad was already under intense scrutiny at work. He managed to retain his faculty position but was now working under additional constraints imposed by the university. Gail had received an e-mail from a former classmate indicating that rumors about Brad's affair were circulating among their colleagues around the country. At home their lives alternated between isolation and heated arguments. They slept in different rooms. Eventually, Gail insisted that Brad move out and find a place of his own, at least for the next semester. Avoiding each other at work proved more difficult. In the initial session, they agreed to meet separately with their department head to rearrange respective responsibilities so they would not overlap on various committees. Gail wanted to draw on the support of her family by sharing information about Brad's affair but, upon Brad's request and encouragement of the therapist, she agreed for now to tell them only that she and Brad were having marital problems and were going to counseling together.

Assessing the Outside-Affair Relationship

Evaluating both previous and current contact with the outside-affair person is critical to understanding factors that potentially influence the nature of the affair trauma, ongoing sources of continued turmoil, and the likelihood of restoring emotional security in the couple's relationship. Obtaining relevant information can be complicated because, in some cases, the participating partner has not yet disclosed this information to the injured partner. It is important to consider the possible impact of eliciting new disclosures in the initial session because these could exacerbate the couple's turmoil before they have decided whether to continue with couple therapy. Balancing efforts to obtain information and protect the couple from escalations they are not yet prepared to handle may follow the format used by Gail's and Brad's therapist in the initial interview:

THERAPIST: Brad, I'd like to ask you some questions about your relationship with Jill, but if there are things you aren't ready to talk about yet, let me know that. We likely will need to address them in time, but I want to establish an atmosphere of honesty and truthfulness, so only tell me about what you can address truthfully.

GAIL: There's a lot he still hasn't told me, and I'm not so sure what he has told me is the truth.

THERAPIST: Well, my concern is that there's certain information about Brad's involvement with Jill that I'm going to need in order to understand where things stand at this point, but I don't want to take us down a path that will throw the two of you into further turmoil before we're prepared to deal with that.

BRAD: I've pretty much told Gail everything: how it started, how it ended, how stupid it was for me to get involved with a student . . .

THERAPIST: Well, for now, Brad, let me go ahead and begin getting some of the information I'll need from you about that relationship. If at some point I ask you something that you're not ready or willing to answer today, then simply let me know and—for today—I'll accept those limits. Okay?

Invite the participating partner to share basic information about the outside relationship, for example, when and how it began, how long it continued, and whether it has ended. Having the first name of the outside person (if known to both partners) can be helpful as a way of referencing that person in sessions. Encouraging the participating partner to take the lead in providing details, and asking for additional information along the way, can avoid the risks of making the process feel like an interrogation. Set limits on the injured partner's intrusions while trying to obtain this information, particularly if those intrusions are attacking of either the participating partner or the outside person. You may acknowledge how difficult this portion of the interview is likely to feel for both partners. Information you are eventually going to need includes the following:

- When did the affair begin? Was it primarily emotional, primarily sexual, or both? When did it become sexual, if it was sexual?
- Has the affair ended? If the affair has ended, is it over temporarily or

permanently? What contact has either partner had with the outside person since then? What steps, if any, have been taken to ensure that no further contact takes place or has been limited in certain ways?

- What does the outside-affair person want from the participating partner? Is the other person married or in a committed relationship? Does that person's partner know?

- What kinds of contraception or protection against sexually transmitted disease (STD) were used? Were there any times when protection was not used? Have the participating and injured partners or the outside person been tested for STDs?

- Who else knows about the affair? Are there any other consequences the couple needs to consider, for example, any complications at work or other legal problems? Could the outside person or his or her partner make the couple's lives more difficult if either of them wanted to?

Assessing Individual Strengths and Vulnerabilities

Even among individuals with good premorbid individual functioning, emotional and behavioral well-being after the disclosure or discovery of an affair may be substantially disrupted. As noted in Chapter 1, both research and clinical findings indicate that the partner of the person engaging in an affair often experiences strong negative emotional reactions, including shame, rage, depression, anxiety, a sense of victimization, and symptoms consistent with those seen in PTSD. Among persons having participated in an affair, similar reactions of depression, guilt, and acute anxiety are also common, particularly when disclosure or discovery of infidelity results in marital separation or threats of divorce. Such intense feelings can lead to misuse of alcohol or other substances, suicidal thoughts or behaviors, or physical aggression. (For a review of the literature regarding partners' responses to disclosure or discovery of an affair, see Allen et al., 2005.)

Adverse emotional or behavioral consequences may also be seen in the couple's children, even if they have not been informed explicitly about the affair. There is ample evidence linking severe or chronic marital conflict to a wide range of deleterious effects on children, including depression, withdrawal, disrupted social functioning, poor academic performance, and a variety of conduct-related difficulties (Gottman, 1999).

Assessing partners' individual functioning, as well as the emotional and behavioral well-being of their children, can be pursued by asking both partners a series of questions similar to the following:

- What are you (or your children) struggling with the most right now in terms of thoughts and feelings or just getting through the day? What sometimes makes things worse or more difficult?
- Tell me how you (or your children) are continuing to manage despite the challenges. What has been the most helpful to you, considering your own resources, responses from your partner, and support from others?

Assessing and responding to participating partners' distress presents special challenges. Participating partners are often reluctant to disclose their own feelings of depression, anxiety, or even guilt, believing that the obvious pain they have brought to their injured partner precludes legitimate expression of their own distress. They may find it particularly difficult to reveal feelings of loneliness or missing the outside-affair person. Even when participating partners disclose such feelings, allowing empathic understanding from the therapist, the injured partner may display such strong negative reactions as to render continued vulnerable disclosures or therapeutic support quite difficult. Such reactions may suggest two alternative assessment strategies: (1) use of individual sessions to obtain important information regarding partners' functioning or (2) standardized assessment measures of emotional or behavioral well-being. With regard to the latter, we recommend focused and brief measures (e.g., the Beck Depression Inventory–II [BDI-II; Beck, Steer, & Brown, 1996] or the Symptom Checklist-90—Revised [SCL-90-R; Derogatis & Savitz, 1999]).

Expressing empathic understanding toward both partners requires the therapist to recognize partners' respective needs and tolerance for each other's hurt feelings and then to work toward a delicate balance as shown in the following exchange:

THERAPIST: Brad, Gail has been clear today about how much she continues to struggle from the affair, and I can tell from your previous responses that you heard that distress when you expressed your own regrets. But I'm wondering about how you're getting along, too. Can you tell me some about that?

BRAD: I'm fine . . .

GAIL: (*sarcastically*) Sure, what does he have to worry about other than his own career, certainly not about *me*.

THERAPIST: (*to Gail*) Well, he may worry only about his career, but I'm not yet convinced of that, and I think it could be helpful to both of us if we knew more about what's going on with Brad beneath the surface. Would that be okay?

GAIL: I guess . . .

THERAPIST: (to Brad) Brad, it would really help if you could share more about what's going on with you. I suspect that you believe responding to Gail's distress is the main priority right now, and that's fine. But ultimately, if you're not doing okay yourself, it's going to undermine your ability to be there for her in the way that you may want and that she's going to need. So help me understand a little better what's going on with you right now, all right?

BRAD: My job is the least of my worries; things there will be okay eventually. Mostly I worry about us (looking at Gail) and whether we're going to make it through this. I'm confused about how to make things better. If I approach Gail, she pushes me away. If I leave her alone, she accuses me of abandoning her . . .

GAIL: (angrily) Well, maybe I'm confused, too. I think I'm entitled . . .

THERAPIST: My hunch is you're both feeling pretty confused right now, for good reasons. Neither of you want to make things worse, but it's not clear to either of you how to make things better. If nothing else, one thing you have in common right now is not feeling understood by the other, and perhaps not knowing just how to express understanding or concern for the other in ways that work well. But being able to talk more effectively about that confusion may help you avoid making hurtful interpretations that the other one just doesn't care any more. In the meantime, it may also be good for us to talk about how you can each take care of yourself a bit better for now until you're more able to provide each other the kinds of support or encouragement you're needing . . .

In the context of such exchanges, the therapist can follow up by assessing basic self-care (discussed further in Chapter 5). Are both partners attending to their physical needs, getting adequate sleep, maintaining good nutrition, and attending to any health concerns? Are they avoiding alcohol and other drugs? Obtaining emotional support from friends or family members but without disclosing the affair, as well as drawing on spiritual resources either individually or with others, can be important means of self-care. In some cases, severe or persistent emotional distress may warrant referral for collateral individual counseling or psychotropic medications.

It is also important to determine the extent to which the injured partner is experiencing flashback phenomena: painful reexperiencing of the initial trauma of the affair's discovery triggered by situations or interactions associated with that event. Helping both partners to recognize and understand such experiences, and to have both individual and shared strategies for responding to them, may help to limit their adverse impact. Flashback phenomena and therapeutic strategies for dealing with flashbacks are discussed in more detail in Chapter 5.

Finally, it is important to distinguish between "normative" emotional and behavioral turmoil frequently accompanying disclosure or discovery of an affair and more chronic or intense problems that may require interventions beyond those addressed here. Such distinctions require clinical judgment informed by the history and levels of disruption related to these difficulties. For example, as therapist you may need to differentiate (1) feelings of hopelessness or despair from acute suicidal risk, (2) emotional turmoil secondary to the affair from long-term patterns of unstable and intense interpersonal relationships, or (3) current moderate misuse of alcohol from long-standing patterns of substance abuse. In each of these comparisons, the former might be addressed adequately in the context of couple treatment focusing on the affair, whereas the latter may warrant collateral individual therapy or pharmacological intervention. In some cases, intense and pervasive dysregulation of emotion expressed in suicidality, physical aggression, or substance abuse may contraindicate couple therapy targeting the affair until partners' individual functioning improves to a level permitting constructive engagement in conjoint sessions.

Assessing Outside Stressors and Resources

Outside stressors and resources may be revealed in part by inquiring about what influences make partners' current struggles more manageable or more difficult. At other times, these need to be evaluated by a series of questions scanning the broader family and social environment for evidence of stress or support. Common stressors that can interfere with initial efforts to contain the impact of the affair include continued contact initiated by the outside-affair person, excessive demands from work or family responsibilities; or concerns related to finances, physical health, or children's well-being. Common resources that can buffer the adverse impact of an affair or render recovery more promising include a history of strong emotional connection and positive interactions before the affair, shared values or commitment to common goals (including caring for one's children), support for the couple's relationship from family and friends, and healthy patterns of separate interests or pursuits that facilitate tolerance of current disruption in the couple's own relationship.

In assessing outside stressors during this initial assessment, the primary goal is not to evaluate factors that potentially contributed to the affair; that will come later in treatment (as discussed in Chapter 9). Rather, the goal is to identify immediate stressors that undermine the couple's ability to manage the initial turmoil accompanying disclosure or discovery of the affair. For example, ongoing problems with in-laws might have been a stressor contributing to the affair; however, if the in-laws do not currently know about the affair, then this kind of conflict is less likely to be an immediate major focus of this phase of treatment but will be addressed more in Stage 2. However, if the in-laws do know about the affair and are actively trying to force the partners apart, then it is appropriate and probably necessary to focus on these attempts.

A particularly difficult situation arises when the outside-affair person persists in pursuing contact despite explicit requests from the participating partner to stop. When such a situation becomes apparent during the initial interview, the couple may benefit from specific guidelines for how to pursue stronger boundaries involving the outside person. Strategies for dealing with this issue are described later in Chapter 4.

Assessing Expectations for Couple Therapy

The initial assessment needs to determine not only what a couple is currently experiencing but also the partners' thoughts about where they hope to be eventually with their relationship. Sometimes one or both partners may reveal considerable ambivalence about remaining in the relationship or despair about their ability to recover despite their best efforts. At other times, both partners are explicit about their commitment to remaining in the relationship and doing "whatever it takes" to make their relationship succeed. In these cases, their history as individuals and as a couple may offer strong evidence of their ability to overcome difficult challenges; alternatively, their history may reveal critical individual or relationship vulnerabilities, suggesting ways in which recovery from the affair may be particularly difficult, protracted, or constrained. Examples include long-standing individual difficulties (e.g., major psychopathology) or relationship problems (e.g., high levels of conflict or low levels of intimacy) that predate the current affair.

In all cases, unless both partners have definitively and irrevocably decided to end their relationship and are only seeking assistance in ending it with the least adverse consequences for themselves or their children, it is important that, as their therapist, you communicate optimism for the potential to work through the trauma of the affair and reach good decisions about how to move forward, whether together or apart. It is not uncommon for couples who initially despair of ever recovering, and who objectively appear to face overwhelming challenges, to persevere and accomplish tremendous strides in restoring or creating a strong and healthy marriage. Similarly, when couples announce their determination to remain together and initially refuse even to acknowledge alternative outcomes, their convictions initially can be supported as reflecting their strong commitment, but then at the appropriate time in treatment, most likely in Stage 3, you can invite them to reexamine and hopefully affirm their decision once they have explored more fully how the affair came to occur.

Providing an Initial Formulation

The initial assessment should conclude with offering the couple a provisional formulation that integrates the therapist's best understanding of what the partners are currently experiencing, factors that may have contributed to their arriving at this point, and what next steps will likely be required for moving forward. As noted, depending on the format you have adopted for conducting the assessment, this formulation may occur in the last 20–30 minutes of an initial interview lasting 1½–2 hours, or it may be reserved for a separate session after the initial conjoint interview and separate individual sessions with both partners. Regardless of the specific format, the initial formulation should highlight the following:

- Where both partners are currently.
- How they arrived at that point.
- Where they appear to be headed.
- What will be required in order for them to get there.

Partners need a way of understanding what they are both experiencing. For couples in Stage 1 of recovery, this may require normalizing the emotional chaos and intense negativity that frequently characterize the initial response to an affair. For other couples stuck in Stage 2, it may require understanding why, after surviving the initial turmoil and months of relative calm, they are growing progressively more distant and disillusioned. Persons frequently do not understand their own feelings and behaviors after an affair, much less the experiences and behaviors of their partner. Confusion and misinterpretation surrounding these experiences contribute to anxiety, further hurtful interactions, deepened resentments, and feelings of hopelessness. Describing common patterns of recovery can instill hopefulness and also help partners to be vigilant about how to avoid making matters worse.

When summarizing the couple's current functioning, it is useful to begin with the injured partner, move on to the participating partner, and then discuss how their respective experiences likely influence their current interactions. The formulation should be discussed interactively, with the therapist taking the lead but inviting feedback from partners along the way. In the following example, we emphasize the therapist's contributions, but in practice this material would be interspersed with input from the partners affirming, clarifying, or expanding on the therapist's formulation.

THERAPIST: (to Gail) Gail, right now you seem to be really struggling in ways that are very understandable and somewhat typical when someone has just learned of a partner's affair. You're mostly trying to figure out what's happened to you and are reeling from the impact. We think of this as Stage 1 in the recovery process: just dealing with the initial impact. Your whole world has been shaken up, and nothing feels stable or secure any more. Everything you thought you knew about Brad now seems uncertain. Your assumptions about your marriage have been shattered, and it's hard for you to predict what the relationship will be like in the future. All that uncertainty at times likely leaves you feeling anxious as well as deeply hurt and sad. In the past you've looked to Brad for emotional support during tough times, and my sense is that at times you still want to be reassured or even comforted by him. But that also feels scary because Brad's affair is the reason you're feeling so devastated, so that causes you to retreat or pull back if he reaches out to you. It feels extremely painful and confusing, with strong but mixed feelings, and sometimes you just can't figure out where to turn. Is that about right? [Here the therapist might engage with Gail and refine the formulation based on Gail's reactions and feedback.] (to Brad) And Brad, it sounds like you're struggling, too. On the one hand, you describe having considerable regret about your affair and understand what Gail's going through. There's a part of you that wants to reach out to her, to comfort her, and perhaps get some reassurance yourself that things will be okay. But when you do, she sometimes pushes you away and then you're not sure what to do, so you pull back, which leads Gail to think that maybe you don't really understand or care after all. Does that seem to fit?

BRAD: Yeah, that about sums it up . . .

THERAPIST: (*to both*) The initial stage after discovering an affair can be chaotic and really difficult. But as hard as it is, I can reassure you that it won't last forever. There may not be a lot of "recovery" per se during this time, but I think I can help you both get through this and avoid making things worse. If we can get through these next few weeks successfully and get some of this turmoil under better control, I think that will let you work toward a better understanding of exactly what's happened and the impact it's had. Once we accomplish that, we can go on to the second stage of recovery.

GAIL: What's that about?

THERAPIST: Ultimately, for your marriage to be healthy again, you're both going to need to come to a shared understanding of how the affair came about.

BRAD: I already know how it came about – from a dumb choice on my part – and I'm determined not to repeat that mistake.

THERAPIST: Brad, I don't doubt your resolve not to have another affair. And you may be right that your affair with Jill resulted from a "dumb choice." But Gail's going to need a better understanding of how it is you came to make such a choice. Otherwise, she can't feel secure that you couldn't make another poor choice sometime down the road. And that's what Stage 2 is all about: working toward a more comprehensive, shared understanding of all the factors that potentially contributed to a situation in which you chose to have an affair, Brad. Gail's going to need that kind of understanding as a basis for trying to rebuild security in the marriage if you decide to stay together. The two of you aren't likely to recover enduring trust and intimacy until you're both convinced that you've looked at this from all angles, understand everything that potentially paved the way for an affair, and then have addressed each source of vulnerability you've identified. I can tell you that this will be the most important work we do together and perhaps also the most difficult.

GAIL: What happens then?

THERAPIST: Then I think you'll both be in a better position to make good, informed decisions about how to move forward.

BRAD: I already know how I want us to move forward: by staying married.

THERAPIST: Well, that's good that you already know that's the outcome you'd like to achieve. Gail may also know that for herself. But Stage 3 involves not only identifying the desired outcome but also figuring out how to get there. The two of you have a tough journey ahead of you, make no mistake. Already having an idea of where you want to end up can help you keep your "eye on the prize" when the going gets tough. But if we're successful in pursuing the challenges of Stage 2 and taking a comprehensive look at all the factors that potentially made your marriage more vulnerable to an affair, I'm convinced you'll identify some influences that you're not aware of now. The more contributing influences you're able to identify together in Stage 2, the more risk factors you'll be able to reduce, and the more secure your marriage is likely to be in the long run. So, in summary, we first need just to contain the turmoil you're both experiencing now and prevent further damage. Then we need to take a hard look at what was going on both in and outside of your marriage, and with each of you separately, that could have made your marriage more vulnerable to an affair. If we can do these first two stages well, then you'll be able to determine exactly how to move forward to achieve healthy outcomes for each of you, whether together or apart. Does that make sense to both of you? (*Both Brad and Gail nod.*) Good. Then let's talk about the format for how we'll work together and what our respective roles will be . . .

At this point, the therapist can refer to the material described in Chapter 3 to create the optimal therapeutic environment by setting guidelines to limit negative exchanges and develop an atmosphere of safety and trust.

Summary

Working effectively with couples struggling to get past an affair requires that you offer them a road map for recovery, beginning with where they are, offering some hypotheses about how they got there, and outlining the next steps for reaching a place where they can make and implement good decisions regarding how to move on. Developing this road map entails obtaining information about the couple's marriage; factors impacting the marriage from the outside, including the affair relationship itself; and both strengths and vulnerabilities of each of the individual partners. Preparing couples for therapy requires developing a formulation tailored to the couple's own unique situation and then integrating this formulation within a three-stage model of dealing with the initial impact, developing a shared understanding of factors contributing to the affair, and making and implementing healthy decisions for moving forward.

Resources from *Getting Past the Affair*

Our self-help book for couples, *Getting Past the Affair: A Program to Help You Cope, Heal, and Move On—Together or Apart* (Snyder et al., 2007), can be a useful adjunct in treating couples dealing with infidelity. It is based on the same treatment model discussed in the current book. If you decide to have the couple read this self-help book in conjunction with your therapy, encourage them to read both the Introduction and Chapter 1 following the initial session.

The Introduction to the companion book discusses why and how the reader can use this book to work past an affair and summarizes typical experiences and essential tasks of each of the three stages of recovery.

Chapter 1, "What's Happening to Us?," describes common thoughts, feelings, and behaviors that characterize the initial response to an affair, beginning with what is happening with the injured partner and then describing what is likely to be happening in the couple's relationship. A separate section in the chapter specifically addresses the participating partner, discussing what that partner may be experiencing and describing how he or she can be helpful to the recovery process. The chapter concludes with an exercise designed to help partners examine their own reactions to the affair.

CHAPTER 3

Creating a Therapeutic Environment

P am and Tom, a couple in their late 30s, sought therapy soon after Tom became aware of Pam's affair with an office coworker, Mark. Tom had been reluctant to believe rumors of Pam's affair but became increasingly uneasy when Pam began staying late at work but could not be reached by phone. After several weeks of Pam's unusual behavior, Tom began parking outside her building to observe Pam as she left work. One evening he saw Pam and Mark drive up to her building together in Mark's car and give each other a warm and lengthy embrace. Pam then quickly entered her own car to drive home. When Tom confronted Pam later that night, she initially denied a relationship with Mark but eventually confessed to a 6-month romance that had become sexual in the last month.

Both partners entered couple therapy with considerable ambivalence, uncertain about their relationship and what they wanted for their future. Both expressed love and deep concern for their daughters, ages 13 and 10. Although Pam and Tom both wanted to explore the possibility of staying together, neither of them was committed to that outcome.

PAM: You've got to stop hounding me. Day in, day out, you keep badgering me about what I want. I told you—I don't know what I want. I've stopped seeing Mark, but you simply won't believe me. You're so hostile toward me around the house that I don't even want to come home any more.

TOM: Why should I believe you? You lied to me about Mark, even after I caught the two of you that night in the parking lot. Angry? Hostile? You bet I am. And don't blame me for your not wanting to come home. You weren't exactly "Betty homemaker" before I found out about your affair.

THERAPIST: It sounds like right now things are pretty difficult at home . . .

PAM: That's an understatement.

THERAPIST: Let's pause for a moment and consider what needs to happen for now just to ease some of the conflict at home so the two of you don't make things worse.

PAM: He's got to ease up. It's unbearable.

TOM: She's got to cut all ties with Mark. I don't know whether we can pull this marriage back together again or not, but I know darn well that we can't if she continues to see him.

PAM: I'm not "seeing" him. We still work at the same place. I still have to work with him around projects we were both assigned to.

THERAPIST: For now, regardless of what you decide about your marriage in the long run, we need to find ways to decrease the negative interactions you're having. It's clear this is a very difficult time for you both. Let's see if we can identify what you each need just to make it through the next few weeks without doing more damage. For now, we won't try to reach any long-term decisions about your marriage. Instead, let's focus on ways of calming things down a bit in the short run so you can give yourselves and this marriage some rest. Would that be agreeable to each of you?

PAM: Sure. I could use a break.

TOM: Yeah, I guess so. It can't go on like this.

In Chapter 1, we identified numerous reasons why couples struggling with the aftermath of an affair are so difficult to treat. The emotions of both partners typically run hot, and partners may have difficulty regulating their own emotions or coping with the other's intense emotions. Anger, shame, fear, or despair may overwhelm the couple and dominate the therapy if not contained by the therapist. A sense of urgency and yearning for emotional safety can drive either partner to behave in uncharacteristic or unpredictable ways. Less typical but still common, couples can present as distant, cold, and disconnected and yet have a number of angry and bitter emotions underneath the surface, particularly when the affair has occurred in the past but is unresolved. Establishing even a fledgling collaborative alliance between partners in both situations can prove challenging.

Superimposed on this cauldron of churning emotions may be either partner's ambivalence about staying in the marriage. Even if both partners know (or think they know) what outcome they want, they often have no idea how to get there. Not only do couples struggling with an affair typically find themselves in uncharted waters, but their intense emotions often interfere with their ability to think clearly about the multiple dilemmas they face. Even couples managing their own emotions well may struggle because of negative influences from outside their marriage, including the outside-affair person as well as well-intentioned but misguided family members or friends.

Against this backdrop, couple therapists need to be armed with a clear conceptualization of recovery from infidelity and equipped with specific strategies for implementing this vision. When working with couples struggling with an affair, you need to provide a road map for how to move from chaos to understanding and from understanding to good decisions. You need to provide a compelling rationale for both partners to embark on this journey together. You need to know when and how to intervene when the process goes astray, when to linger along the way to ensure that sequential tasks are mastered, and when to nudge the couple past their comfort zone.

In this chapter we describe challenges and basic strategies for creating a therapeutic environment for couples struggling with the aftermath of infidelity. These basic strategies are summarized in Table 3.1. Some of the principles we emphasize apply generally to couple therapy, but they are especially important when working with affair couples. Other strategies we describe are more specific to couples contending with infidelity or other relationship trauma.

Establishing Safety and Trust

For most couples beginning to address an affair, their relationship does not feel safe and partners typically mistrust each other. Therefore, it is critical that you create a safe, trusting environment for them in the therapy room and eventually in their daily lives outside of the session. To begin with, you need to ensure that they feel safe during the sessions by addressing several features of treatment. Almost no one feels safe in a negative or hostile environment; therefore, you must first limit the amount and types of negativity that are expressed during the session. Second, partners must feel that it is safe to disclose the thoughts and feelings that they are experiencing and that these thoughts and feelings will be heard and respected without being attacked or belittled. Third, both partners need to know that you will keep them in "safe"

TABLE 3.1. Strategies for Creating a Therapeutic Environment

Strategy	Descriptions
Establishing safety and trust	
Limiting negative exchanges	Limiting verbal negativity and keeping discussions focused; providing a rationale for therapeutic containment.
Facilitating disclosure	Facilitating disclosure of difficult feelings and responding empathically.
Keeping the couple in safe territory	Monitoring partners' capacity to disclose or discuss highly sensitive or volatile information; balancing levels and timing of emotional discussions.
Promoting confidence in the therapist's expertise	
Promoting a normative context	Describing common responses to affairs for both partners, typical patterns of recovery, and common challenges.
Offering a strategy for recovery	Proposing an overall treatment plan that integrates the three-stage recovery process with specific aspects of partners' individual and relationship functioning.
Affirming ethical practice	
Ensuring physical safety	Addressing issues of physical aggression and risks of sexually transmitted diseases from unprotected intercourse with outside person.
Handling issues of confidentiality	Describing policies regarding information obtained from individual sessions and sharing of information with outside parties (e.g., attorneys, physicians, other therapists).
Affirming fairness to both partners	Discussing policies regarding therapeutic neutrality and handling of potential conflicts of interest.
Encouraging a therapeutic alliance	
Defining your role as therapist	Describing such roles as • Presenting information. • Directing the flow of exchanges in session. • Facilitating partners' self-awareness and disclosures. • Promoting partners' understanding of each other • Advocating for the couple's relationship.
Defining partners' roles	Describing such roles and responsibilities as • Attending and actively engaging in sessions. • Restraining from verbal and physical aggression. • Accepting accountability for own decisions and behaviors. • Being honest. • Providing feedback to the therapist throughout treatment. • Committing to a process of recovery independent of a specific outcome.

territory and will not push or encourage them to disclose things or do things that they are not ready for. Often couples will go where you take them, and they need to know that you will not take them into territory that is too dangerous or volatile when they are not yet able to negotiate that potentially treacherous terrain.

Limiting Negative Exchanges

Couples struggling to recover from an affair typically experience deep and painful feelings. Intense angry exchanges between partners may run rampant if left unchecked by their therapist, or they may erupt only episodically or at unpredictable moments. In establishing therapeutic safety, it is important to achieve a balance between obtaining a sample of partners' interaction patterns and imposing control over destructive interactions. Similarly, you need to obtain basic information about the affair (e.g., when it began, who the outside person is, whether the affair has ended) but prevent the couple from becoming derailed by irrelevant or highly contentious details that detract from the initial goals of regaining equilibrium and identifying immediate next steps toward recovery. As the therapist, you need to firmly but respectfully limit antagonistic exchanges and help partners focus their discussion on matters most important at that moment in their recovery. Offering a rationale for interrupting and redirecting partners' destructive exchanges helps to promote tolerance for such interventions, as exemplified here:

THERAPIST: Tom, talk some about what you need to get through the coming week.

TOM: I need her to talk with me.

PAM: Then you need to listen . . .

THERAPIST: Tom, describe what it is you most need to know from Pam.

TOM: I need to know how she could have done this to me and our daughters. How could she betray the whole family? How did she let this jerk come into our lives and screw everything up? Why doesn't she care about anyone but herself?

PAM: How am I supposed to answer questions like that?

THERAPIST: Tom, what are you most worried about right now?

TOM: I'm worried that she's already given up—that our marriage is over.

THERAPIST: Try asking her that in a way that doesn't leave her feeling so attacked by you. I know that you're really hurt, and you're angry. But my sense is that what you'd really like right now is some reassurance from Pam that there's still a chance for the two of you. But when you confront her with questions like you did a moment ago, it pushes her further away rather than inviting reassurance.

TOM: (*to Pam*) Why can't you see how you're destroying me and our daughters?

THERAPIST: If you want to know if Pam is still open to working on your marriage, then let's deal directly with that. Try it this way, "Have you already given up?"

TOM: (*to Pam*) Have you given up?

PAM: No, Tom. That's why I'm here.

THERAPIST: (*to Tom*) Ask her if the marriage is over.

TOM: (*to Pam*) Well, is it? Is our marriage over?

PAM: No, Tom.

THERAPIST: (*to Pam*) Try to offer more about whatever you're feeling. I don't want you to commit to anything more than you're ready to, but I'd like to see whether the two of you can at least find a common foothold that will allow you to look at the marriage and examine some really difficult issues together.

PAM: Tom, I haven't lost all hope. I don't know yet what I want in terms of the marriage—that's why I'm here. We haven't been a healthy couple lately, even before my involvement with Mark. I don't know if we can get it right. We need to figure that out—for our daughters' sake if not our own. We can't go on the way we have been for the past few years.

Facilitating Disclosure

Some injured partners feel such profound hurt or despair that they are left without words to describe what they are experiencing. Participating partners may also be so overcome by guilt, shame, or fear of divorce that they are unable or unwilling to disclose their thoughts or feelings to their partner. With such couples, establishing safety involves facilitating disclosure, listening empathically, and acknowledging each partner's distress. Both people need confidence that if they do disclose their thoughts and feelings, the therapeutic environment is a place where it is safe to do so and where understanding and respect, from both the therapist and the partner, are the norm.

Responding empathically to both partners—always a challenge in couple therapy—can be particularly difficult when working with affair couples. The implicit roles of injured and participating partner as victim and perpetrator, respectively, can make it difficult to offer compassionate responses to the participating partner's own feelings of hurt or sadness, especially if the latter relates to loss from ending a deep relationship with the outside-affair partner. In managing this implicit imbalance in partners' roles, it is sometimes helpful to acknowledge or overtly infer possible feelings of the participating partner but to postpone their exploration until later in the therapy when the therapeutic alliance with both partners is stronger. Early in therapy, the injured partner often cannot tolerate seeing the therapist being empathic toward the participating partner, who has already caused such damage. Consider the following exchange involving Vicki and Bill, a couple introduced in Chapter 1:

THERAPIST: Bill, I'm wondering in what ways this is difficult for you, too.

BILL: I'll be okay.

THERAPIST: Well, that's good to hear, but it might be useful for Vicki to know about how you're struggling, too.

VICKI: He doesn't say much.

THERAPIST: It may be hard to describe your own feelings of distress if you don't think you're entitled to have them, or if you don't believe your partner is willing to hear them.

BILL: It's just that I know how deeply I've hurt Vicki, and I can hardly stand that. I wish I could make it better for her, and I know I can't. So I don't know what to say. I know I caused this, and I'm not about to look for any sympathy.

VICKI: You're not about to get any either, at least not from *me*.

THERAPIST: (*to Bill*) I'm wondering if you're feeling alone right now.

BILL: (*after long pause*) More than I can say . . .

THERAPIST: Bill, I won't suggest that you ask Vicki for sympathy. But by your being stoic, Vicki's left without any sense of whether this is difficult for you, too. It leaves her wondering whether you care.

BILL: Of course I care.

THERAPIST: Okay, then try sharing with Vicki, for just a bit, how you're struggling with this, too.

BILL: I have trouble finding the words. I'm hardly sleeping, and I feel sick to my stomach most of the time. I can't stand to face myself in the mirror. I'm terrified she's going to leave, and wouldn't blame her if she did. I'm lost like I've never been lost before, and I have utterly no idea what to do next.

VICKI: Bill, I'm not just going to leave. That's not what I want.

Keeping the Couple in Safe Territory

In facilitating disclosure, it is important to be sensitive to information that a partner may not yet be willing to share because of uncertainty about where the marriage is headed or information that may be volatile or could produce additional turmoil before a couple is equipped to deal with it. For example, the injured partner may have consulted an attorney but not yet be willing to disclose to whom he or she has spoken. Or the participating partner may not have yet disclosed the identity of the outside-affair person or specific details of the affair relationship and may not yet be ready to do so. It can be helpful to preface discussion of the affair, especially in the first session, by acknowledging this potential constraint on what can be discussed at this time:

THERAPIST: Sam, is there anything that I might ask you regarding your affair that might come as a surprise to Diane?

SAM: There are some things she doesn't know yet.

DIANE: He won't tell me who the other woman was.

THERAPIST: Let me explain why I asked that and what implications it has for us. At some point, if you're going to move forward as a couple, it will probably be important for Diane to have more information about your affair than she has now, not all the gory details but more than she knows now. But for today I don't want to introduce new information that's potentially explosive or more than you can handle at this time. It goes along with the immediate goal I described earlier: not making things worse before we have a chance to make them better. So for today if I ask you questions that you're not yet willing to answer, just tell me so and I'll respect that. If we continue to work together, at some point that will change and I'll probably push harder. But not today. Does that make sense to both of you?

SAM: Sure.

DIANE: I guess so. But at some point we're going to have to talk about these things.

THERAPIST: Yes, I think you're right. But I appreciate your willingness to let me structure the sessions in a way to protect your marriage from exchanges that the two of you may not be able to handle just yet.

Promoting Confidence in Your Expertise

Fostering safety and trust by containing negative exchanges, facilitating effective disclosure, and postponing dangerous topics are key ways of promoting partners' confidence in you as a skilled couple therapist. Additionally, couples struggling with the aftermath of infidelity need to feel confident in your expertise specific to treating such relationship trauma as an affair.

Providing a Normative Context

Couples struggling after an affair need a way of understanding what is happening to them. For many, nothing makes sense any more. Partners' beliefs about themselves, each other, and their relationship have been shaken. They may by consumed by emotional turmoil and desperate for a vision of how to move forward. Or they may be separated by a wall of silence and despair of ever becoming close again. Following an affair, couples must make many decisions about how to get through the day, how to interact with the children, whether to eat together or even continuing living together, where to turn for help, or how to find occasional respite. They may be unable to deal with any of these issues without help.

Couples gain confidence in you as their therapist, and frequently experience profound relief, when you provide a normative context for their individual and relationship experiences. Hearing you describe common responses to affairs for both injured and participating partners allows them to make better sense of their own and each other's current behaviors. Your descriptions of typical patterns of recovery can instill hope as well as vigilance about what to avoid. Such descriptions also begin to prepare the couple for realistic expectations for what the course of recovery may involve and how much time is likely to be required. For most couples, the aftermath of an affair is an unfamiliar and terrifying time. They need to know they are in the hands of someone who has seen couples in this situation before and knows how to structure and guide them through a therapeutic process.

The normative context you provide needs to be integrated with acknowledgment of what you learn to be unique about this couple: their individual and shared histories, their strengths and liabilities, and influences contributing to their current struggles. You will promote confidence in your expertise by conveying what you know about recovery from affairs in general, what you already have begun to understand about this couple in particular, and what you are eager to learn from them in the course of working together. As you provide a sense of what they can expect, there are also times when you might be directive or make strong recommendations from a position of confidence, explaining why you are making those recommendations.

> "It sounds like these last few weeks have been really chaotic. You've decided to live in the same house for now, but sleep in separate rooms. It's not unusual for couples to struggle with these kinds of decisions following the disclosure or discovery of an affair or to wrestle with additional decisions you haven't mentioned yet, such as how to maintain interactions with the kids, how to handle the upcoming holiday and visits to relatives, or whom to tell about your situation. Dave, you said earlier that you were undecided whether to tell anyone in your family about Beth's affair. My best advice is that, for now, you continue with your earlier decision to keep this private between the two of you for the time being until we have a chance to talk about the possible impact of telling family members. We can revisit this issue in a few weeks. The two of you describe a good history of working together as parents, but right now you're finding it hard to do this. My best guess is that you'll recover that ability before long, but for now I trust that you can each continue to honor the principles that have guided your parenting in the past, even if you need to do so separately for now . . . "

Offering a Strategy for Recovery

In addition to providing a normative context for what the couple is currently experiencing, you also need to provide a broader, overall treatment plan. Not only does such a plan instill confidence in your expertise, but it also gives the couple a sense of predictability and a course to follow when their lives seem out of control. Therefore, it is important to give the couple a clear overall strategy for working together to recover from this affair, preferably before the first session ends. This strategy includes a summary of the three stages of recovery described in Chapter 1 and a conceptualization of how this model applies to the couple's own situation. The more the couple is embroiled in turmoil and destructive exchanges, the more you may emphasize challenges and strategies specific to Stage 1, but it is important to offer a brief description of each stage. Similarly, if a couple has entered treatment months after the affair has become known or demonstrates regulation of emotions through disengagement or overcontrol of negative feelings, your conceptualization may give greater attention to understanding how the affair occurred through Stage 2 interventions. However, it is important to note that, even in these cases, some Stage 1 strategies may still apply, as we discuss in later chapters. Alternatively, when one or both partners express deep ambivalence about their marriage and uncertainty about whether to invest in couple therapy, you might emphasize that the goal of treatment is not to keep the partners together at all costs but rather to help both partners reach a good decision about how to move on, either together or separately.

Occasionally, one or both partners enter therapy with strong beliefs or expectations regarding the course of recovery that differ from the process advocated here. For example, they might believe that a decision to stay together in the long term needs to be achieved at the outset as a condition for working together on their relationship. The injured partner may believe that every microscopic detail of the affair needs to be revealed in the spirit of full disclosure, whereas the participating partner may believe that any further disclosures will only promote additional turmoil. Some partners may resist the idea that exploring a broad range of potential contributing factors is important to recovery in the long term, even if it prolongs or increases distress in the short run. We gently but persistently convey our experience in working with many different couples, which affirms the benefits of the three-stage model advocated here. In responding to specific components of partners' apprehension or reluctance, we are careful to label such feelings not as "resistance to treatment" but rather as well-intentioned concerns about how best to move forward. We ask partners to trust our experience in the short term on a trial basis, affirming our willingness to revisit the issues of treatment goals and processes along the way and asserting our commitment to be mindful and responsive to both partners' concerns throughout therapy.

Affirming Ethical Practice

Couple therapy is fraught with ethical challenges extending beyond those generic to psychotherapy generally. These challenges become magnified when working with couples after an affair (Snyder & Doss, 2005).

Ensuring Physical Safety

Physical safety assumes increased importance not only because of the intensity of angry exchanges that frequently occur after discovery of an affair but also because of unique risks posed by sexual exchanges with an outside person. Hence, it is important to evaluate (1) whether the affair relationship involved sexual contact and, if so, what type; (2) more specifically, whether there was intercourse and, if so, whether there was even one occasion of intercourse in which a condom was not used; and (3) whether both partners have been tested since the affair for HIV or other STDs. Limiting aggressive behaviors both within and between sessions is also critical to couple therapy. Guidelines for addressing the latter are addressed in greater detail in Chapter 4, but clear expectations precluding tolerance of any physical aggression should be noted from the outset.

Handling Issues of Confidentiality

Your policies regarding confidentiality should be discussed at the outset of treatment and thereafter as new circumstances may warrant. Gottlieb (1996) identified four approaches to handling confidentiality when working with couples or families: (1) Treat information disclosed individually as confidential to that person; (2) set a policy that no information is to be confidential to one partner; (3) agree that certain information will be kept confidential as a matter of personal privacy; or (4) agree to keep certain information confidential temporarily with the understanding that it will be disclosed at a later date. Although cogent arguments can be made for each of these approaches, ethical practice requires you to convey a clear policy on confidentiality from the outset.

There are occasions (addressed later in this book) when individual sessions with either partner may be warranted (e.g., to provide an opportunity to discuss information about past or present experiences that the person finds difficult or threatening to discuss in front of the partner). We advocate informing participants in the initial session that anything revealed outside of conjoint sessions becomes a part of the couple therapy and, *at the discretion of the therapist*, may be disclosed in subsequent sessions involving both partners. The qualifier regarding the therapist's discretion permits clinical judgments concerning the potential consequences for all participants of sharing or withholding specific information on either an interim or a permanent basis. However, we do not disclose volatile information provided by one partner without advance discussion. Instead, we typically meet with that person and clarify why we believe the information needs to be shared, deciding together whether that person or the therapist will raise it with the partner. If the person insists that it not be disclosed, then the therapist must decide whether to continue therapy under that condition or whether to terminate treatment. We have found such circumstances to be rare, but it is important to make your policy clear for those few occasions when it does arise.

Affirming Fairness to Both Partners

When working with couples after an affair, it is important that you convey as soon and as fully as possible your conceptualization of who comprises the client and your stance regarding therapeutic neutrality as components of informed consent to treatment. You need to remain vigilant to real or perceived emerging conflicts of interest and to ensure that multiple roles and professional responsibilities are clarified as often as necessary. Even when two partners present simultaneously for couple therapy and agree to identify their relationship as the "client," conflicts of interest may be unavoidable (e.g., when partners differ in mental or physical health or when caring for one partner requires decisions with negative consequences for the other). Challenges in ensuring fairness to both partners can sometimes be addressed, at least in part, by clearly articulating the nature of this challenge to both partners.

THERAPIST: Micah, you've described your concern for Sarah and your regret that she learned about your affair, but you've also been pretty clear that it is her discovery you regret, not so much the affair itself.

MICAH: I know she's hurt by my affair, and I do regret that. But I'm not so certain that the affair itself was all that wrong. Sarah and I haven't been intimate for years ever since her accident, and I continued to treat Sarah with kindness, even more so during the affair.

SARAH: It was wrong because you didn't tell me. We made vows to be faithful . . .

MICAH: I understand that, Sarah. But how was the situation fair to me? I didn't mean to hurt you, but I'm only 34, and you expect me never to have sex again. From your perspective, any kind of sex other than intercourse is wrong, and if we can't do that then we'll just have to do without. How is that fair?

THERAPIST: There's no doubt that you both have reasons to feel hurt. What's happened doesn't feel fair to either one of you. You've faced a real dilemma, and the choices you make will need to be based on the different values you bring to the situation. At least for now, I'm not inclined to try to convince either of you about what values to have in those respects. But in fairness to each of you, I *am* going to advocate your honesty in articulating those values—and your willingness to be accountable in adhering to them—so that you can each reach an informed decision about whether, or how, to stay in this marriage.

Committing to a Therapeutic Process

There is a difference between committing to a therapeutic process and committing to a specific outcome. The former should be pursued from the outset, and the latter should be avoided. It is important to articulate a conceptual model describing the process of recovery from an affair and the roles of each participant without assumptions about informed decisions either partner may eventually make for the future of the relationship.

> "I spoke earlier about the stages of recovery: dealing with the initial impact of this affair, understanding more fully how it came about, and then reaching informed decisions about how to move on. I don't presume to know at this point whether you'll decide to move on together or separately. You may have already reached a tentative decision on your own, but I'm going to encourage you to hold that decision aside while we're working through this process so that we don't leave important issues unexamined. If we're successful in our work together, you'll each gain a more balanced view of this affair and each other, be less consumed by your hurt or anger, and be able to move forward without seeking further punishment or restitution. The affair won't be forgotten, but it will have less control over your lives. I'm committed to working toward those outcomes for both of you, whether you decide to stay together or move on separately."

It is also important to note that being fair to both persons does not always mean maintaining neutrality and letting the couple decide how to proceed, without the therapist expressing any views about healthy versus unhealthy choices. For example, we worked with a couple in which a domineering husband had persuaded his pregnant wife that, because she could not respond to his sexual needs during the final trimester of pregnancy, it was appropriate for him to have sex with her best friend, someone whom she could trust. In this instance, being fair did not mean allowing the husband to use his dominance to convince his wife to agree with an idea that the therapist saw as highly destructive.

Encouraging a Collaborative Alliance

Your Role as Therapist

After an affair, many couples recognize that they need help to recover, but they do not understand what kinds of help they need or what kinds of assistance you are prepared to offer. You can foster a collaborative alliance by describing the multiple roles you are likely to have with them as you work together toward recovery.

Educator

You have information about couple processes in general and about recovering from an affair specifically, which will help the couple move forward. Depending on your therapeutic approach, you might also help partners develop specific relationship skills, such as emotional expressiveness, empathic listening, and effective decision making. You will be providing a blueprint for reconstructing their lives and sharing critical tools for doing so. To gain partners' trust in your expertise, you need to be clear about possessing such information and demonstrate your ability to impart it effectively.

Conductor

As a conductor, you direct the flow of exchanges: when to stop, when to go, when to change directions. Couples contending with deep hurt and confusion need assistance in interrupting their negative exchanges and redirecting their efforts toward more productive interactions aimed at disclosing useful information and reaching good decisions. Disengaged couples need support in tolerating discomfort and reengaging in ways designed to work through painful feelings as a means of healing and moving forward. Therapists differ in their levels of directiveness in working with couples; while respecting these differences in therapeutic approaches, we believe that the nature of treating couples recovering from infidelity frequently calls for therapists to assume a more active and directive role.

Facilitator

Couples rely on their therapist to facilitate two kinds of processes. First, the therapist facilitates partners' self-awareness as the therapist listens empathically, not only to what is said but also to what is not said, and reflects or clarifies thoughts and feelings beneath the surface to bring them to light. Couples also rely on therapists to facilitate a process enabling partners to listen to and understand each other, recognizing each other's vulnerability and offering a softened or more compassionate response to each other as a step toward emotional closeness.

Interpreter

To make sense of the information they acquire about themselves, each other, and their relationship, partners need an "interpreter" or "processor" of the information. Rarely are the causes or consequences of an affair simple. Some information can be understood from an individual perspective, but other disclosures only make sense when viewed from interactive perspectives between partners or between the couple and other members of their extended family or social system. Influences identified from recent events may conflict with those stemming from a more distant past. In the midst of their own turmoil, it is unrealistic to expect partners to be able to distinguish among predisposing, precipitating, and perpetuating influences related to the affair or partners' recovery. You will need to work collaboratively with the couple as all three of you contribute to this process. However, as the couple's therapist, you are uniquely equipped to serve this integrative, interpretive role, and ideally you are able to draw on multiple theoretical perspectives as appropriate. In the process, you will share your understanding with the couple, who can then accept, reject, or revise the information and integrate it in a way that is meaningful for them.

Advocate

Couples need someone to believe in them and in their relationship, particularly when they are not confident in themselves. It is important to reassure couples that some of the most profoundly distressed couples you have worked with in the past not only have recovered but have found ways to create a new and stronger relationship. Out of the ashes often comes new growth, healthier, with deeper roots, unimpeded by the decayed underbrush of old, ineffective patterns. While being an advocate and at times a cheerleader, you must always remain honest, avoiding reassurances that are unrealistic or that suggest strengths that are absent. Thus, the principle of creating an atmosphere that is safe, trusting, and realistic is always present.

"I'm encouraging you to have trust in this process and confidence in yourselves to work through it to reach good decisions by the end. In my experience, about a third of the couples who use this process to work through an affair restore a strong marriage and move on, feeling as strong as or even healthier than before. Another third stay together but continue to struggle, sometimes because they never address some of the problems that may have put their relationship at risk in the first place. Of the one third of couples who decide to move on separately, many do so in ways that permit both partners to develop new, satisfying intimate relationships with someone else. Others move on in ways that leave one or both partners wounded. However, my experience suggests that if you'll both commit to working through this process together, you'll be able to reach a decision about your relationship that makes sense and will take you where you need to go as a couple."

Partners' Roles

You can also encourage a collaborative alliance by conveying clearly to partners their own roles in therapy, in terms of both how they interact with each other and how they engage in the treatment process.

Mutual Involvement

It is critical that both partners commit to attending regularly, actively participating in sessions, and engaging in exercises you may provide for working between sessions, whether separately or together.

Commitment to Safety

Both partners should be asked to commit to restraint from verbal and physical aggression both within and between sessions. It may be useful to acknowledge that the pledge involving restraint from verbal aggression can sometimes be difficult to honor; however, partners' commitment to this principle includes disclosing in the therapy sessions times and specific ways they have struggled or fallen short of this goal and inviting you as their therapist to focus on these events as a means of restoring both physical and emotional safety.

Accountability for Self

Both partners should be asked to take responsibility for their own decisions— past, present, and future. It is useful to distinguish between "reasons" and "excuses" for behaving in any particular way. Emphasizing this concept from the outset of treatment has two key advantages: (1) It encourages partners to take responsibility for their own contributions to current interactions rather than focusing primarily on what they would like the other person to do differently, and (2) it paves the way for interventions in Stage 2, which will explore a broad range of factors potentially contributing to vulnerability to the affair, including potential influences from the injured partner.

Honesty

Further deceit by either partner, regardless of the intention or rationale, will undermine efforts toward recovery. The couple should be reassured that they will receive some guidance on what to discuss and in what ways. Partners should be informed that, for now, they will not be required to disclose or talk about everything, but whatever they say must be honest.

> "Susan, I understand that there are details about your affair that you're not yet willing to share with Vince, just as I understand, Vince, how important it feels to you to discuss these details. For now, Susan, I advise you to handle this in the following way: If Vince pursues specific aspects of the affair you're not yet willing to discuss, I want you to say, `I know this is important to you, but I'm not yet ready to talk about this. It doesn't feel safe enough yet to do that. I don't want to avoid the truth by lying. But I'm asking that for now you accept that I'm not yet ready to discuss this part of the situation on our own. I'm willing for you to raise that question in our next session to see if we can handle it better there. I know we'll probably need to talk about those questions eventually.' Can you do this? That way, whatever you say, Vince can start to believe that you're telling him the truth, and the two of you will begin restoring a basis of trust in your relationship. Let's try it now, just to make sure you understand what I'm asking of you."

Feedback to the Therapist

Therapists foster a deeper therapeutic alliance when they invite feedback from partners about the therapy process along the way. This includes partners' responses to the initial conceptualization of the treatment process, reactions to specific formulations or interpretations along the way, experiences of confusion or frustration with either the pacing or content of sessions, or other potential intrusions into the therapeutic alliance. As therapist, you have a unique opportunity to model effective communication and input by inviting partners' concerns about the therapeutic process, listening empathically, and working to create mutually acceptable ways of collaborating.

Commitment to the Process, Not to a Particular Outcome

Similar to the therapist's own commitment to the therapeutic process rather than to a specific outcome, neither partner should be asked to commit to staying in their relationship or moving on separately either by the therapist or by the other person. However, both partners should be encouraged to adopt a shared goal of moving on in a healthy way, free of disabling hurt, anger, or shame.

Fostering Hope

Hope undergirds commitment and sustains efforts, fostering resilience in the face of frustrations, disappointments, or enduring pain. Encourage both partners to remain hopeful, noting that they may already have survived the worst and now have the opportunity to build something better.

Summary

Establishing and maintaining a therapeutic alliance with couples struggling to recover from an affair presents unique challenges. Both partners may exhibit intense emotions of depression, anxiety, hurt, guilt, and anger, impairing their ability to engage constructively in interactions with each other and with you as their therapist. The potential for rapid escalation of negative exchanges within sessions is particularly high with affair couples. The perceived imbalance of partners' roles as perpetrator and victim may further complicate efforts to build and maintain a therapeutic alliance.

An essential task in working with affair couples is establishing an atmosphere of safety and trust. The therapist must contain the partners' negative exchanges while facilitating their disclosure of vulnerable feelings. Because these couples so frequently struggle with difficulties in managing their own turmoil, they need to experience confidence in their therapist's expertise early in treatment. You can promote this confidence by demonstrating your understanding of affair-related trauma and recovery through providing a normative context for partners' respective experiences and describing an explicit three-stage model for recovery. Confidence in your expertise is further enhanced by clarifying policies for ensuring partners' physical safety, handling issues of confidentiality, and affirming a commitment of fairness to both partners.

Couples need to have clear expectations about your roles as therapist and their own roles as participants in the therapeutic process. You should describe ways in which you will function as an educator about couple- and affair-related processes, a conductor and facilitator of constructive exchanges, a translator of partners' respective experiences, and an advocate for their relationship. Partners also need to understand their own responsibilities for engaging actively in therapy both during and between sessions and being accountable for their own behaviors, particularly restraint from verbal and physical aggression. Both partners need encouragement to retain hope and to commit to a therapeutic process rather than a specific relationship outcome. They need confidence that although the journey ahead may be difficult, with sustained effort they can expect to experience relief.

PART TWO

STAGE 1 OF TREATMENT

Introduction to Stage 1 of Treatment

As we described in Chapter 1, individuals' responses to infidelity often unfold in three stages. Although progress through these stages may be unsteady and marked by occasional lapses or steps backward, recognizing the stage that each person is experiencing when the couple comes for treatment provides a help-ful conceptual framework for you as the clinician, both for understanding the couple's dilemmas and for planning treatment. When the injured partner first learns that the other partner is having or has had an affair, the injured individual often is overwhelmed by this new knowledge. Although there is variability among couples, this immediate awareness sets the stage for a wide range of experiences that are typical in Stage 1.

During this stage, the couple is grappling with the new shared information and trying to understand how it fits into their lives, which feels quite different than it did before the affair. As we discussed in Chapter 1, the injured partner typically is confused, emotionally overwhelmed and dysregulated, and uncertain how to behave. Often both partners feel misunderstood: The injured partner feels betrayed, and the participating partner feels that he or she is being portrayed as evil or psychopathic without any understanding or empathy for the difficulties that he or she has been experiencing. Either inadvertently or intentionally, one or both partners often behave in ways that make matters worse once the affair is known. You need to address all these experiences in Stage 1 of treatment.

GOALS FOR STAGE 1

As a therapist, you will individualize the treatment to each couple based on a careful assessment, as described in Chapter 2. Within this context, however, if a couple is in Stage 1, there are three overarching goals that you, as a clinician, will help them achieve before moving to additional goals in Stages 2 and 3:

- Damage control.
- Restoring equilibrium and order.
- Understanding and validating each person's experiences.

Damage Control

The mantra for a couple in Stage 1 should be "First, do no further harm." When the two partners initially confront the reality of an affair, their emotions often rise to an extreme level, at times involving a great deal of anger and hostility. During such times, we have seen individuals who were previously kind and gentle become physically abusive toward their partners. In addition to obviously unacceptable acts such as physical abuse, some partners say or do less extreme things that can have damaging long-term consequences, such as asserting that the other individual has never been sexually appealing because of being overweight. Thus, it is critical during this stage to ensure that the partners interact in ways that do not inflict further damage on the relationship.

In addition, partners sometimes behave in ways that create difficulties with other individuals around them. For example, upon learning that her professor husband had had an affair with a female graduate student, a wife sent an e-mail to his faculty colleagues informing them of his behavior. Although it was intended as retaliation to hurt the husband, this act could also complicate the partners' lives in the future as a result of unintended consequences, such as disciplinary action or even termination of employment for the husband. Similarly, a wife who tells her parents that her husband has had an affair may irreparably damage the relationship between her husband and parents, even if she and her husband eventually work through the affair and decide to stay together. Therefore, you should work with the couple to stop detrimental behaviors that will impact interactions with the outside world, along with educating the couple to prevent such behaviors from beginning.

Restoring Equilibrium and Order

During Stage 1, not only are the partners confused and emotionally distressed, but their typical patterns of behavior break down as well. The two partners might have worked well together as a team before the affair, but now they may be unwilling to provide needed help to each other. Thus, routine chores that keep the family moving forward are no longer maintained. Similarly, partners may no longer demonstrate caring and openness to each other. For example, they may not want to eat dinner together or discuss the day's events. This breakdown of interaction patterns can be further complicated when one or both partners become so distressed that individual adaptive behaviors are altered as well; that is, their sleeping becomes disrupted; they stop exercising, or they lose their appetite. Therefore, important goals early in treatment are to provide some sense of order and to establish acceptable patterns of interaction between the partners.

Understanding and Validating Each Person's Experiences

When couples arrive for treatment and are experiencing Stage 1, each person often feels terrible and needs to be understood and validated. Both people need to be able to tell their "story" and be heard by a thoughtful, understanding therapist: you. In addition, each person needs to be heard and understood by the partner. Often during this time of heightened distress, the partners understandably react to each other in extremely negative ways. Either they justify, defend, and blame rather than validate each other, or they withdraw from each other and refuse to express feelings and related thoughts about the infidelity. An important goal of therapy during Stage 1 is to validate both partners yourself while also providing them with resources to help them talk effectively with each other.

CHALLENGES AND RISKS FOR THE THERAPIST DURING STAGE 1 OF TREATMENT

Dealing with couples who have experienced an affair is very challenging work, and the therapeutic context is complicated. However, it can be mitigated to some degree if you understand the potential pitfalls and challenges that are likely at different stages of the treatment. We have already briefly alluded to some of these challenges that are present throughout treatment but are particularly pertinent to Stage 1:

- Getting lost in the chaos.
- Taking sides with one partner.
- Encouraging unrealistic commitments from either partner.
- Attempting to exert influence over persons not in the therapy room.
- Failing to differentiate between normative distress versus danger.

Getting Lost in the Chaos

As noted, couples in Stage 1 often are confused, feel out of control, and have no idea how to proceed in their lives or during the therapy sessions. Negative emotions are at a fever pitch. It is critical, therefore, that you, as the therapist, avoid becoming swept up in their experience of chaos and confusion. You need to provide structure and direction during this time of confusion and distress for the couple. Having unstructured sessions and allowing the couple to guide the sessions will likely result in their continuing to jump from one topic to the next and interact in destructive ways that mirror their conversations and interactions at home. Many couples comment on the comfort and relief they experience from the structure and direction of the therapy session, when the therapist explains where the session is headed and the reasons for it. Some of the most common concerns we hear from therapists who are inexperienced in this kind of work are that the sessions seem out of control and the therapists are uncertain how to proceed. They have become caught up in the chaos. In writing this book, we have attempted to provide you with a road map that you can share with your couples.

Taking Sides with One Partner

In addition to expressing care and concern for both partners, the therapist must decide how to respond to behaviors that have been destructive to the couple, including lies, deceptions, and sexual behavior outside of the relationship. Although it may feel natural to side with the injured partner, if a therapist responds to destructive behaviors in a highly moralistic and judgmental fashion, the therapist will likely alienate the participating partner, and run the risk of imposing the therapist's own value system on the couple. On the other hand, responding to such behaviors in a neutral manner can put forth the message that the therapist considers these behaviors to be acceptable. Hence, we have found it most useful to evaluate with the couple whether a given set of behaviors has a detrimental impact on either partner, the relationship, or others around them. In addition, we help couples evaluate whether a given behavior is consistent or inconsistent with their own standards and values and how it relates to their implicit or explicit "relationship contract" for acceptable behavior. By using such strategies, usually we have found it possible to create a common agreement about what behaviors are detrimental and need to be addressed, typically without siding with either partner.

Encouraging Unrealistic Commitments from Either Partner

In an attempt to minimize further damage and create a sense of safety and predictability, therapists may be tempted to ask partners to make commitments about how they will behave toward each other and with other people in the future. For example, if a couple has been having endless conversations about why the affair occurred, you might be inclined to ask them to agree to terminate such conversations outside of the therapy sessions for the time being. Although this approach might be optimal for the couple, you must consider whether it is realistic. The injured partner often feels obsessed with the question of "why" and is likely to be unsuccessful in totally avoiding conversations about the affair. Consequently, you might find it more productive to discuss the overall goals for the couple and decide together about a realistic set of expectations. To set expectations and reach agreements with the couple that are then not respected can lead to further discouragement and hopelessness for the couple, and can create doubt about the utility of treatment.

Even more damaging can be unrealistic commitments made about interactions with the outside-affair person. It might be optimal for the participating partner to terminate all interactions with this person immediately, but in many instances such a step is not realistic at the beginning of therapy. Making an ill-advised commitment with subsequent failure to honor it will likely compound the couple's problems. It is essential to begin developing a pattern of trust and openness between the injured and the participating partners as treatment begins. Therefore, as a therapist, you might work with the couple to establish a long-term goal of no future interaction with the outside person and then discuss realistic intermediate strategies for reaching that long-term goal.

Attempting to Exert Influence over Persons Not in the Therapy Room

It is always a therapeutic challenge when people not present in the therapy room can have a major impact on the therapy process. With highly emotional issues such as infidelity, family and friends are quick to offer advice, which may run counter to your therapeutic plan. Friends are often generous in their conclusion that "You should take all the money out of the bank, grab the children, and leave that sorry creature tomorrow morning when he goes to work, and don't let him ever find you!" Perhaps even more demanding is dealing with an outside-affair person who does not want to end the relationship. Some outside-affair partners might continue to initiate interaction with the participating partner or suggest maintaining the relationship in total secrecy. Or, confronted with the reality that the relationship is ending, the outside-affair person might threaten to commit suicide or engage in some other destructive behavior. Not having had direct contact with this person, as a therapist you will be working with the couple to help them make decisions regarding how to respond when there are potential major consequences and yet you are receiving only second-hand information about the individual and the situation.

Differentiating between Normative Distress Versus Danger

When an affair comes to light, one or both partners are likely to become overwhelmed and make statements such as "I can't take it. I think I'm going crazy. I would rather die than live like this." Although you always want to take such expressions seriously in terms of how the person feels, it is more complicated to assess whether the person is likely to act on these thoughts and feelings. This is one reason why a careful assessment of current functioning and each person's history is important. Even with such information, it is often impossible to predict precisely, particularly given that many individuals have never been in such an extreme situation. Thus, as a therapist you must assess the danger that is suggested by such statements. At the beginning of treatment, you might want to see the couple frequently, more often than the traditional one session per week. At the same time, you do not want to overreact to every statement of distress. It is important to help the couple begin to develop a sense of individual and couple efficacy, as you reassure them that they can tolerate the distress and that you will provide them with the structure and direction to help them through the process.

CONCLUDING COMMENTS

Chapters 4, 5, and 6 provide detailed descriptions of how to help couples address the issues that you and they are likely to confront in the immediate aftermath of learning about an affair: Stage 1 of treatment. Consistent with the goals described previously, Chapter 4 provides a series of strategies and specific interventions that can be used to minimize further damage. Chapter 5 offers strategies and techniques to help the couple restore a sense of equilibrium and control in their individual lives and relationship. Chapter 6 elaborates on ways to help both people feel understood and validated both by the other partner and by you without alienating the other individual present in the therapy room. Throughout these chapters and the remainder of the book, we provide detailed discussions of how to address the challenges and risks encountered by couples as they struggle to recover from an affair.

CHAPTER 4

Damage Control

PAM: You did *what*? You actually told your mother that I got involved with Mark? I can't believe it. Were you just trying to get back at me? Even if we get through this, how am I ever going to face your parents again? Telling your mother means telling everyone in your family—your father, sister, brother, and whoever else she considers "part of the family." Nothing is private in your family; you know that.

TOM: No, I wasn't trying to get back at you. If I wanted to do that, you would know it, believe me. I've always talked to my mother when I have a problem, and this certainly qualifies as a problem. You know that about me. Maybe you should have taken me and how I operate into account before you got involved with Mark. You caused this mess, and I'm not going to lie to cover up for you.

THERAPIST: Let's stop for a moment. I know you're both really upset, and things seem terrible already. Let's talk about how you want to handle discussing the affair with other people so that you don't make things worse and still are respectful of needs that one or both of you might have, such as Tom's wish to tell someone and get support.

When couples are struggling with an affair, they typically have strong emotions and are not thinking clearly. As a result, at times they respond to these strong emotions in order to lower their distress or feel better in the short term, without recognizing or caring about the long-term consequences of their behavior. Even under the best of circumstances, dealing with an extramarital affair is extremely difficult, and it becomes increasingly complex when one or both partners compound the problem by responding in hurtful ways. Thus, a major goal early in treatment is to avoid or minimize further damage to either person and to the relationship.

In this chapter, we discuss ways in which partners often complicate matters by their responses to the affair, along with therapeutic strategies you can use to help them avoid such complications. In doing so, we explore two major areas of potential damage:

- Damage within the relationship involving either individual or their relationship.
- Damage between either individual and the outside world.

In both instances, the additional damage might be intentional or inadvertent. In the prior example, Pam and Tom are debating why Tom told his mother about Pam's affair. Did he tell her in order to get back at Pam or punish Pam in some way for having hurt him so deeply? Although clearly angry, Tom responds that he simply needed to talk to his mom. What responsibility does he have for potential negative consequences for Pam or for their marriage from seeking this support from his mother? What responsibilities does the therapist have?

Minimizing Additional Damage to Partners and the Relationship

Intentional Hurtful Acts Directed toward the Partner

At times, one or both partners are so angry or distressed about the affair or the couple's interactions after the affair that they strike out at the other person in a variety of ways to be hurtful. As the therapist, your major goals are to stop such behaviors immediately when they occur to avoid escalation and to help the couple develop strategies to avoid such behaviors in the future. Although partners in these circumstances find many ways to hurt each other, we discuss typical patterns as well as strategies you can use to help couples in these circumstances.

Destructive Couple Interactions

After an affair, partners often are most destructive when they are interacting directly with each other. Although both partners might initiate or at least contribute to these interactions, often these destructive interactions are initiated by the injured partner. At times, the mere presence of the participating partner is enough to trigger strong feelings of anger and a desire for revenge. As a result, many couples dealing with affairs have angry and destructive conversations, both at home and during the therapy sessions. For example, Pam and Tom reported a conversation they had the night before their therapy session:

THERAPIST: Why don't you briefly bring me up to date on how things have been since I last saw you?

PAM: Things have been terrible. We had a horrible argument last night. Tom just won't let up. He tries to make me talk about it constantly, and last night he started pushing every button he could think of. What I did with Mark was bad enough, but if Tom keeps this up, he's going to put the final touches on destroying our marriage. He started laughing at me, saying that Mark and I must really have a strong intellectual connection because Mark certainly couldn't be responding to my big thighs and small breasts. That was *so* hurtful. I was tempted to let him have it, but I managed not to sling mud back at him.

TOM: You know, for years you've complained that I'm too mild mannered and not assertive enough, and that's one of the things you found appealing about Mark. Well, I'm going to assert myself from now on and tell you exactly what I think.

THERAPIST: Okay, thanks for updating me. It sounds like things got pretty bad during some of your conversations. I think we need to establish some guidelines about how you two are going to talk with each other and stay out of these types of interactions . . .

Although these hurtful statements often come from the injured partner, participating partners can make equally hurtful comments, particularly if they feel pushed to talk about the affair and become exasperated with what they experience as a constant barrage of questions. For example, earlier in the week Pam felt "worn out" by Tom's endless questions about why she "did it." Finally, she responded:

"Okay, if you want to know, I'll tell you. I have huge respect for Mark. He's bright and ambitious, and he knows how to get where he wants to go. I happen to find that very appealing; he's confident and believes in himself. Unlike you, he's not going to sit in the same job for years, particularly when he's not happy with it. I just can't respect you when you act like that; you come home and complain but you never do anything about it. Why can't you stand up and be a man? Maybe then, I'd want to lie down with you."

Some hurtful behaviors extend beyond the verbal level. For couples who have used physical force or have been physically violent with each other in the past, the discovery of an affair is a particularly high-risk situation for more aggression. In essence, some couples have allowed themselves to use physical force such as hitting, shoving, slapping, or more violent strategies as ways of expressing their anger or as ways to control the other person. For such couples, an affair seems to justify such a response of physically hurting the other person. Even among couples who have never shown physical violence, discovery of an affair can trigger an escalation of conflict, culminating in hitting or harming a partner physically. These expressions of aggression after an affair are consistent with broader findings that traumatic experiences in a wide variety of contexts are associated with high levels of both verbal and physical partner aggression among both men and women (Taft, Watkins, Stafford, Street, & Monson, 2007).

Destructive Behaviors in the Partner's Absence

Not all hurtful behavior aimed at a partner occurs during interactions between them. For example, Andrea had eagerly supported Will's recent decisions to buy what seemed like a whole new wardrobe. She was delighted that he seemed to be taking more pride in his appearance. When she learned that this new pride in his appearance coincided with an affair he was having, she took each piece of his new clothing, burned a hole in it, and then neatly hung the clothes back in his closet.

In such instances, it seems clear that the upset partner is knowingly and willfully behaving in a destructive manner. Some people seem to operate on the principle of retribution: "When you hurt me this badly, I'll hurt you back." The presumption is that the magnitude of the payback should be consistent with the original injury, and that an affair warrants a huge response.

There are a variety of strategies that you might use to stop or prevent such destructive behaviors. Some of these strategies involve structuring the environment and the couple's interactions to lower the risk of destructive behaviors. On many occasions, you might want to directly target one or both partners' strong emotions that contribute to the destructive behavior. At other times, you might conclude that the destructive behavior follows from a partner's beliefs about how to respond to being hurt. In those instances, you'll need to explore those beliefs and help the person develop new ways of thinking about how to respond to being harmed. Next we note strategies that we have found to be effective, recognizing that therapists might use other strategies as well, in order to achieve the goal of helping stop destructive interactions at this highly volatile time.

Therapeutic Strategies to Address Hurtful Behaviors Aimed at the Partner

DISSECTING DESTRUCTIVE INTERACTIONS. One of the most effective ways to minimize destructive behaviors that are triggered by strong emotions is to restructure the couple's environment and the ways they interact in order to keep emotions at a low level or to help the partners alter their responses when emotions do escalate. Before attempting to help them restructure their environment, first it is important to know exactly what happens when they interact: what one person says or does, what the other person thinks and feels in response, how the partner then responds, and so on. That is, you can have the couple describe the situation within which emotions escalate and subsequent destructive behaviors occur (Kirby & Baucom, 2007a, 2007b). The goal is to interrupt this sequence of behaviors, thoughts, and emotions as early in the interaction as possible before the couple escalates. For example, the therapist helped Pam and Tom discern that Pam frequently made hurtful comments about Tom's character when Tom repeatedly asked her what she found so appealing about Mark. They reported that at first Pam would avoid responding, but if Tom persisted eventually she would describe something that was a strength of Mark's and a weakness of Tom's. Her thinking went something like this, "If you're going to keep pushing me, I'll tell you something that will shut you up." In essence, she wanted Tom to stop asking her these questions, so she punished his response by making hurtful statements. The therapist pointed out this pattern, and for the short term Tom agreed to stop asking Pam this question at home.

THERAPIST: I think we're starting to get a handle on what happens that results in Pam saying things that really hurt you, Tom. Let me see if I understand it, okay? Tom, it sounds like you're really trying to understand why Pam got involved with Mark, and you can't get it out of your mind. So you ask her to help you understand, and the way you do that is by asking her to compare you directly with Mark—why she preferred him over you—is that right?

TOM: When I hear it, it sounds pretty stupid, but I guess that's right.

THERAPIST: So a part of you sees that this is not the best way to go about understanding what happens, but you don't know what else to do, and when you're upset, you probably aren't thinking that clearly anyway. So we need to figure out how you can do this more effectively. Then it sounds like Pam tries to avoid answering, either by saying nothing or that she doesn't want to talk about it. Tom, you keep pushing, and then, Pam, you feel angry and hurt and respond in some very hurtful way yourself, talking about Mark's strengths and Tom's weaknesses in order to stop his questioning. Is that right?

PAM: Well, yes. But that's exactly what Tom is asking me, so if he won't let up, I finally tell him.

THERAPIST: Right, but am I correct that you tell him in a way that you know is going to really hurt or upset him?

PAM: Sure, but at that point I'm not worried about him. I'm angry myself, and I want to get him off my back. If he didn't push me, I wouldn't respond that way.

THERAPIST: Exactly. The two of you are caught in a vicious cycle where both of you end up doing the opposite of what you intend. Tom, you want to understand, but the way you try to understand hurts and angers Pam and pushes her away. And Pam, when you get angry and lash out at Tom, it makes his confusion and pain worse, and he pushes more. So what we're trying to do is get an understanding of what each of you does and how that triggers the other person's response. Let's go back and look at each step along the way and what you might do differently so that you don't repeat these hurtful conversations.

THERAPIST DIRECTIVES/RECOMMENDATIONS. In the prior example, the therapist had a conversation with the couple in order to gain some understanding about hurtful behaviors that were happening at home. At other times, as the therapist, you might have a clearer picture of what needs to happen for a couple to end their destructive behaviors, even though they are not clear on what would be helpful. Therefore, at times you might decide to give the couple explicit directives or recommendations about what to avoid outside of the session. For example, you might request of a couple, "I think that right now things are simply too volatile for you to have any discussion that involves Mark outside of our sessions. For now, let's restrict those conversations to our therapy sessions." Therapists from different theoretical orientations vary in terms of how directive they typically are with couples, yet the crisis nature of this time creates in many couples a need for structure and direction from the therapist.

TIME-OUT PROCEDURES/TAKING A BREAK IN THE ACTION. The prior procedures attempt to minimize the likelihood that the couple will have certain interactions that lead to escalating emotions. During this time of crisis and emotional instability, it is almost impossible to avoid high-risk interactions and escalating emotions altogether. When these interactions do occur, it is important to terminate them as quickly as possible. In these situations, you might help the couple use a time-out procedure in which they stop their interaction and each person does something alone to lower the emotional intensity. The important elements of the time-out procedure are that the partners stop interacting with each other, use the time apart to de-escalate their emotions rather than preparing a new battle strategy, and come back to interact in a different way following the time-out. Table 4.1 offers guidelines for conducting a time-out that you can discuss with the couple. (Some couples like the term "time-out" because of its clear, direct meaning, but others associate it with strategies for parenting young children and can find the term demeaning. Therefore, alternative terms such as "taking a break" or "cool-down period" can be used to communicate the idea that the couple needs to stop the interaction before it becomes too heated.)

Although time-outs typically are viewed as short-term breaks in interactions between the two partners, you might conclude that, at least for the time being, continuing to live in the same house with each other would create a high risk of escalation into serious psychological or physical aggression between these partners. At such times, it is important to raise this concern with the couple, discuss it, and reach a mutually agreeable strategy to maintain the physical and emotional safety of both partners. In some instances, you might conclude that the partners need to be apart for the immediate future and, therefore, you would recommend that they live in different settings for now. You can then discuss with them different strategies for accomplishing this goal. In contrast to most other situations, during this crisis period when the partners might not be thinking clearly and the physical or emotional well-being of one or both persons is at stake, it is appropriate to be active and directive in establishing a safe environment for the couple.

FREQUENT THERAPY SESSIONS AND TELEPHONE CALLS TO THE THERAPIST. The above strategies involve actions the partners can take on their own

TABLE 4.1. Guidelines for Constructive Time-Outs

Recognize when your feelings may be getting out of control. Some signs might be
- You're yelling or getting louder as you speak.
- You're having "hot thoughts."
- You're slamming doors or throwing things.
- You can't listen to what your partner is saying.
- You're cursing or using other hurtful language.
- Your muscles are getting tense or your stomach feels upset.

Acknowledge your feelings without blaming your partner.

Share the responsibility. Either one or both partners can call for a time-out.

Develop a plan. Be sure you and your partner are clear about the following:
- Who leaves the room? Both of you? The one who calls the time-out?
- How long will the time-out last?
- When and where will you get back together?

Use time-outs to get your feelings in better control. Techniques that can be helpful include
- Meditation and relaxation techniques.
- Moderate physical exercise.
- Going for a walk (but clarifying with your partner when you'll be back).
- Writing a letter to "vent" your feelings (but then throwing it away).
- Organizing your thoughts so they feel less overwhelming.
- Deciding how to interact with your partner more productively when you get back together.

During a time-out, things you should not do include
- Replaying the earlier argument in your mind and blaming your partner.
- Doing things that could possibly be hurtful to yourself or others (e.g., drinking alcohol, driving when you're upset).

After the time-out is over, you should get back together and try discussing the problem again.

If you're still not able to discuss the problem without either one of you getting out of control, then
- Take another time-out.
  Or:
- Suggest another time (e.g., the next day) to continue discussing the problem.

Note. Adapted from Holtzworth-Munroe, Marshall, Meehan, and Rehman (2003). Copyright (2003) by The Guilford Press. Adapted by permission.

between sessions to minimize destructive behavior. Another way to decrease the chances that emotions will spiral out of control is to schedule frequent treatment sessions during the early crisis period. With frequent sessions, the therapist can provide prompt, corrective feedback to the partners if they are becoming destructive as well as a therapeutic context for addressing volatile issues that need to be discussed. Likewise, you might invite either partner to call you if the partner becomes concerned that the interactions are becoming highly destructive or dangerous. If you do provide the option of telephone calls, you need to ensure that neither partner takes advantage of this offer simply to complain about the other person, share secrets, or express routine distress during this difficult time. Partners should be encouraged to call *only if* they believe that their interactions are becoming dangerous or destructive and they are unable to change the interactions. You also may want to set additional limits or ground rules for the content of these crisis calls; Linehan (1993) provides useful examples of preemptive ground rules for crisis calls in her treatment manual for working with emotionally dysregulated individuals; these same guidelines apply to working with couples in times of crisis.

PROMOTING EFFECTIVE COMMUNICATION AND SHARING OF EMOTIONS. The strategies just discussed are aimed primarily at avoiding high-risk situations or terminating them quickly. Because partners typically have strong negative feelings after the discovery of an affair, they need ways to express their feelings to each other adaptively. The ability to express emotions adaptively is important in almost all couple therapy but takes on particular significance after a trauma such as infidelity. Verbally expressing hurt, confusion, anger, and disappointment in appropriate ways can lessen the likelihood that either partner will lash out destructively. One way to achieve the goal of effective communication is to teach the couple communication skills for expressing their feelings and thoughts about the affair, and a significant portion of Chapter 6 is devoted to communication training and other strategies for emotional expression. Several therapeutic approaches that have empirical support for their broad utility in treating relationship distress assist couples in expressing deep emotions without an emphasis on skills training. For example, a primary focus of Johnson and Greenberg's (1995) emotionally focused couple therapy involves helping couples express important feelings about their relationship without skills training. Likewise, integrative behavioral couple therapy (Jacobson & Christensen, 1996b) and insight-oriented couple therapy (Snyder & Wills, 1989) place a heavy focus on adaptive expression of emotion without emphasizing communication skills. What seems to be important is to provide sufficient structure in the session along with a safe environment and guidance from the therapist to assist partners in expressing strong emotions in an adaptive way, regardless of the specific interventions used to achieve this goal.

ADDRESSING DESTRUCTIVE THOUGHTS AND BELIEFS THAT CONTRIBUTE TO DESTRUCTIVE BEHAVIOR. Not only do destructive behaviors result from certain interaction patterns that trigger strong emotions, but some partners behave destructively because they believe they *should* behave that way. It can be difficult to convince partners to stop behaving in hurtful ways when they believe that such behavior is appropriate. Therefore, at times it is important to address the partners' thoughts and beliefs that lead to subsequent hurtful behavior. For example, injured partners often feel justified in hurting participating partners in a wide variety of ways based on beliefs about retribution: "If you hurt me, I should hurt you back." Such beliefs form a relationship rule or standard regarding how one should behave in this circumstance. Altering such beliefs or standards can be complex and time consuming but fundamentally involves helping partners see the negative implications of the standards and behaviors. Epstein and Baucom (2002, pp. 352–356) provide a detailed discussion of how to work with partners in couple therapy to alter important relationship standards for how one should behave toward a partner. The basic steps in addressing a person's standard for responding to hurt are provided as follows:

- Clarify the person's standard for how to respond after being hurt by the partner.

    "If you hurt me, I should hurt you back."
- List advantages and disadvantages of that standard, with input from both partners.

    "You might be less likely to do it again if you know there is a big price to pay."

    "If I hurt you badly, you might feel justified in your own behavior, retaliate, or decide you don't want to be with someone like me."
- Search for some shift in the standard, however slight, that might accomplish the same goals without the destructive impact.

    "If you hurt me, I should let you know how destructive you have been but do it in a way that doesn't make things worse between us."

- Translate the shared standard into specific behaviors that each person will enact.

    "Rather than call you names, I'll tell you directly how much you hurt me and how much I continue to hurt and am disappointed in you."

- Try behaving according to the new standard for a trial period, and evaluate its impact on each person and the relationship.

    "For the next week, I will not call you any names but will tell you at agreed upon times how I am feeling about the affair."

- Engage in problem solving about any difficulties that arise during the trial period, recognizing that shifting long-standing personal standards is likely to be difficult for each individual.

    "When I don't say hurtful things to you and instead express my hurt directly, you don't seem to take it as seriously, as if things are going to be just fine. We need to have a way for you to understand how horrible it is for me without my having to escalate."

- Modify the new standard and try another trial period.

This series of steps is based on a detailed strategy for analyzing one partner's thinking about appropriate ways to respond to hurt. Approaching relationship standards might be done in a more informal way as well, in which you and the couple discuss their beliefs about ways to respond after being hurt and treated in ways that seem unfair. Such a discussion can include alternative ways to think about betrayals and appropriate ways to respond, including what would be realistic for these specific partners. Regardless of the specific strategies used, it can be important to clarify whether destructive behavior is driven by beliefs regarding what is appropriate and then helping the couple consider alternative ways to think about how to respond when needed.

Standards for how one should behave after being hurt by a partner often correspond to a prediction or expectancy of what will happen if the injured person does not respond by punishing the participating partner: "If your partner has an affair and you don't punish him strongly for it, you're just asking for him to do it again. Make him pay a price; otherwise, you're weak and deserve more of the same." In such circumstances, you might find it useful to discuss the notion of reciprocity with the couple (Gottman, 1979). Research indicates that negative behaviors from one partner greatly increase the likelihood that the other partner will respond in a negative manner as well. However, this sequence in which both people have now responded negatively does not usually terminate the interaction. Instead, it increases the likelihood that additional negative behaviors will occur. Over time, not only does this pattern establish an atmosphere of ongoing negative interactions, but also the intensity of the negativity often escalates. Therefore, "paying back" the participating partner usually sets the stage for continued destructive behaviors by both partners. The issue here is not whether the injured partner has the right to hurt the participating partner in return; instead, the issue is the consequences that result from such ongoing destructive behavior. Helping partners see how their behaviors ultimately hurt *themselves or make matters worse* can help to shift beliefs and behaviors involving retribution.

Naturally, the injured partner wants to make certain that the participating partner never has another affair. You can show them alternative ways to try to achieve that goal without engaging in destructive behaviors. Typically, both partners acknowledge that their interactions have become destructive and that life is feeling increasingly unbearable. Consequently, it is important that they make a strong effort to stop these hurtful interaction patterns. The basic message is: "Don't respond to a hurtful or destructive behavior by engaging in a destructive behavior yourself. Either don't respond at all, do something more neutral, or, when possible, respond to a negative behavior with a positive one, recognizing that the latter response might not be likely during a time of such distress.

Similarly, it can be helpful to appeal to each partner's "good side." During highly stressful and difficult times, you should emphasize to the partners the importance of maintaining their self-respect and avoiding being pulled into destructive behaviors that are uncharacteristic or inconsistent with their values. Rather than "preaching" messages to the couple to be virtuous, it is important to raise these ideas if needed, have a discussion with the couple, and have them decide for themselves how they want to behave during these stressful times.

Unintended Hurtful Acts Directed toward the Partner

Some destructive behaviors, such as those described previously, are intended to hurt the other person. In addition, at times the partners interact in ways that are harmful, even though they are not intending to be destructive. This pattern frequently happens through discussions about the affair. As we discussed in Chapter 1, one devastating consequence of an affair for the injured partner is that it destroys his or her basic assumptions about the participating partner and their relationship. Typically, the injured partner is confused, cannot make sense of what happened, and subsequently feels out of control. As a result, the injured partner often appears obsessed with wanting to know everything possible about the affair, which has felt so confusing. In part, the injured partner hopes that this information will help clarify what has happened. Gaining information is one way of restoring a feeling of control; therefore, the injured partner seeks all possible information as a way of trying to reestablish some sense of control over his or her personal life. We agree that having a full understanding of the *factors that contributed to the development and maintenance of the affair* is critical for the couple to move forward. Establishing this broad context is the central focus of Stage 2 of treatment.

However, understanding the factors that contributed to the development and maintenance of the affair is different from knowing all the details about what the participating partner did with the outside-affair person. For example, knowing details about the sexual behaviors of the two people contributes little or no understanding in most instances; instead, it merely enhances disturbing mental imagery that continues to upset the injured partner. Therefore, besides obtaining information about potential STDs, there is little reason to seek specific, detailed information about sexual behavior. Likewise, knowing detailed information about how the partner experienced the sexual interaction emotionally or physically is unlikely to be productive and will only produce further hurt or emotional distress. Rather than focusing on detailed discussions of the sexual interaction in the affair, it can be much more productive at the appropriate point in therapy for the couple to discuss their satisfaction with their own sexual relationship before the affair and what they might do to enhance it should they decide to stay together.

The parallels between responses to infidelity and posttraumatic stress disorder (PTSD) raise the issue of how to think about the concept of exposure, which is often used successfully in the treatment of PTSD and other anxiety disorders. It is most important to consider what you want to expose the couple to and for what goals. Having the injured partner visualize or rehearse the specific sexual behavior of the participating partner and outside-affair person has little value, and it is not appropriate to set a goal of helping the injured partner have a nondistressed response to such affair-related sexual behavior. However, it is critical that both partners be fully exposed to understanding what happened in general during the affair and the factors that contributed to the affair. Thus, Stage 2 of treatment places a major focus on discussing in detail the factors that contributed to the affair. One or both partners might prefer to avoid such extensive discussion because of the distress it creates; however, we teach them how to have these conversations without engaging in destructive responses. Thus, the partners learn that they do not need to avoid discussing these issues with each other. In essence, they benefit from a form of exposure and response prevention that is effective in treating PTSD.

Given the potential destructive impact of learning about detailed sexual behavior during the affair, we routinely have a conversation with couples early in treatment regarding how to discuss the affair outside of the therapy sessions. It particular, we advise that they not discuss detailed information about sexual behaviors that occurred, statements of affection or endearment that were exchanged between the participating partner and the outside-affair person, or other behaviors that would primarily serve to upset the injured partner without having beneficial consequences. Our concern is that this additional detail will retraumatize the injured partner with little benefit. We do emphasize that it is important for both people to develop a broad understanding of the factors that contributed to the development and maintenance of the affair, and we help them to establish that understanding. Conversations should be geared toward that end rather than an indiscriminate seeking of detailed information. If the injured partner persists that he or she "still just wants to know" about details, we ask that person to wait until later in the therapy to seek this information. Almost never have we had partners persist late in treatment requesting this detailed information.

Unfortunately, by the time they sought treatment, Brad and Gail had already discussed his sexual relationship with Jill in detail:

THERAPIST: . . . So for those reasons, I'd recommend you stay away from really detailed conversations about Brad's sexual relationship with Jill. Does that make sense?

GAIL: Yes, it makes a lot of sense. I only wish we had come to see you sooner. I asked Brad about what happened between him and Jill sexually. He was trying to be honest, and he told me. Now I'm stuck with it. As you know, she's a graduate student in the department where Brad and I both work. So now every time I come into his office, I can visualize the two of them fondling each other. I literally avoid even walking down that hallway now.

THERAPIST: I'm so sorry that happened. Although we can't undo what you already know, I have some ideas of how we might try to make it as bearable as possible; I'll discuss that with you later. Right now, you can see how the types of conversations you've already had can be really destructive. But that doesn't mean we're going to avoid talking about the affair. In fact, we're going to talk about it a lot, but in ways that hopefully will be helpful to you. Most importantly, we're going to explore a wide range of factors that might have influenced Brad's decision to have an affair with Jill. You need to know how it came about so that you can decide whether you want to stay together, what would need to change if you did so this doesn't happen again, and so on.

In addition to making suggestions to couples about what not to discuss, you might also provide guidance about what kinds of conversations might be productive and contribute to the overall therapeutic goals. In Table 4.2 we provide a list of topics about the affair and the couple's relationship subsequent to the affair that might lead to productive conversations. Some couples might be prepared to have some of these conversations on their own, whereas others might need to discuss these topics during therapy sessions. Also, many of these issues will be raised as a part of the treatment described in the remainder of this book. Therefore, rather than merely giving this table to the couple as a handout for them to select what to discuss, you might share it with them, review it together, and decide what would be productive for them to address on their own at this point and what should be discussed later or only in therapy sessions.

Minimizing Additional Damage during Interactions with the Outside World

The prior discussion focuses on how partners interact with each other and how their responses to the affair can create further difficulties for them and damage their relationship. In addition, other individuals in both partners' lives need to be taken into account as the couple attempts to move on from the affair. First, there is the outside-affair person. In situations in which the affair has ended, the participating partner might believe that nothing more needs to be done regarding this person: the affair has ended, and the couple should move on with their lives. However, even if the affair has come to a close, there typically are a number of issues that need to be resolved regarding the outside-affair person. If the injured partner learns of an affair that is ongoing, there are important, immediate decisions that need to be made regarding the relationship with the outside person.

In addition to the outside-affair person, who is usually perceived as a threat by the injured partner, other caring individuals such as friends and family must be considered. Will the couple tell their parents what has hap-

TABLE 4.2. Talking about the Affair

What happened?

- When did the affair begin? Is this person someone you've known for a while? How long had you been feeling attracted to the other person before to the affair? When did it first become flirtatious? When did it become sexual, if it was sexual?

- Who initiated the affair? Did either one of you try to stop it? If so, how? What prevented those efforts from working?

- Is the other person married or in a committed relationship? Does that person's partner know? If so, what was the partner's response? If not, do you or the affair person intend to tell the other partner?

- When and where did you get together? How long did the affair last? How many times did you and the other person engage in sexual activity?

- How much emotional involvement was there? How frequently did you and the outside person talk with or write to each other? What else did you do together?

- What kinds of contraception or protection against sexually transmitted disease (STD) were used? Did you sometimes not use protection? Have you or the other person been tested for STDs?

- How much money was spent on the affair? Were gifts exchanged? What do you intend to do with gifts or other mementos from the affair?

- Has the affair ended? If so, when and why? Who ended it? If the affair has ended, is this just for now or permanently? What contact have you had with the outside person since then? What steps, if any, have you taken to ensure that no further contact takes place? What does the outside-affair person want? What are your plans if the outside person contacts you first?

- Who else knows about the affair? What do others know, and how did they find out?

- Are there any other consequences we need to consider? Could there be any complications at work or other legal problems? Could the outside person make our lives more difficult if he or she wanted to? Could the outside person's partner cause more difficulties? Are we in physical danger?

Why did you do it?

- Why do you think this happened? What was going on with you? What else was going on in your life? What was going on between us?

- What were you thinking about me and our family?

- Why didn't you tell me? (Or why did you wait to tell me?)

(continued)

TABLE 4.2. *(continued)*

Where does this leave us?

- What about us? Should we continue to live together?

- Do you know what you want? How did you reach that decision, and how certain are you that your feelings won't change?

- What do you think it would take for us to get through this? How willing are you to make these changes, and for how long?

- Have you considered divorce? What steps, if any, have you already taken? Have you talked with anyone about moving in with him or her? Have you contacted an attorney? Have you set up a separate bank account?

- How do we deal with the basic tasks of managing the relationship and our household? Do we continue to do laundry together, cook meals, or clean up afterward together? Do we go to church or the kids' ball games together?

- What acts of caring feel okay right now? Should we still call each other during the day just to chat? Do we still have our morning coffee together?

- What other expressions of intimacy do we want? Is it okay to touch one another or to hold hands? Are hugs okay? Do we still sleep together? Do kisses feel okay? What about making love together? What do we do if it starts to feel uncomfortable for either one of us?

- How do we make sure that we talk about the things that need to be talked about?

- How should we handle it when our discussions start to get out of control? Can we set limits on what we say to each other? For how long do we talk at any one time? On when and where we talk about the affair? How should we handle other arguments that get out of control?

- What commitments, if any, does either of us feel prepared to make at this time? Are we ready to make commitments about this relationship? About how to work toward moving on? About our own relationships with our children?

---

pened? How about their children, best friends, and work colleagues? At times, one or both partners might decide that some of these individuals deserve to know what has happened because they are central in the couple's life. Likewise, some of these people can be potential sources of support to one or both partners as they deal with the affair. At the same time, if these individuals become aware of the affair, it might damage the relationship between that person and one of the partners. For example, Pam might be correct that once Tom's parents know about her affair, they will never accept her again. Likewise, one of Tom's friends may lose respect for him if he stays with Pam after she has treated him so poorly. Numerous negative consequences can result from telling friends and family members, even if the intent was to gain support.

Setting Boundaries on Interactions with the Outside-Affair Person

Important Issues to Address When the Affair Has Ended

Whether or not the affair has ended will, in part, determine the kinds of discussions that the couple will need to have about the outside-affair person. Ending an affair typically means that the sexual relationship is over, but it does not necessarily clarify if, how, and under what circumstances the participating partner might interact with the outside-affair person in the future. It is important for couples to address these issues early in treatment. Almost all injured partners experience the outside-affair person as a major threat to the relationship. Continuing to worry about interactions with the outside person can lead the injured partner to experience strong painful emotions, a sense of danger, and a reluctance to become vulnerable and explore the possibility of rebuilding the couple's relationship. In essence, it runs the risk of being retraumatizing. In Table 4.3, we list a number of issues that are valuable for the couple to discuss and make decisions about regarding interactions with the outside-affair person. In discussing these issues, we recommend that you share the following guidelines with the couple:

- The stronger and firmer the boundaries with the outside-affair person, the better for the couple's relationship.
- The couple should only make agreements that they can realistically keep so that they can begin to rebuild their relationship based on honesty and trust.
- Discussing and establishing boundaries is a process that takes time, and decisions might change as time passes.

As noted in Table 4.3, it can be helpful for the couple to decide what, if any, forms of interaction are allowable between the participating partner and the outside-affair person. This issue has become particularly important as modern means of communication have expanded to include more private and convenient forms of communication such as cell phones and e-mail. Given that many affairs occur with friends and colleagues, at times it may be difficult to set absolute limits. Therefore, it also can be helpful for couples to address this issue in terms of the setting or context in which the limits apply.

**TABLE 4.3. Setting Limits Regarding Interactions
with the Outside-Affair Person**

When the affair has ended

- Establish clear expectations regarding limits on any future contact:
  Face-to-face interaction.
  Phone calls.
  Letters or notes.
  Indirect messages through a third person.
- If contacts are to take place, clarify what topics of conversation are acceptable and what are not.
- Develop specific guidelines for how the participating partner is to inform the injured partner of any violations or inadvertent interactions.
- Agree on a plan for how to respond if the other person initiates contact.
- If necessary, reaffirm to the outside person that the affair has ended:
  A letter to the outside person, written or discussed by both partners.
  A phone call, with the injured partner present or participating.
  A face-to-face meeting in a public setting, perhaps with *both* partners present.
- Address special circumstances that require continued contact, such as working in the same office. Specify both the setting and focus of any interactions.
- Specify a trial period and date for reevaluating any agreements, if necessary.

When the affair is ongoing

- Distinguish between intermediate and long-term goals. Be realistic about what to expect in the short term.
- Agree on a time frame for the participating partner to reach a decision regarding the affair.
- Define the limits, if any, on the nature of continued contact.
- Develop specific guidelines for communicating with each other about either partner's contact with the outside person.
- Be clear about next steps to pursue when
  The participating partner decides to end the affair.
  Either partner decides to end the marriage.

When the outside person doesn't want to let go

- Discuss additional strategies for reinforcing to the outside person that the affair is over.
- Examine any potential sources of "mixed messages" to the outside person and take steps to eliminate them.
- If necessary, seek assistance in limiting contact by the outside person from
  Supervisors at work.
  Police or other legal assistance.
- In extreme circumstances, consider moving to another community.

For example, the couple might decide that there is to be no personal e-mail contact, but e-mail contact with the outside person who is a business colleague might be allowable if the e-mail addresses only work-related matters and is written in a way that it would be sent to any other business colleague. This last point implies another area that the couple needs to discuss: specifically, the types of conversation with the outside person that are acceptable. For example, most injured partners do not want the conversations to include any discussion of a personal or relationship nature, including feelings that the participating partner and outside person might still have for each other, expressions of affection or "insider" references, or discussions of the relationship between the participating and injured partner.

It is hoped that the participating partner will be able to abide by all agreements. However, the couple also needs to agree on how the participating partner will inform the injured partner if any violations of the agreements do occur. The following is an example of how Brad and Gail handled contact from the outside-affair person, Jill.

BRAD: We agreed that I would let you know if either Jill or I made any contact with each other. I got an e-mail from her today asking me how I was doing. It was brief, just a few sentences about her new job and then literally asking, "How are you? Jill." As we agreed, I didn't respond, and I hope that will be the end of it.

THERAPIST: Gail, what's your reaction to what Brad just told you, including the e-mail from Jill, how he responded to it, and the fact that he just told you?

GAIL: Well, the e-mail makes me furious. She still hasn't given up and is after my husband. I'm very glad that Brad didn't respond, just as we had agreed. And, although I hate to hear that she's still after him, I am really pleased and relieved that you told me. When you do that, I don't have to wonder if you are in contact with her. I can start to trust that unless you tell me otherwise, nothing is happening. But I also have to be honest; the whole thing really upsets me even though Brad handled it well.

THERAPIST: It's really upsetting to find out that Jill has made contact again, and we can discuss whether you need to take any additional actions regarding her. But what I think is most important is that you two are working as a team on this. Brad didn't respond to her, and it's so important, Brad, that you told Gail about the e-mail. That's exactly what will help to rebuild trust in your relationship.

Important Issues to Address When the Affair Is Continuing

Discussing interactions with the outside-affair person is usually very difficult and emotionally arousing, even if the affair has ended. However, it can become excruciatingly painful and difficult if the injured partner has discovered an affair that is ongoing. In some cases, the participating partner immediately ends the affair once the injured partner has learned of it. If this happens quickly, it is particularly important to ensure that the couple makes agreements that both of them can follow through on, particularly the participating partner. If the participating partner has strong feelings for the outside-affair person, agreeing to end the relationship immediately without ever speaking to, or having any interaction with, the outside person again is likely unrealistic. Rarely does anyone bring a caring relationship to an end so abruptly. Making unrealistic agreements can set the couple up for additional betrayals and deceptions rather than helping them to potentially rebuild a relationship based on honesty.

If the injured partner discovers an ongoing affair, often the participating partner is unwilling to end the outside relationship immediately. Some therapists refuse to work with couples in this circumstance until the participating partner either ends the outside relationship or the current committed relationship. However, we do *not* take this approach. We believe that it is extremely difficult for couples to address this situation, make good decisions, and move forward in a thoughtful way. Therefore, we believe that it is important to assist couples at this painful time rather than telling them to work out this difficult issue first on their own and then come back to see us.

In helping couples address this difficult issue, we make an important distinction between short-term goals and long-term solutions. We directly address a partner's wish to maintain the long-term committed primary relationship while at the same time continuing with another relationship, which is a violation of the couple's implicit or explicit contract. First, we acknowledge and explore the difficult choice that the person faces in giving up a potentially gratifying relationship. Yet, at the same time, we also point out that continuing in a second romantic relationship will make it extremely difficult for the couple to move forward in their own relationship, decide whether to stay together, and explore how to rebuild their relationship and develop a sense of trust. The continuation of the outside relationship almost always makes the injured partner feel extremely vulnerable, results in dysregulation of emotion, and creates barriers between the two people that further complicate their relationship. In essence, there are strong negative consequences for the couple's relationship if the participating partner continues in a relationship with the outside-affair person. By addressing the issue in this way, it is usually possible to help the couple make good decisions without introducing your own moral values about affairs into the therapy.

Without condoning such an arrangement, as the therapist, you will have to help the couple confront the reality that, on an immediate basis, the participating partner may be unwilling to make a decision between the two relationships, and if pushed to make a decision immediately between the two, the decision might be ill informed. Therefore, you and the couple will have to negotiate what forms of contact with the outside-affair person are acceptable on a *short-term basis*, perhaps with time lines for ending either the outside relationship or the current committed relationship or, at the least, a time to revisit the current decisions. When working with a very ambivalent participating partner, it may be useful to adopt motivational interviewing strategies to help the partner him- or herself recognize why making a decision is critical (Miller & Rollnick, 2002). In some cases, it might be useful to conduct some individual sessions focused on exploring and resolving this ambivalence.

It is difficult to know what decisions are reasonable in this context; some injured partners can and are willing to tolerate much more contact than others. The injured partner must not agree to behaviors that constitute continued abuse of the injured partner or the primary relationship or that will come at too great a personal cost, such as precipitating a clinical depression. On the other hand, providing some time and opportunity for the participating partner to bring the outside relationship to a close or decide between the two relationships also is important. In our experience, decisions that couples make about continued contact with the outside person have to be revisited frequently because each person may believe rationally that a particular solution is workable, but after attempting to live with it one or both partners may find the solution unacceptable: "I thought I could do it short term, but I just can't. Knowing you're out with her, supposedly just talking, is destroying me." As the therapist, you need to monitor this issue continually with the couple so that they do not live in an ambiguous and painful state for too long, almost always slowing down or halting the progress they achieve on their own relationship in therapy. For some participating partners, avoiding making a decision between the two relationships is the preferred outcome, but one that must not be allowed to continue indefinitely.

Thus, a number of topics need to be discussed about the outside affair partner, whether the affair has ended or not. Often the injured partner will raise some of these issues early in treatment, providing a natural context for discussion. However, if neither partner raises these issues, it is important for you to raise them early in treatment in order to avoid potential complications in the future. Typically, these issues are most productively addressed through problem-solving or decision-making conversations during the therapy sessions or as homework if the couple can have these discussions without the therapist present. In Chapter 5, we present guidelines to help couples problem solve or make decisions about a wide range of topics, including dealing with the outside-affair person.

Dealing with Family, Friends, and Colleagues

It might seem obvious that the couple needs to discuss the outside-affair person because that individual is such a threat to the current relationship. However, it might not be obvious to the couple that they also need to make decisions about whether and how to address the affair with family, friends, and business associates or colleagues. Some partners conclude that these are important individuals in their lives and, therefore, they deserve to know what has happened. That is, these are people with whom they typically share personal information so either partner might understandably decide to tell them about the affair as well. Moreover, some of these people might be regular sources of support, and a relationship crisis might seem like a particularly important time to draw on that support. Whereas venting, informing people who should know, or seeking support might seem useful in the short run, it also can have some negative consequences that the couple must consider. In helping partners decide whom to tell about the affair, you might share with them the following guidelines:

- Be cautious in telling someone about the affair if it is likely to damage the relationship between that person and either partner in the future (e.g., your parents or your children).

- In discussing the affair, talk with someone who has an exclusive or primary relationship with you (e.g., a single friend who is not a potential romantic partner for you) rather than someone with loyalty to both partners, who could feel torn hearing information from only one of you and might feel uncomfortable taking sides.

- Seek support only from people who are in appropriate roles where support should be requested. Typically, your own children are not appropriate people to turn to for support for such highly personal matters between you and your partner.

After providing these guidelines, have problem-solving discussions with couples about whom they will and will not inform about the affair. In addition, we generally recommend that each person let the other know whom they have told about the affair so that both people will be clear on what information has been shared with other people. We believe it is also important to help both partners be honest in their motivation for telling other people about the affair. For example, Vicki initially insisted that she wanted to tell her 10-year-old daughter from her first marriage about Bill's affair so that her daughter would understand why there was so much distress in the home. However, with further discussion, it seemed clear that Vicki wanted to punish Bill and wanted her daughter to side with her against her stepfather. Once she acknowledged her motivation, Vicki was able to explore whether it was in her daughter's best interest to know about Bill's affair, knowledge that might seriously disrupt her daughter's relationship with him.

Summary

The discovery or disclosure of an affair typically is overwhelming on an individual level, and the couple's response to their distress can either help to set the stage for a productive therapeutic process or create additional difficulties for them. Therefore, early in the treatment it is important to set ground rules and make good decisions so that greater harm does not result from their treatment of each other or their interaction with other people. There is no exact order for addressing these issues, and you will need to individualize this component of treatment according to which areas have the most potential to be destructive to the couple. Later in the treatment, you and the couple will devote increasing energy to exploring ways to build positive interactions between the partners, but the focus of this chapter is how to minimize damage or destruction to the relationship and the partners. As we have discussed, a wide variety of strategies can be used to accomplish these goals, and you should select the ones that seem appropriate for a given couple. We also have identified communication skills such as teaching couples how to share their thoughts and feelings and how to problem solve and make good decisions. These guidelines are discussed in upcoming chapters within the context of other topics, but they can be very useful at this stage in helping to minimize relationship damage. Therefore, you might decide to bring these or other skills into the therapy process early to achieve specific goals.

Resources from *Getting Past the Affair*

If you are having the couple read our self-help book in conjunction with your therapy, information related to the topics discussed in the current chapter can be found in *Getting Past the Affair* on the following pages:

Minimizing damage between partners: Chapter 2 (pp. 29–39) includes a discussion of what the couple should and should not talk about regarding the affair. Exercise 2.1 also provides a conversation that the couple might have during a therapy session or at home related to this topic.

How to deal with other people, including the outside-affair person and friends, family, and colleagues: Chapter 4 is devoted in entirety to dealing with people outside of the partners' relationship. The chapter also includes three exercises that can be used in or outside of the therapy sessions.

CHAPTER 5

Restoring Equilibrium

THERAPIST: So how have things been since we got together earlier this week?

BILL: It hasn't been quite as bad as it was before, but it still isn't good at all; everything feels so awkward and out of kilter. The hurricane has died down, but what's left is devastation with everyone wandering around in a daze not knowing what to do. Nothing seems normal now. We don't eat together; we certainly don't sleep together, and it's hard even to discuss who's going to pick up the children. We've had so many arguments that we're both reluctant to say anything for fear it will blow up, and to be honest, I'm not sure what to talk about anyway.

VICKI: I agree; things are a little better and I think we're arguing less. But when you destroyed me emotionally, it killed the part of me that was happy to do things for you. So, if something hasn't been taken care of and we can't talk about it, you might want to take care of it yourself or else it's not likely to happen.

THERAPIST: Well, it sounds like things really aren't flowing well at home, but the good thing is that you've decreased saying or doing harmful things to each other, and that's critical. And, Bill, as you said, you're both now dealing with the aftermath of the trauma and don't know what to do about it. What happens in a relationship is that over time, you develop ways of interacting, taking care of chores and so on, that become automatic and often aren't even discussed once they're in place. They're merely part of the routine. But after an affair, almost everything is called into question, and your routines are thrown off. It might be helpful if we spend some time talking about what's been disrupted for you as a couple and for each of you as individuals. At times like this, you need to be able to rely on some predictability and routines so that your whole world doesn't seem confusing or destroyed.

As Vicki and Bill were experiencing, there are multiple negative consequences of an affair. In the last chapter, we discussed numerous ways in which a couple can make matters worse through with each other and their interactions with the outside world. It is critical to stop these negative behaviors so that the couple does not compound their problems beyond what the affair itself has created. However, even if partners are successful in decreasing or terminating these negative interactions, the trauma of an affair often leads to a continued sense of confusion and turmoil, including a disruption of couple and individual routines. Hence, partners need to regain some sense of equilibrium, order, and predictability. Otherwise, their focus and energy become divided between the effort needed to move on and the work necessary to address daily responsibilities and interactions for both individuals and the family as a whole. In addition, if individual self-care routines such as exercise, eating, and sleeping become disrupted, then the couple's ability to address consequences of the affair becomes further compromised. In this chapter, we discuss some of the major ways that partners' lives become disrupted after an affair, along with strategies for helping the couple to develop a new equilibrium on a short-term basis while contemplating longer term decisions about their relationship.

Disruptions in Relationship Functioning

Although an affair can disrupt a couple's relationship in almost any area, we have identified three broad domains that frequently show negative impact from the affair. For some couples, one or more of these areas was already a source of difficulty before the affair. For such couples, the additional stress of an affair often leads to severe dysfunction in that same domain. If a couple quarreled before the affair about who would complete which household tasks, they are likely to experience even more conflict in this area after the affair because either partner may feel less motivated to contribute or compromise. On the other hand, couples who have been completing household chores smoothly before to the affair can still have a breakdown in that area as a result of the trauma itself; for example, no one checks to make certain they have food for the children's lunches for the coming week. Consequently, almost all couples need to address the issue of how to regain some sense of equilibrium in one or more of the following areas, which vary on a continuum of vulnerability from instrumental/task-oriented activities to more emotional/intimate activities:

- *Daily tasks* that are integral to helping the partners, their relationship, and the broader family system function at an optimal level.
- *Companionship activities* such as going to movies, attending children's school and extracurricular activities, and having casual conversations.
- More *intimate activities* such as physical and verbal expressions of affection, support, and love, sleeping in the same bed, or disrobing in front of the other person, along with explicitly sexual interactions.

Disruption of Daily Tasks

Many couples report that after learning about an affair, they experience a breakdown in daily routines, household chores, and patterns of interaction. This disruption can happen for a number of reasons. One or both partners might be so emotionally distraught that they are distracted, inefficient, or unmotivated in many aspects of life. Alternatively, one person might be so angry that he or she becomes uncooperative and vengeful. Even if not explicitly deciding to be vengeful, many individuals, particularly injured partners, no longer put forth the same effort for the well-being of the relationship that they had made previously. Typically, both partners contribute to the relationship and complete various tasks for the well-being of the couple or the other person. After an affair, however, motivation to expend extra effort to benefit the other partner or the relationship is often significantly compromised. Consequently, shopping for and preparing meals, doing laundry, cleaning the house, filling the cars with gas, and many other tasks are no longer carried out in a typical manner. If partners are so upset or angry with each other that they cannot even discuss these issues, then their lives become more stressful as bills go unpaid and daily needs are not addressed.

In the prior excerpt, Bill and Vicki raised this issue themselves, providing the therapist with an opportunity to address it in the session. However, if a couple does not raise the issue of how daily tasks and other aspects of couple and individual functioning have become disrupted, we typically raise this issue early in therapy, as demonstrated next.

"I'd like to get a sense of how things are going for the two of you in terms of your daily routines, both as a couple and for each of you individually. For many couples at a time like this when there's a lot of turmoil, their daily lives can become disrupted, even in terms of fairly mundane routines and tasks such as cooking meals, doing the laundry, and so forth. For all these things to get taken care of, both partners need to be motivated to work for the well-being of their relationship, and I know that at times like this you can be distracted or your motivation can really suffer. What has been your experience lately? Are there areas of your daily lives that have been thrown off by the situation you're in?"

Disruption of Companionship Activities

In addition to being an efficient team that takes care of tasks, another important aspect of most intimate relationships is the companionship that partners share, engaging in a wide variety of enjoyable activities together. Every couple has routines for relaxation or play, such as going to movies together, enjoying a play, exercising together, inviting friends over for the evening, or taking short weekend trips out of town; however, these activities are frequently disrupted in the aftermath of an affair. The injured partner might feel too upset and angry to propose that the couple go to a movie together. Likewise, the participating partner might believe that it is too presumptuous to suggest that the couple continue with their previously planned trip to the mountains for the weekend. On the other hand, one or both partners may retain a strong wish for such activities. The participating partner might want to show how much he or she wants to be with the injured partner, thus suggesting a lot of "togetherness" activities. Likewise, some injured partners seek reassurance from shared activities or fear that they have not been a "good enough" companion and now try to make up for it by suggesting lots of ways to spend time together.

Offering clear directives regarding companionship behaviors after an affair may initially seem inappropriate because companionship activities typically arise from wanting to be with the other person. However, because there may be some confusion between the partners about what is acceptable, it is important to raise the issue of companionship activities with them if they have not raised it, and ask what each person wants at this time. We also discuss with couples that their desire for companionship with the other person is likely to change over the course of treatment, and the two of them might have different desires and preferences at various times. We also caution them that often it is hard to know what they will experience emotionally once they are in these circumstances. Therefore, while making a good-faith effort to be positive during these interactions, they should tell the other person if such an activity becomes unpleasant or aversive.

Disruption of Intimate Interactions

The activities described previously are ones that someone might do with a friend. Other activities that couples enjoy involve more intimate interactions typically reserved for a romantic, committed relationship. This category includes certain types of conversation that are experienced as intimate, either because of the vulnerability that is involved in the conversation or because of statements of love, affection, and caring. Other intimate behaviors include undressing in front of the other person, physical displays of affection, and explicitly sexual interactions. All of these intimate interactions can become disrupted after an affair, because the partners may feel distant from each other and the injured partner often feels vulnerable after a betrayal. Moreover, given that the trauma of an affair involves sexual interactions with a third person, sexual interactions between the participating and injured partner may seem meaningless or even aversive. Some injured partners convey an implicit or explicit message, "If you're going to have a sexual relationship with another person, don't expect to have one with me." However, at the other end of the continuum, either the participating partner or the injured partner might seek a significant increase in intimate or sexual interactions after an affair, fearing the relationship might end and, therefore, initiating intimate behaviors, hoping to prevent this loss.

Given the wide range of responses and motivations regarding these intimate behaviors, there is no single recommendation to make to couples regarding intimate or sexual interactions. Again, if couples do not raise this issue, we raise it with them during a therapy session. We encourage couples not to engage in intimate behaviors that make either person highly uncomfortable at this time. Instead, we try to help couples understand that, after an affair, they have many decisions to make, including how to interact with each other, as they assess whether to maintain their relationship long term. The primary goal at this early stage in recovery is to settle the situation, regain some sense of order and predictability, and make certain that day-to-day functioning is acceptable. While working with Vicki and Bill, their therapist raised the issue of physical and sexual interaction as follows:

THERAPIST: We've talked some about trying to get some order and regularity in taking care of daily tasks, and that's important to help make life run smoothly. And we talked about trying to find ways that you might want to do some pleasant or fun things together, just to enjoy each other in a nonpressured way, so that you aren't always focusing on these very difficult issues. I think it might also be useful if we talk a bit about how you do or don't want to relate to each other in more caring, loving, or even romantic ways. We don't want to push you beyond what either of you is comfortable with right now, and that's likely to change over time. But you've both told me this has been such an important part of your relationship in the past, and I'm not sure where both of you are on this right now. Vicki, what are your thoughts and feelings about this area?

VICKI: Well, we really haven't talked about it since Bill's affair, and there isn't much happening in an affectionate way, either verbally or physically. We certainly don't have any physical relationship, and right now the thought of him touching me just makes me sick to my stomach.

BILL: I think it's more accurate to say it's all one way right now. I tell you every day how sorry I am and how much I love you, and you just ignore it. There have been a couple of times when I've touched your shoulder or something, not in a sexual way, but just sort of reaching out, and you freeze, it seems to me. For me, I'm ready to start trying to see if we can rebuild our marriage, but it takes two of us. I get a very bright red light from you that says, "Don't even think about any kind of caring or loving interaction!"

THERAPIST: It isn't surprising to me that this whole area has been thrown off track for you. Vicki, often people in your position want to go really slowly or not even think about expressing caring because it feels too vulnerable or reminds them of the affair. Again, I don't want to push either of you, but are there ways that you would like to show caring, concern, or affection for each other that would feel genuine and not too risky or upsetting? And this is something we'll continue to check on over time. You might want to wait on this altogether for now, or if you do try something, we'll want to see how it goes because often people can't anticipate what it will be like.

As noted earlier, it can be helpful to think about these various domains, including daily tasks, companionship, and intimate interactions, as occurring on a continuum of vulnerability. From this perspective, we try to help couples think about rebuilding by starting with activities that involve less vulnerability and moving toward more vulnerable interactions as they become more comfortable and trusting of each other. Consequently, we typically begin by focusing on daily responsibilities that are essential for smooth individual and relationship functioning and that typically involve little threat to vulnerability. If both partners are interested and motivated, we then help them rebuild some companionship activities that involve pleasure and enjoyment, but still with little vulnerability to the other person. Finally, as they progress through treatment, if couples have decided that they want to stay together or want to actively explore that possibility, at some point they need to take more risk with each other in a variety of ways, including more intimate ways of relating. Both partners need to experience directly whether they can trust the other individual and their relationship with these more vulnerable parts of themselves, but they should not do so until they feel ready.

Therapeutic Strategies to Address Disruptions in Relationship Functioning

The primary goal of interventions in this context is to help the couple establish interaction patterns appropriate to their current stage of response to the affair that will provide them immediate stability and predictability, recognizing that any solution might need to be revised as the couple proceeds through the recovery process. Therefore, a major focus involves helping the couple make good decisions and solve problems. One approach is to teach them decision-making or problem-solving skills. Next we describe a series of steps that can assist couples in this process. At times, this process can be straightforward; for example, you might help a couple renegotiate how to accomplish daily chores. However, before making decisions about companionship and intimate interactions, often it is valuable to explore in more depth partners' thoughts and feelings about these domains in order to clarify their desires for interacting with each other.

For example, recall Brad, a university professor, who had an affair with Jill, his graduate student. While discussing the affair with his wife, Gail, Brad clarified that he and Jill had often been physically affectionate in his office. Brad was distraught that, after his affair, Gail seemed to want to spend little time with him. In particular, he had really valued how they used to drop in and see each other in the department, with Gail popping her head in his office just to say hello or to have a cup of coffee together midmorning. Brad and Gail had not discussed this change, but Brad assumed that Gail's reason for no longer coming to his office was that she simply did not want to be around him. It was important to explore whether he was interpreting Gail's behavior appropriately and how they might respond accordingly.

Challenging Dysfunctional Thoughts Regarding Changes in Behavior

In the previous chapter, we discussed how important beliefs or standards for how to respond to being injured can lead to further complications for the couple. In addition to standards that individuals might hold for how one *should* respond, other types of distorted thinking can interfere with couples' ability to make good decisions. Epstein and Baucom (2002) provide a detailed discussion of how to address these different types of cognitions in couple therapy more generally. More focal to the current discussion, the therapist needed to help Brad and Gail explore Brad's explanations or attributions for why Gail no longer dropped by his office. In the following excerpt, the therapist uses a strategy called *guided discovery*, in which the therapist guides the couple through a conversation or assists them in gaining new information as a way of rethinking their interpretations.

BRAD: I really miss the little rituals that Gail and I used to have in the department. She knew my schedule and was aware of times when I would be alone in my office. So every day, she would pop her head in the door just to say "hi," and sometimes she would say something very suggestive or scandalous, just so we could rebel and be inappropriate in the midst of a formal academic department. She would then suddenly become very formal and professorial, continuing to walk down the hall. It was so funny, but now that's all gone. She never comes by. It's clear that she just doesn't want anything to do with me beyond what's necessary.

THERAPIST: That's a possibility, Brad. But it's important to realize that you've given an important interpretation for why Gail doesn't stop by any more: that she really doesn't want to have anything to do with you. You might be right, but I think it's important to check that out with her. So many things in your relationship are disrupted right now, and how you interpret each other's behavior can have a strong influence on how you feel and then how you respond to each other. Have you and Gail talked about why she doesn't stop by any more?

BRAD: No, not really. I didn't think it was necessary since it seemed pretty obvious to me. Also, I didn't feel like I had the right to ask her to stop by, given what I've done.

THERAPIST: Well, how about if we take a few minutes to have a conversation and let Gail tell you why she doesn't stop by any more. Then, based on what she tells you, the two of you might want to decide how you're going to interact at the department for the immediate future.

BRAD: Sure. Gail, I assume that you just don't want to talk to me in general, particularly at the department with Jill being a student there and all. But I don't really know since we don't talk about these things. So I'd really like to know what's going on from your side.

GAIL: Well, you're partly right, but it isn't that simple. It's so awkward to try to talk, and also I don't know what to say to you most of the time. Actually, I feel very lonely in the department now, but I don't want to come to your office and peek in to say "Hi." You and Jill went there together, and any time I get near your office, I start to feel faint and think that I'm going to throw up or pass out. So I just can't do that. But if we could find another place or way to speak at the department, I'd actually welcome it, I think. At least, I'd be willing to give it a try and see what happens.

THERAPIST: Great, let's stop for a moment. That was a really nice interaction. Brad, you straightforwardly asked Gail why she no longer comes by, and, Gail, you were open and honest with Brad. And it sounds like you might want to continue the conversation about how you can interact at the department since you both seem to value that. What I want you to notice is how easy it is to assume that you know why the other person is behaving in a certain way. You might be correct some of the time, but I can almost guarantee you that there will be many times when you're misinterpreting each other's behavior, so it's critical to ask each other directly so that you don't respond based on your misinterpretation. Would you both agree to do that and be honest with each other? If the other person is behaving in some way that seems hurtful or that you don't understand, would you be willing to ask about it rather than interpreting it on your own?

Decision-Making and Problem-Solving Skills

Couples routinely face a wide range of issues requiring joint decisions, for example, how to manage couple- and family-focused daily responsibilities, engage in companionship activities, and consider more intimate interactions. One way to approach helping the couple make decisions is from a skills-based approach. For example, decision-making skills have been widely researched with couples and described clinically, both for treating distressed couples and for couple education and enhancement programs. These general decision-making skills can be helpful for many couples confronting difficult issues after an affair. Epstein and Baucom (2002, pp. 314–325) provide a detailed consideration of decision making that is consistent with our approach to working with couples addressing infidelity. Table 5.1 provides decision-making guidelines

TABLE 5.1. Guidelines for Decision-Making Discussions

State the issue clearly and specifically.
- Phrase the issue in terms of behaviors that are currently occurring or not occurring or in terms of what needs to be decided.
- Break down large, complex problems into several smaller problems, and deal with them one at a time.
- Make certain that both people agree on the statement of the problem and are willing to discuss it.

Clarify why the issue is important and what your needs are.
- Clarify why the issue is important to you, and provide your understanding of the issues involved.
- Explain what your needs are that you would like to see taken into account in the solution; do not offer specific solutions at this time.

Discuss possible solutions.
- Propose concrete, specific solutions that take both people's needs and preferences into account. Do not focus on solutions that meet only your individual needs.
- Focus on solutions for the present and the future. Do not dwell on the past or attempt to attribute blame for past difficulties.
- If you tend to focus on a single or a limited number of alternatives, consider brainstorming (generating a variety of possible solutions in a creative way).

Decide on a solution that is agreeable to both of you.
- If you cannot find a solution that pleases both partners, suggest a compromise solution. If a compromise is not possible, agree to follow one person's preferences for now.
- State your solution in clear, specific, behavioral terms.
- After agreeing on a solution, have one partner restate the solution.
- Do not accept a solution if you do not intend to follow through with it.
- Do not accept a solution that will make you angry or resentful.

Decide on a trial period to implement the solution, if it is a situation that will occur more than once.
- Allow for several attempts of the new solution.
- Review the solution at the end of the trial period.
- Revise the solution if needed, taking into account what you have learned thus far.

Note. Adapted from Epstein and Baucom (2002). Copyright 2002 by the American Psychological Association. Adapted by permission.

that we hand out and discuss with couples. Once the partners understand the principles of effective decision making or problem solving, we ask them to use these guidelines in making decisions, such as whether they want to engage in companionship activities with each other, and if so, what kinds of activities, under what circumstances, and so on.

For each step in the process, there are points of emphasis focal to affairs that we recommend you discuss with the couple:

1. *State what the issue is clearly and specifically.* It is critical that the issue be presented in a relatively straightforward, specific manner without casting blame on either person. When the problems occurred because the participating partner violated sexual boundaries, it is easy for issues to be presented in a blaming manner. Given that the typical response to feeling attacked is either to counterattack, withdraw, or freeze, such a statement sets the stage for an unproductive interaction. In the prior example, the therapist might encourage Brad and Gail to have a decision-making conversation about whether they want to spend time interacting with each other at the department, and if so, how.

2. *Clarify why the issue is important and what your needs are.* Although they were not having a decision-making conversation in the prior example, both Brad and Gail provided some understanding of how they felt and what was important to them. They both clarified that they would like to see each other casually in the department, and Gail indirectly suggested that she needed to do it in a way that would not remind her of Brad's affair. Understanding how both partners experience the situation and what they need for a good solution is crucial because it lays the groundwork for good decisions. Once Brad understood that coming by his office was a significant part of the difficulty for Gail, the two of them began thinking of alternative ways to interact in the department.

3. *Discuss possible solutions and decide on a solution that is agreeable to both of you.* It is important to consider both partners' preferences and needs when proposing various solutions. Frequently after an affair, the participating partner feels in a "one-down" position, needing to agree to whatever the injured partner wants in order to restore the relationship. Consequently, it is not uncommon during decision-making conversations for the injured partner to make strong demands of the participating partner, who then feels obligated to comply. Such a strategy might demonstrate the participating partner's commitment to restoring the relationship, but it is unlikely to lead to good long-term solutions unless both persons' needs are considered.

On the other hand, at times injured partners also feel that they are somewhat powerless, worried that the participating partner might leave them. Therefore, the injured partner is sometimes willing to do whatever the participating partner wants in order not to threaten the relationship further. In essence, affairs often create various power imbalances in the relationship that can be played out during decision-making conversations. Although this imbalance may not be eliminated entirely, as the therapist you should help the couple avoid making bad decisions because of one person's feeling disadvantaged or powerless in the situation.

4. *Decide on a trial period to implement the solution.* In deciding how to interact with each other after an affair, partners frequently experience strong emotions, some unanticipated, when they implement the solutions. They may not know how they will feel if they go out to dinner together until they actually experience it. It might be a lovely occasion, or they might feel awkward and not know what to say to each other. At worst, one person might experience a flashback-like phenomenon, as described later in this chapter. Therefore, once they have implemented the agreed-upon solutions, a couple might find that they need to discuss the issue again and revise their solution. On many occasions when a couple returns to the next therapy session, one of them says, "It really didn't work. When we sat in here and discussed it, I thought it would be fine. But when I got in the situation, it was really upsetting."

These guidelines for decision making can be used with a couple in at least two different ways. First, you can teach the decision-making guidelines as a set of skills, discussing the importance of reaching effective solutions as a major form of couple communication. Following this rationale, you would hand out and discuss the guidelines with the couple, answer questions, and then invite the couple to have a decision-making conversation on a relevant topic. Your role during that conversation would be to help them stay focused on the topic and use good communication skills while providing input about the content of their proposed solutions if what they are suggesting seems contrary to their broader goals. You are teaching them communication and decision-making skills that they then implement with your assistance.

However, there may be occasions when you help the couple make decisions that serve to restore equilibrium without using decision-making skills. (In fact, many therapists who work with couples do not use a skills-based approach.) Or you might plan to teach them such skills, but when you are in an early stage of therapy, you may not have taught these decision-making guidelines yet. In this instance, there may not be sufficient time to focus on skill building before the couple needs to reach a solution. Alternatively, in later sessions, you may not want to disrupt the couple's discussion of a critical issue to focus on communication skills. At such times, you might decide to take a second approach, in which you join with them in a three-person conversation as you informally guide them through a decision-making process. For example, you might suggest, "Brad, why don't you clarify for Gail what your concerns are about the way the two of you interact in the department? Try to avoid mind reading Gail's thoughts or feelings. Just state your concern; let her know what you'd like to discuss, and then in a few minutes we'll talk about possible solutions you both might find to be acceptable."

At present, there are no research findings that indicate which couples benefit most from a skills-oriented approach to decision making versus a guided discussion with the therapist. It seems likely that a skills approach might be particularly useful if a couple has generally lacked the ability to discuss issues and make good decisions, and such difficulties have contributed to relationship distress and the participating partner's decision to have an affair. Regardless of which strategy you use to have a decision-making conversation, during Stage 1 you need to remain particularly attentive to helping the couple reach solutions that promote a sense of equilibrium and predictability and disrupt escalation of negative interactions.

Disruptions in Individual Functioning

After an affair, not only are partners' interactions with each other disrupted, but each person's individual functioning can be adversely impacted as well. In part, this disruption occurs because individual functioning exists within the broader context of the relationship. Consequently, as the relationship deteriorates and the couple's interaction patterns are interrupted, individual behaviors can change as well. For example, Fran had typically bought groceries for her and Tim, but she stopped grocery shopping after Tim's affair. Previously, Tim had taken his lunch to work, but now he often found little to eat in the refrigerator. In response, he began skipping lunches and found that he was irritable and tired by mid-afternoon. Individual functioning also can become disrupted as a result of the strong moods that are evoked by the affair. Fran stopped buying groceries not to get back at Tim, but because she felt sad and depleted by his affair. In addition, she did not enjoy exercising but had typically pushed herself to work out regularly. After learning about Tim's affair, she could not make herself go to the gym and found that her mood worsened, which lowered her motivation even further, and a vicious cycle ensued.

Therapists need to be aware of the importance of focusing on disruptions in individual functioning after an affair. Not only is the well-being of each individual important for its own sake, but both partners are confronting a difficult and demanding task for their relationship. If either person is suffering from sleep deprivation, lowered self-esteem as a result of weight gain, or other factors related to individual functioning, it can become more challenging for them to address the difficult issues involved in the treatment process. These physical depletions also can cause problems in partners' abilities to regulate themselves emotionally, leading to diminished resources and decreased inhibitions during stressful couple interactions.

These disruptions in individual functioning often occur in the following domains:

• *Physical functioning:* Individuals often remark that their sleep, exercise, and eating behaviors change after an affair. In addition, some people begin or increase their use of alcohol or drugs to cope with their distress.

• *Social functioning:* Because of feelings of depression, guilt, shame, or embarrassment, some people withdraw from their friendships and other social interactions, leaving them even more isolated at this critical time. Alternatively, either partner may actually seek out more social support but in maladaptive ways. For example, injured partners may begin to flirt or behave inappropriately to prove to themselves or the participating partner that they are still attractive to other individuals; such behaviors can lead to further relationship complications.

• *Spiritual functioning:* Partners may find that their spiritual lives are altered after the affair; for example, they might withdraw from religious institutions or feel more distant from God or a higher power or question how they fit into a broader world. Such disruptions of spiritual beliefs can then lead to a broader sense of confusion, because not only is the couple's relationship threatened but the person's broader worldview and spiritual beliefs are compromised as well. For couples who are part of religious organizations, participating partners might believe that their behavior is so contrary to their own spiritual beliefs or the standards of their religious group that they withdraw from this potential source of support. Likewise, injured partners may withdraw as a result of embarrassment or out of anger that they have been treated so badly in spite of trying to live in a manner consistent with their spiritual beliefs.

Sometimes individual issues can be handled during conjoint couple sessions. However, it may also be beneficial to address these issues in an individual session with one partner. Whereas concerns of confidentiality during individual sessions must be taken into account, we have held individual sessions with each partner during the treatment when either or both partners appear to be struggling individually. When conducting individual sessions, it is important to emphasize that the goal is to address individual functioning and not the concerns of the couple.

We have found that such individual sessions also can be beneficial in establishing rapport with each person, particularly the participating partner. During conjoint sessions, often the injured partner is so angry and distressed that he or she can tolerate little empathy or support by the therapist for the participating partner. Therefore, individual sessions with the participating partner can provide an opportunity to show care and concern, without suggesting approval of the infidelity. When conducting such sessions, we routinely schedule individual sessions with both partners so that neither partner feels marginalized or experiences a sense of alignment between the therapist and the other individual. During these sessions, the primary goal is to clarify how each person is functioning individually, followed by self-care, decision-making, and problem-solving strategies to minimize destructive patterns that are evolving and to optimize individual quality of life during this difficult time. In addition, we use these sessions to prepare the partners for the difficult emotional work that they still have ahead of them and problem-solve with them on how they will cope emotionally with these difficult sessions and interactions with their partners in ways that do not further damage themselves or their relationship.

We have successfully conducted individual sessions during couple therapy for infidelity, but we also refer partners for individual therapy when appropriate, for example, if the level of individual distress or maladaptive behavior is extreme or persistent or if there are complicated alliance issues between the therapist and the two partners that would be exacerbated by individual sessions.

Flashbacks and Reexperiencing the Trauma: A Special Case of Individual and Relationship Disequilibrium

THERAPIST: Vicki, you look pretty upset. What's going on?

VICKI: It's awful. It all fell apart this weekend. I thought that we were starting to make some progress; the arguments had decreased, and we had had some pleasant conversations, just discussing the events of the day. So we decided it was time to take the next step and do something together over the weekend. In the past when we've gone out dancing, we've always had a great time, so we thought that would be a safe thing to do. And it was fun; I think we both were having a good time until they played a slow dance. We were dancing, and suddenly I felt flooded and overwhelmed. I really don't know if Bill ever took her dancing, but suddenly it was as if I was looking at him holding her tight. That image was too much. I started to cry, and I tried my best to hold it back. I was so hurt and angry that I didn't know what to do. We sat down, and I know I got very quiet. Bill kept asking me what was wrong, and I kept telling him nothing, just that I thought it was a little hot in the room. It pretty much ruined the evening. The next day Bill kept asking me what happened. So I finally told him, and we had a big argument. It seems like we're right back at square one where we started, or maybe even worse. In spite of all the effort, it seems really hopeless at this point.

BILL: I don't know what to do. I feel so discouraged. Vicki knows that the affair is over, and I've sworn to her I'll never do that again. I can't take it back, and I'm doing everything that I know to make it better. She was the one who suggested going dancing. And then, out of the blue, she has a meltdown. As far as I know, I didn't do anything to bring it on, and I haven't gone out dancing with anyone but her in years. Either she's let her imagination go wild, or in the middle of our fun time out together, she decided to punish me. Maybe *you* understand it, but I sure don't.

What Bill and Vicki experienced was deeply upsetting to both of them, and neither person seemed to understand exactly what happened or how it came about. However, we believe that infidelity is often experienced as an interpersonal trauma; therefore, some partners, particularly injured partners, experience symptoms consistent with PTSD. One defining characteristic of PTSD is that the traumatic event is reexperienced in a variety of ways: (1) recurrent and intrusive distressing recollections of the event that include images, thoughts, or perceptions; (2) distressing dreams about the event; (3) acting or feeling as if the traumatic event were recurring at the moment; (4) intense psychological distress when exposed to either internal or external cues that symbolize or resemble the event; and (5) physiological arousal when exposed to internal or external cues that symbolize or resemble the traumatic event (American Psychiatric Association, 2000).

The kinds of visual images and physical distress that Vicki experienced are common after an affair, and these reactions can have an immediate, intense negative impact on both partners when they occur. In addition, because partners typically do not understand these events, they can feel confusion and despair about their progress. In essence, these flashback and reexperiencing phenomena have a significant dysregulating effect that requires therapeutic assistance.

Our approach to addressing these reexperiencing events involves two major intervention components: (1) psychoeducation or explanations regarding the nature of flashbacks and reexperiences and (2) guidelines for addressing these phenomena when they do occur. When possible, we spend time with the couple addressing these issues before they occur in order to minimize the confusion and resulting emotional distress when they are experienced. However, because there can be so many issues that require attention early in the intervention, sometimes couples such as Vicki and Bill reexperience the trauma before it is discussed in session. The following is an example of how you might introduce the concept of reexperiencing a trauma to a couple:

"Let's spend some time talking about what happened to you this weekend. First, I want you to know that although it was extremely upsetting, it's quite common for this sort of thing to happen, and it does *not* mean that you're not making progress. This is almost expected—we don't want it to happen, but it shouldn't be a surprise if and when it does. As we've discussed, learning of your partner's affair is often traumatic, in many ways like the experiences that people have in wartime or during natural disasters. And the reaction to an affair can include symptoms that people show after other traumas, what we call posttraumatic stress disorder. [You might ask the couple if they are familiar with this term and what they know about it.] People who experience PTSD tend to be extremely sensitive and reactive to things that remind them of the traumatic event. I'm not saying that you have PTSD, but some of the reactions to trauma are similar. That's why a strange number on the phone bill or being at a restaurant where your partner went with the other person can so easily set you off. What happens is that the person has started to associate certain experiences, memories, and so on with the traumatic event. As you experienced, it really doesn't matter whether the specific event actually occurred or not. As long as Vicki is able to visualize Bill dancing closely with the other woman, that's what is important. We call these reexperiences of traumatic events 'flashbacks.' I think that's what happened when you went dancing this weekend; does that make sense?"

The second part of the intervention involves providing guidelines and recommendations to the couple regarding how to deal with flashbacks when they do occur. We have created a handout of these guidelines that we typically share with couples (see Table 5.2). Next, we describe how you might discuss these guidelines with a couple. To conserve space, we present this discussion as if it is a monologue that you might present. In actuality, you will want to have a conversation with the couple at various points, make a major point, check to be certain that the couple understands, and ask for possible examples from their own experiences.

"Now that you understand that flashbacks or reexperiences may occur, let's discuss how the two of you want to handle this kind of situation when it happens. We have a few suggestions on this handout. [Give them the guidelines.] First, we suggest that when you become aware that you're feeling extremely upset, you take a few minutes to think about what might have triggered these feelings again: For example, did you remember a certain scene, did you drive by a motel, did you see someone who reminded you of the other person? Taking time to step back and think may help to bring you back to a calmer frame of mind, and even if it doesn't, it might give you important information about what triggers the upsetting feelings. In other words, if you notice yourself feeling upset, panicky, or accusatory toward your partner, take a minute to evaluate whether this reaction is realistic or not; is it one you would have had even if the affair hadn't occurred?

"If your reaction seems appropriate even in the absence of the affair, then you should address this issue with your partner. For example, if Bill tells you he'll be home at 5:00 and doesn't show up until 7:00, almost anyone would be upset. Of course, it might be worse for you given that this may stir up memories of when he didn't come home during the affair. But even without those additional feelings from the affair, you might want to discuss and make decisions about informing each other about when you'll be home and what to do if you're going to be late.

"On the other hand, if you decide that your reaction isn't based mainly on the present situation but instead is a reaction to the past, then we suggest that you tell the other person what's happening. Explain briefly what you're feeling and why you think it is happening. This will be helpful because often the other person is confused and frustrated by these sudden switches in emotions. Everything seems to be going well and then all of a sudden you're angry, crying, and so forth. If you both can understand it as a flashback, it may help lessen some of the confusion and

TABLE 5.2. Guidelines for Coping with Flashbacks

If you recognize that you're responding to your partner in a panicky, worried, accusatory, or angry manner, then step back and evaluate the situation and your reaction.

If you decide that your reaction is realistic given the immediate circumstances, then express your feelings to your partner and work to find a more acceptable solution to this problem.

> EXAMPLE: "When you're an hour late getting home from work and haven't called, it disrupts my schedule and doesn't feel respectful. I'd like us to agree on how to handle occasions when you are unexpectedly delayed."

If you decide that your reaction is most likely a reaction to a memory of the affair, let your partner know what is happening by describing your feelings and linking them to the memory that has been activated.

> EXAMPLE: "Driving by that motel just triggered memories of your affair, and I feel hurt and frightened all over again."

Be specific about what would be most helpful at this moment to cope with these feelings.
- Do you simply want your feelings to be understood and acknowledged?

> EXAMPLE: "I've just been feeling sad today and have had trouble shaking off thoughts about the affair. I'll be okay. But I need you to understand if I'm not as cheerful tonight as you'd like."

- Do you want your partner to respond to your feelings by offering to hold you, reassure you, or provide you time and space to be alone?

> EXAMPLE: "I've been feeling more alone and distant from you today. I really need you to be with me and just hold me for a while."

- Do you want the two of you to find a way to reduce the likelihood or frequency of the memory-trigger occurring again?

> EXAMPLE: "Watching movies together used to be fun, but right now I really need us to avoid movies about romance, infidelity, or other reminders of your affair. How can we manage that?"

Balance discussions with your partner about flashbacks with efforts to cope with these experiences on your own to avoid overwhelming your relationship or wearing down your partner with these difficult exchanges. Draw upon self-care strategies you've used successfully in the past or heard described by your therapist.

frustration. In this kind of a situation, how would you let the other person know what's happening? [After discussing with the couple, continue.]

"Another important step is to let the other person know what you want or need at that time in order to make it better or get through the situation. For example, you might want to be held, or reassured that you're cared for. Or you might need some space or just some quiet time, either alone or together. You might prefer talking about something else or doing something else. Of course, what you need might vary according to the specific situation, but often people have general preferences for what they want at such times. Do you have some sense of what you generally might want in these situations and how you might ask for it? [After discussing with the couple, continue.]

"After you've talked about the particular situation that happened and what you need, you'll probably find it helpful at some point to discuss how you'd like to handle this kind of event in the future. You might decide to avoid certain situations for now if that's realistic, or you could think about a supportive way to approach the situation together in the future.

"As you'll notice from the handout, we also think that it's important that the two of you pay attention to balancing the amount of time that you talk about these flashbacks. If they're happening very often, it can become wearing on both of you to have long, drawn-out discussions on these topics, and because it gets so tiring, the two of you are likely to be unsuccessful in dealing with them. So to protect you from disappointment and increase the likelihood of your success, we suggest that you also think of additional ways to deal with the flashbacks that don't involve your partner or require only minimal involvement from the other person. It's important that the two of you be able to talk about these upsetting situations. I'm merely saying there needs to be some balance and that you should have other ways to manage your feelings without your partner at times if you need to. [Follow up with these questions, allowing discussion in between.] How do the two of you want to address this issue of balance? What would feel unbalanced to you? Is one of you likely to need a lot more time to process this together than the other person would? What could you do in addition to discussing the issue together? [Help the couple develop a plan for how to deal with these flashbacks without relying solely on discussing it with the partner—some of the strategies for individual coping discussed earlier in this chapter might be of help here.]

"Finally, we suggest that the two of you try to communicate as effectively as possible while sharing thoughts and feelings about these flashbacks. For example, Vicki, try to avoid attacking Bill in order to get the empathy and understanding that you want. Similarly, Bill, work at not being defensive and do your best to really listen to what Vicki is saying. Attacking and defending are more likely to get you into a vicious cycle of more attacking and defending, and you're unlikely to resolve any issues or feelings successfully. Communicating well might be hard because we're talking about doing it while you're very upset. Knowing your own communication styles, in what ways will you need to be particularly careful in addressing these issues, and what does each of you need to focus on in communicating to make it work well?"

Summary

When a couple is in Stage 1 of responding to an affair, life feels unpredictable and out of control. The therapist's task is to help the couple regain a sense of consistency and equilibrium. In this chapter, we point out how disequilibrium can occur at both individual and relationship levels. In both cases, the primary therapeutic interventions involve helping partners make sound decisions. At times, this goal can be facilitated by helping the couple think differently about their interactions. However, because the couple is in such a state of flux, whatever decisions are made often are temporary, and couples need to understand that they may need to revisit decisions later. One particular form of disruption involves flashbacks and reexperiencing of affair-related events. Hence, some explanation of flashbacks can be invaluable, along with guidelines for how the couple might respond to such situations.

Interventions aimed at helping the couple minimize destructive interactions and regain some sense of stability may require several weeks of work with considerable structuring and support from you as the therapist. Although we have laid out these tasks and sessions in a sequential manner, you should use flexibility in achieving these goals. In Chapter 6, we describe guidelines that can help couples share their thoughts and feelings, a different yet equally important type of conversation. If you use a skills-based approach, you might decide that you need to teach these emotional expressiveness skills earlier in treatment, based on the particular experiences of the couple. Rather than adhering to a predetermined order of interventions, we have found that emphasizing the particular interventions that the couple needs in an order individualized to the couple is optimal for assisting them during Stage 1.

Resources from *Getting Past the Affair*

Our self-help book for couples, *Getting Past the Affair*, includes information related to the topics discussed in the current chapter. If you use that book in conjunction with the couple therapy, you might find the following pages useful to assign to the couple to read, along with relevant exercises:

Disruptions in relationship functioning: Chapter 2 (pp. 39–40) includes a discussion of stabilizing couple interactions. Exercise 2.2 also provides a conversation that the couple might have during a therapy session or at home related to this topic.

Disruptions in individual functioning: Chapter 5 is devoted entirely to self-care. Chapter 5 also includes two exercises targeting self-care that can be used in or outside of the therapy sessions.

Flashbacks and reexperiencing the trauma: Chapter 2 (pp. 40–46) focuses on addressing flashbacks and reexperiences of the trauma. Exercise 2.3 provides the couple with ways to discuss flashbacks.

Decision-making and problem-solving: Chapter 3 (pp. 69–73) presents guidelines for decision making that we addressed in the current chapter. In addition to your own presentation of the guidelines and points of emphasis, this section might help couples consolidate decision-making guidelines into their own conversations.

CHAPTER 6

Addressing Emotional Upheaval

THERAPIST: Pam and Tom, what's been going on with you since our last session?

PAM: We haven't been doing very well at all. We're still struggling trying to find ways to talk about what happened. Tom has gotten stuck on the idea that I'm attracted to assertive men, and he's right; that is one quality that made Mark so attractive. So now Tom is "asserting" himself in ways that are ridiculous; he's become hostile and aggressive. We even had a blowup last night at 11:30. We were lying in bed and I was trying to go to sleep, but apparently Tom wanted to talk about the affair. He started bombarding me with one accusatory question after another, even though it was obvious to me we weren't going to get anywhere at that time of night. And, as I've told you, if I had only one wish in the world, it would be that we would never discuss this again. It's over with Mark; I feel terribly guilty about what I did, and I want to move on. You can bet I'm not going to have a conversation about it at almost midnight.

THERAPIST: Can you both tell me more about what happened, without trying to make the other person look bad?

PAM: Well, as I said, Tom started asking me accusatory questions, and I wasn't going to answer them. So I just lay there quietly. He started yelling at me, and I put the pillow over my head. I guess he decided he wasn't going to let me sleep, so he turned the television on and literally turned the volume up all the way. Well, he got what he wanted. I finally turned toward him and yelled as loud as I could so he could hear me over the television. Then it disintegrated into a yelling match.

THERAPIST: Tom, what was this like for you?

TOM: I don't know what to do or how to interact with her. Up to now in our relationship, I've allowed her to control things the way she wanted, and she tells me that my lack of assertiveness is one thing that drove her to Mark. I hear that and I've decided to assert myself from now on, particularly about this affair. So she's not going to get her wish; we are going to talk about it whether she wants to or not. And I wasn't accusing her; I was just trying to get her to explain to me how it happened. When she tried to ignore me, I decided she would never ignore me again, no matter what I have to do. As I got louder, she continued to ignore me, so I turned up the television so she would at least have to acknowledge my existence in the room.

In the prior example, Tom and Pam are continuing to struggle to find a way to discuss Pam's affair. The heightened emotionality and difficulty in communicating about the affair apparent in this excerpt must be addressed directly before they can move forward. Tom and Pam's experiences are not unique. After the discovery of an affair, hyperarousal, strong negative emotions, and verbal aggression are common experiences (Taft et al., 2007). In the current chapter, we focus directly on helping the couple manage their experiences and communicate their emotions in a more constructive fashion.

Although the most common pattern is for one or both partners to express strong negative emotions frequently in a somewhat uncontrolled manner, other individuals respond to an affair in a more distant, intellectualized fashion with little emotional response, similar to the emotional numbing and avoidance experienced in PTSD. Therefore, we discuss how to help couples (1) regulate and contain excessive emotions as well as (2) heighten emotional experience and expression, as appropriate. For most couples, this experience of emotional dysregulation is not part of their everyday lives; instead, it is a unique response to a relationship trauma. In a small number of instances, however, one or both partners have significant ongoing deficits in emotion regulation that become significantly heightened in the context of an affair. Given that many people demonstrate situationally based emotion dysregulation during Stage 1, it can be difficult to differentiate dysregulation that is focal to the affair versus ongoing deficits in emotion regulation. However, making this distinction is important because working with individuals with general deficits in emotion regulation is a clinical challenge for therapists when such a person experiences infidelity.

Guidelines for Sharing Thoughts and Feelings

Couples responding to an affair must be able to talk about a wide range of issues related to that experience. The most pressing issue from the injured partner typically takes the form, "I just can't understand it. Why did you do it?" A great deal of conversation during treatment and outside of the sessions is devoted to addressing that question. More generally, understanding what both people were thinking and feeling before, during, and in the aftermath of the affair is central to their overall progress and the various therapeutic tasks that you and they will explore in treatment. Consequently, it is critical that the couple be able to communicate their thoughts and feelings effectively, whether partners' general tendencies are to avoid their thoughts and feelings on these topics or whether they are prone to express strong emotions in an unproductive fashion.

Almost all approaches to couple therapy emphasize equipping couples to express their emotions and related thoughts in an adaptive manner. Our approach is to address expressing emotions from a communications, skills-based perspective, which we explain later. Other effective forms of couple therapy, such as emotionally focused couple therapy, integrative behavioral couple therapy, and insight-oriented couple therapy, help guide couples in expressing their feelings without an emphasis on communication training. In particular, Johnson and Greenberg (1985) developed emotionally focused couple therapy as an approach that gives strong and direct emphasis to the role of emotions in couples' interactions. A detailed description of their nine-step approach, which can easily be adapted for addressing emotional components of infidelity, has been provided by Johnson (1996). Whether a particular therapist prefers our skills-based approach or other therapeutic strategies to assist couples in expressing emotions, the following issues and guidelines highlight domains that are important to keep in mind when helping couples respond to an affair. Thus, as the therapist, you might share our handouts with couples and systematically discuss guidelines for speaking and listening, or you may keep these guidelines in mind and raise specific points when they are pertinent to a given couple.

It is also important to differentiate between (1) couple conversations that have the goal of sharing one's own thoughts and feelings and understanding the other person's perspectives versus (2) decision-making or problem-solving conversations as described in Chapter 5. Some couples are naturally aware of whether the goal of a conversation is to reach a decision or to share ideas and feelings and, therefore, do not need information regarding these matters. However, others seem to lose focus within their conversation and move from one type of interaction to another. Therefore, they might benefit from a discussion about differentiating between sharing thoughts and feelings versus making decisions. Next we provide an example of how you as a therapist might introduce this type of communication when needed and help to ensure that both partners are having the same type of conversation. In presenting this information to a couple, the therapist might speak more than usual. We suggest that you encourage as much dialogue and response from the clients as possible while you are conveying this information. However, because of space constraints, we provide a condensed version here.

"To help you start discussing your feelings and thoughts about this affair, I want us to spend time today discussing some guidelines for talking to each other effectively. And although we're focusing on the affair right now, these guidelines can be valuable as you discuss any topic when you want to share your thoughts and feelings.

"We find that couples typically talk to each other for two important reasons. First, at times you need to make decisions or solve problems; these are the kinds of conversations we talked about last week. With all the upheaval caused by the affair, you have many decisions to make about how you interact with each other and with other people, both immediately and long term.

"Second, you also need to talk to each other when you want to share your thoughts and feelings about something. At these times, you aren't trying to resolve anything; you merely want to let the other person know what you're thinking or feeling, and you want the other person to hear and understand you. It's also important for the other person to let you know that you've been heard; therefore, we include listening skills as well as speaking skills. We call this kind of conversation *emotional expressiveness,* and that's what we're going to focus on today.

"It's important to distinguish between these two types of communication because people can become frustrated with each other when they are having different kinds of conversations at the same time. For example, assume a wife is trying to express her feelings about something that has upset her, and her husband tries to give her advice about what to do. If they are like most couples, they become upset with each other. She becomes frustrated because he isn't focusing on her feelings, and he becomes upset because she isn't paying attention to his ideas for improving the situation. So when two people have a conversation, it's important that they have the same type of conversation. If you're unsure about what the other person wants, you can ask, `Do you just want to discuss the problem and share your thoughts and feelings, or do you want to think of a solution or make a decision?' How effective do the two of you think you are in recognizing whether the other person wants to problem solve or share feelings? Which of these types of communication do you feel you do more effectively? [Discuss with couple and then continue.]

"These guidelines for sharing thoughts and feelings and listening will help your interactions move forward more smoothly. The primary goal is for each of you to be able to express your thoughts and feelings in a way that your partner will be able to hear and understand, without becoming defensive or angry. This is important when communicating in general, and you can see how hard it is when you are discussing the affair. Strong feelings are triggered easily, and expressing them can sound condemning or accusatory.

"The second goal is for the other person to listen carefully to the speaker and communicate that you heard what the speaker said. Your job as the listener is to push aside your own feelings and point of view for the time being so that you can really understand what your partner is experiencing and show that you understand. Doing this can go a long way in helping to break negative cycles, but listening well is often hard. Sometimes there's a strong pull to respond by rejecting what your partner has just said. You might think that your partner is minimizing the issue when speaking or, at the other extreme, you might think that your partner is exaggerating the magnitude of what has occurred. When those situations happen, it's difficult to listen well to what the other person is saying.

"So you have very important jobs, whether you're the speaker or the listener. Before we go further, I'd like for each of you to reflect on your own skills: First, how good are you at sharing your thoughts and feelings effectively, and, second, how well can you listen to what your partner has to say, even if you experience a situation differently? [Have each person briefly speak for him- or herself regarding how well he or she expresses and listens; then continue.]"

After providing this introduction for conversations that emphasize sharing thoughts and feelings, we typically give couples a handout of our guidelines as presented in Table 6.1. When discussing these guidelines with a couple, we individualize the discussion based on what we have observed directly in the sessions or what the couple reports about their interactions outside of the sessions. These guidelines are general principles that couples might adopt in almost any context, not just infidelity. However, there are some particular ways that couples struggle when applying the guidelines in response to infi-

TABLE 6.1. Guidelines for Sharing Thoughts and Feelings

Skills for sharing emotions

- State your views *subjectively,* as *your own* feelings and thoughts, not as absolute truths.
- Express your *emotions or feelings.*
- When talking about your partner, state your feelings about your partner, not just about an event or a situation.
- When expressing negative emotions or concerns, also include any *positive feelings* you have about the person or situation.
- Make your statement as *specific* as possible, both in terms of emotions and thoughts.
- Speak in "paragraphs." That is, express one main idea with some elaboration and then allow your partner to respond. Speaking for a long time period without a break makes it hard for your partner to listen.
- Express your feelings and thoughts with *tact* and *timing* so that your partner can listen to what you are saying without becoming defensive.

Skills for listening to partner

Ways to respond while your partner is speaking
- Show that you *understand* your partner's statements and accept his or her right to have those thoughts and feelings. Demonstrate this *acceptance* through your tone of voice, facial expressions, and posture.
- Try to put yourself *in your partner's place* and look at the situation from his or her perspective in order to determine how the other person feels and thinks about the issue.

Ways to respond after your partner finishes speaking
- After your partner finishes speaking, *summarize* and restate your partner's most important feelings, desires, conflicts, and thoughts.
- While in the listener role, *do not*
  o Ask questions, except for clarification.
  o Express your own viewpoint or opinion.
  o Interpret or change the meaning of your partner's statements.
  o Offer solutions or attempt to solve a problem if one exists.
  o Make judgments or evaluate what your partner has said.

delity. Next we provide suggestions for helping both the participating partner and the injured partner express thoughts and feelings to each other in the aftermath of an affair. These points of emphasis are important, whether you are working from a skills-based approach or otherwise.

Guidelines for Sharing Thoughts and Feelings: The Speaker Role

1. *State your views subjectively, as your own feelings and thoughts, not as absolute truths.* Two key points need to be emphasized: (1) Speak for

yourself and (2) be subjective. It is critical that the speaker present only his or her own perspective and avoid expressing the thoughts and feelings of the partner or listener (do not try to read the partner's mind); the partner will speak for him- or herself when that partner is in the speaker role. The tendency to speak for the other person, which can happen at any time, frequently occurs when the couple is discussing why the affair happened.

Each person is encouraged to speak *subjectively*, relating what he or she thinks and feels emotionally: "This is what I think; this is what I feel; this is what I remember." Often discussions of an affair occur in a climate of suspicion and mistrust that has been created by the incident. Consequently, there is a tendency to attempt to reconstruct past facts, with the goal of clarifying what actually did and did not occur. It is reasonable for couples to try to reestablish a realistic general picture of what happened, but there usually is little value in trying to establish the truth of specific events or arguing at length about what did and did not happen. A more productive discussion would focus on how each person felt about what happened and the meaning that each partner gave to the event.

These emphases on subjectivity and speaking for oneself are not intended to provide either person, particularly the participating partner, with the opportunity to avoid addressing difficult issues: "Our therapist said I should speak for myself, and I must decide what I say and when I say it. I do not want to talk about it." Frequently, the participating partner must be strongly encouraged to address painful aspects of the infidelity, and we emphasize that doing so will reestablish a climate of trust and truthfulness. Therefore, if one partner prefers to avoid discussing an issue at a particular time, we encourage that person to state that preference directly rather than seeking other ways to avoid the topic, such as minimizing what happened in the affair or claiming to have a lapse of memory about it. If the topic is important, the couple should decide when they will have a conversation about it so that important issues are not avoided permanently.

2. *Express your emotions or feelings.* When an affair occurs, typically many feelings emerge; yet certain emotions such as anger are more likely to be expressed, particularly by the injured partner. Specific feelings are linked to different thoughts, and anger often results from an experience of being treated unjustly. Consequently, it is understandable that an injured partner might be consumed by anger when values and moral principles have been broken through infidelity. In addition, anger is a "strong" and invulnerable emotion. Such a powerful stance might be appealing after the discovery of an affair because the injured partner experiences a need to maximize safety and

minimize vulnerability during this time. Consequently, expressions of anger and hostility can dominate conversations about the affair with little attention to other emotions. Therefore, at a time when both partners need understanding and acceptance as they try to rebuild a climate of trust and honesty, the tendency to use anger as a way to attack or defend undercuts their ability to discuss the affair constructively.

In helping couples explore the full range of emotions that they are experiencing, it can be helpful to differentiate between primary and secondary emotions, as discussed by Johnson (1996):

> *Primary emotions* are here-and-now direct responses to situations; *secondary emotions* are reactions to, and attempts to cope with, these direct responses, often obscuring awareness of the primary response. For example, angry defensiveness is often expressed in marital conflict, rather than hurt, fear, or other primary affects. (p. 40)

Obscuring primary emotions serves two important purposes that are particularly pertinent in the context of infidelity: (a) avoiding the experience of an emotion that is uncomfortable or unacceptable to the individual having those feelings and (b) avoiding communication of the primary emotion to the partner in order to escape some negative consequence. Often the injured partner wants to deny feelings of hurt, sadness, or disappointment even to him- or herself; instead, he or she may engage in feelings of anger and righteous indignation to help maintain an experience of personal strength and self-esteem. Likewise, expressing hurt, sadness, and fear to the participating partner can increase a sense of vulnerability that feels unsafe, given that the participating partner already has engaged in hurtful behaviors.

The participating partner often is reluctant to demonstrate vulnerability as well. The injured partner frequently is punitive and vengeful in response to the affair; thus, the participating partner wants to avoid providing any more ammunition or expressing a sense of vulnerability to further attack. Thus, a participating partner might minimize his or her shame, guilt, and remorse.

Finally, it is important to note that some couples may ignore or deny their anger in their rush to recover from the affair. In particular, women may feel it is unacceptable to express anger openly and, therefore, avoid or circumvent their feelings of outrage over the affair in an attempt to offer forgiveness. By failing to engage in a full exploration of the negative impact of the affair, the couple is less likely to put the affair to rest, nor will they gain the information necessary to protect their relationship from future harm. Many writings on forgiveness argue against the dangers of this "hasty" forgiveness (e.g., Murphy,

2005), and we strongly suggest that clinicians be alert to this possibility early in treatment as well.

In addition to avoiding certain emotions because they seem unsafe, either partner might also have difficulty experiencing or expressing certain thoughts and emotions for other reasons. During this time of heightened arousal, individuals frequently do not think or process information clearly. In addition, clarity can be undermined if the individual's sleep, eating, or exercise has become compromised, as discussed in Chapter 5. Moreover, some individuals struggle generally with differentiating or labeling emotions. For these various reasons, we have constructed a handout of "feeling words" that can be shared with couples (see Table 6.2). Even if the couple has the skills to differentiate and label emotions, this list can be helpful in drawing partners' attention to more vulnerable emotions that they might be avoiding. For example, we might say to one partner, "In addition to the anger you're experiencing, what other emotions on this list do you feel when you think about the affair?" For therapists who do not use handouts in their work with couples or for couples for whom such lists might seem patronizing, the therapist can verbally suggest a list of additional emotions that might be experienced during a given interaction.

3. **When discussing a situation, state your feelings about your partner and/or the relationship, not just about the event, situation, or other people.** Although some individuals, particularly injured partners, are quick to focus on the other partner, sometimes a different pattern of discussion evolves. For example, to maintain a positive image of the participating partner and hope for the relationship, some injured partners focus solely on the outside individual or external circumstances that contributed to the affair. Although these are often important contextual factors in understanding why the affair occurred, when the two partners are talking to each other, it also is important to help them maintain a focus on their thoughts and feelings about each other and their relationship.

4. **When expressing negative emotions or concerns, also include any positive feelings you have.** It is much easier to listen to and process negative emotions and concerns from the partner if they are balanced with a discussion of positives. Understandably, subsequent to the discovery of an affair, many of the ideas and emotions expressed are negative. However, some positive emotions and thoughts often underlie the negative reactions, but they frequently are omitted or deemphasized in conversations about the affair. We urge therapists to uncover these underlying positive emotions and encourage

TABLE 6.2. Words for Describing Common Feelings

Positive moods

Happy/joyful	Cheerful	Happy	Excited
	Pleased	Amused	Joyful
	Delighted	Thrilled	Glad
Close/warm	Loving	Warm	Devoted
	Affectionate	Secure	Tender
	Sexy	Close	
Energetic/vigorous	Active	Lively	Peppy
	Vigorous	Energetic	Enthusiastic
	Adventurous	Friendly	
Relaxed/calm	Gentle	Peaceful	Calm
	Relaxed	Contented	
Other positive	Agreeable	Ambitious	Confident
	Inspired	Lucky	Fortunate

Negative moods

Depressed/sad	Sad	Bored	Blue
	Gloomy	Unhappy	Grim
	Discouraged	Low	Miserable
	Dejected	Hurt	
Anxious	Shaky	Tense	Restless
	Nervous	Anxious	Fearful
	Panicky	Insecure	Terrified
	Frightened	Worried	Shy
	Bashful	Confused	
Angry	Angry	Frustrated	Resentful
	Enraged	Furious	Irritated
	Disgusted	Outraged	Annoyed
	Mad		
Contemptuous	Critical	Disdainful	Contemptuous
	Hostile		
Fatigued	Exhausted	Fatigued	Tired
	Listless	Sluggish	Weary
	Wilted		
Other negative	Bewildered	Lonely	Jealous
	Guilty	Ashamed	

Note. Adapted from Epstein and Baucom (2002). Copyright 2002 by the American Psychological Association. Adapted by permission.

their expression by the partners. Doing so can help to change the tone of the conversation into one with more caring and concern. For example, when an injured partner expresses anger about the affair, underlying that anger might be a sense of loss based on many years of caring about the participating partner. The following is an example of how the therapist worked to encourage the expression of this latter sentiment.

THERAPIST: Tom, I understand that you're furious with Pam for getting involved with Mark. And that makes a lot of sense; people typically feel angry when they believe they've been treated badly. When people become really angry, it usually is because what has happened is extremely important to them, and the injustice often involves something valuable that has been taken away unfairly. I wonder if that's what has happened to you. What have you lost; what has been taken away that you have valued so deeply?

TOM: I've lost everything: my wife, my dreams, and my dignity. There's almost nothing else that I can lose.

THERAPIST: Exactly. It feels like you've lost Pam. What emotions do you feel when you think about losing Pam, of her not being there with you or for you?

TOM: It's unbearable, awful. She is, or has been, my world—my reason for being. I don't care that much about my career or anything else. She really is all that matters to me.

THERAPIST: And what emotion do you feel when you think about losing Pam, the most important person to you in the world?

TOM: It feels like my gut is being ripped out. I feel overwhelming sadness and panic. I don't know what to do.

THERAPIST: And if you could determine what to do to make things right between you and Pam again, how would that feel, knowing that you have her back?

TOM: It would be amazing, like a miracle. I've always loved her so much that I almost can't contain it.

THERAPIST: Okay, I want you to tell Pam two things you just shared with me. First, that you love and cherish her more than anything in the world, and second, that the idea of losing her gives you a sense of sadness that is completely overwhelming. For now, focus just on those two things and nothing else. And, Pam, your role is only to listen and try to understand what Tom is telling you; let him know that you accept what he's feeling.

When he's finished, I want you to reflect what you heard him share with you, and stop there, okay?

In the prior excerpt, the therapist guided Tom to discuss his positive and vulnerable emotions. It is important to note that in developing this conversation, the therapist addressed Tom directly rather than having Tom and Pam engage in a conversation initially. Asking Tom to express feelings of tenderness and caring to Pam directly at the beginning might have been quite difficult. In the dialogue between the therapist and Tom, several interventions were used. First, the therapist validated Tom's anger and acknowledged his feelings. Then the therapist guided the conversation to focus on other emotions, responding empathically in order to establish a safe environment for Tom. Only at the end of the dialogue did the therapist ask Tom to speak directly to Pam. In doing so, the therapist must have some degree of confidence that Pam would not use Tom's disclosure as a basis for attacking him. In addition, the therapist structured Pam's response carefully in order to keep the conversation on track and minimize the likelihood that Tom would be punished by Pam for expressing his love for her.

5. *Make your statement as specific as possible in terms of both emotions and thoughts.* This guideline applies to almost all communication and is especially valuable when discussing infidelity. Emotions as words carry a range of meaning, and the expression of specific emotions conveys clearer information than the expression of general ones. For example, being generally "upset" can imply a multitude of different meanings. However, the more specific emotion of anger typically conveys an experience of injustice; sadness indicates an experience of loss; fear typically accompanies a concern about something dangerous in the present; and anxiety conveys a similar worry about future negative consequences. Likewise, hope is about a better future, and feeling calm and at peace conveys that things are okay, at least for now.

6. *Speak in "paragraphs." That is, express one main idea with some elaboration and then allow your partner to respond. Speaking for a long time period without a break makes it difficult for the partner to listen.* Individuals vary in the amount of detail that they generally want to discuss during conversations. Compared with participating partners, injured partners frequently desire longer conversations with more discussion and detail from both people. Often injured partners are overwhelmed and flooded with ideas, emotions, and images, with a resulting need to "get it out." At times, they try to express everything at once with no opportunity for the other person

to respond. They can become more emotional as they speak; their speech becomes more pressured, and they implicitly or explicitly convey the message, "You did this. Now you need to sit there, keep quiet and listen." Unfortunately, the participating partner may be incapable of listening to what sounds like a lengthy barrage of attacks and complaints. In addition, injured partners frequently want the participating partner to provide extensive detail about what happened or explanations for why the affair occurred. The message is, "Keep talking. You're nowhere close to being finished yet."

Therefore, to facilitate effective communication, we encourage both partners to speak in "paragraphs," expressing one major idea with brief elaboration. As described next, the listener then is asked to respond by reflecting the speaker's most important thoughts and feelings. After the listener reflects, either the same speaker can continue if the speaker has more to say immediately, or the two partners can switch roles, and the listener becomes the speaker.

7. *Express your feelings and thoughts with tact and timing so that your partner can listen to what you are saying without becoming defensive.* As Pam mentioned in the excerpt at the beginning of this chapter, few conversations about infidelity are likely to be successful late at night once the couple has gone to bed. Similarly, it is difficult to have conversations about such highly emotional topics during transitional times during the day. Therefore, couples should generally avoid trying to address such topics when getting up in the morning, leaving for work, returning home, or going to bed at night. Moreover, important conversation should be minimized when either person is engaged in another activity or is significantly distracted or stressed by other life situations. Of course, conversations about the affair cannot be relegated to the back burner in order to proceed with the rest of life's demands, but the couple should seek the most opportune times and settings possible for their conversations in order to maximize success.

Guidelines for Sharing Thoughts and Feelings: The Listener Role

When a couple has a conversation in which partners share their thoughts and feelings, there is a flow to the interaction that revolves around a cycle of communication. That cycle is defined as follows: (1) one partner assumes the role of speaker and talks, perhaps using the guidelines described previously; (2) the other partner listens while the first partner speaks; and (3) after the speaker finishes talking, the listener reflects the most important thoughts and feelings that the speaker conveyed. After the cycle ends, the first speaker can continue in the speaker role, or the two partners can switch roles. The listener role is conceptually straightforward: Listen and then reflect. Although many nondistressed couples do not communicate in this manner, following these guidelines can be particularly helpful when a couple is discussing an affair because this approach slows the interaction and helps partners listen well. However, these guidelines can be difficult to implement when the conversation involves strong emotions and different perspectives or when the relationship is in a vulnerable state. Therefore, we provide more detailed guidelines to help both partners become good listeners.

Ways to Respond While Your Partner Is Speaking

1. *Try to put yourself in your partner's place and look at the situation from his or her perspective to determine how the other person feels and thinks about the issue.* This first guideline involves a mind-set or perspective rather than a specific behavior. The partner in the listener role has one single goal: to understand the speaker's thoughts and feelings *from the speaker's point of view.* Frequently, the listener attends to the speaker from the listener's perspective, evaluating whether the speaker's comments are correct or justifiable and whether the listener agrees or disagrees with the speaker's comments. If the listener disagrees, then the listener often begins to prepare a rebuttal while the speaker continues to talk. Our message to the listener is simple, "For now, just listen. Put yourself in the other person's place to understand how he or she feels from the speaker's perspective. You don't need to agree or disagree or prepare a rebuttal. Your only goal for now is to understand what the other person is experiencing."

2. *Show that you understand your partner's statements and accept his or her right to have those thoughts and feelings. Demonstrate this acceptance through your tone of voice, facial expressions, and posture.* The key to this guideline is the word "acceptance." The listener is not being asked to agree with what the speaker says but rather to listen attentively and respect that person's right to have his or her own thoughts, feelings, and perspective. In essence, the person is being asked to adopt the following stance, "What you think and feel is important to me. I will try to understand your perspective and respect it, even though I might disagree." The listener is asked to convey this acceptance nonverbally while listening, for example, by making eye contact, facing the speaker, and maintaining an open posture. Distinguishing between (1) respect and acceptance versus (2) agreement is critical when discussing

infidelity. Often the partners disagree about factual information or the other person's thoughts and interpretations regarding the infidelity.

In addition, one person might consider it inappropriate for the partner to "feel" the way he or she feels. For example, a participating partner might say, "You have no right to be furious with me about a stupid one-night stand. Look at how you've treated me during our entire relationship. If anyone broke our vows, it was you. You promised to love and respect me and to care for me, and you didn't do that. If anyone should be furious, it's me; you've abused me for years. I hurt you for only one night." The listener needs to disregard his or her evaluation of the speaker's message, at least momentarily, in an effort to respect the speaker's right to have his or her own thoughts and feelings. Thus, eye contact, head nods, and other nonverbal forms of acknowledgment convey respect and acceptance but do not necessarily imply agreement.

Ways to Respond after Your Partner Finishes Speaking

1. *After your partner finishes speaking, summarize and restate your partner's most important feelings, desires, conflicts, and thoughts.* At that point, the listener role is straightforward: While summarizing and paraphrasing in the listener's own words, restate the speaker's most important thoughts and feelings. This form of communication can sound artificial and contrived if done in a "parroting" manner that repeats verbatim what the speaker has just said. Instead, the listener should use his or her own words to summarize the speaker's comments. The goal is to maintain an emphasis on what the speaker has said; therefore, the listener is asked to refrain from making statements that would shift that focus. For example, the listener should not ask questions that would take the speaker in a new direction or suggest that the speaker was being dishonest. An example of counterproductive questions might be, "I know that you said that while you were with her, you really were not thinking at all about what you were risking with your family and profession. But do you really expect me to believe that? How could you not be thinking about those things?"

We noted previously the importance of distinguishing between acceptance and agreement. This distinction is particularly important when the listener is asked to reflect the speaker's most important thoughts and feelings. Some listeners are reluctant to follow this guideline because they think that in reflecting they are acknowledging agreement with the speaker. When discussing an affair about which the two partners have vastly different thoughts and feelings, often the listener wants to make clear his or her strong disagreement with what the speaker has said, both while listening when the speaker talks and while responding. As a result, we often make the following type of statement and repeat it in different words throughout the sessions.

> "Tom, when Pam finishes speaking, I want you to summarize the most important things she has told you, both her thoughts and the emotions she is expressing. I know that many times the two of you see things very differently, particularly about the affair. So, when you reflect back what she has told you, we all understand that you are not expressing agreement with what she has said. Instead, what you are saying to her is this: `I understand that this is what you're thinking and feeling, and I respect your right to have those thoughts and feelings.' [At this point, you might inquire about the listener's reactions to this guideline and process those reactions. Then proceed to the next point.] Very soon, you will become the speaker, and at that point you can express your own thoughts and feelings. In fact, when you become the speaker, you might even begin with some statement such as, `I understand what you thought and felt, but I experienced it differently.' Then you can continue with your own perspective. This is a respectful way of talking about differences. Instead of telling the other person that he or she is confused, wrong, or being dishonest, you are acknowledging that the other person had a different experience and then expressing your own perspective once you become the speaker. To return to my major point, when Pam finishes speaking, merely summarize and restate her most important feelings and thoughts that you heard. This does not suggest agreement; instead, it reflects your understanding of what she told you. Are you ready to try it?"

When reflecting the speaker's most important thoughts and feelings in words, the listener should use a tone of voice and body posture that also reflect understanding and acceptance. For example, reflecting while rolling one's eyes or using a sarcastic tone of voice can undermine the listener's reflection. These undermining strategies can be seen any time a couple is discussing a difficult topic. They are particularly likely when an injured partner is in the listening role and feeling a strong desire to demonstrate disapproval of the infidelity and the participating partner's presentation of it. Ironically, the injured partner often pushes the participating partner to explain and provide some understanding of how the infidelity came about, but then responds punitively when the participating partner complies. Therefore, as a therapist, you need to help the injured partner realize that understanding and acceptance can encourage the participating partner to be more disclosing, which will ultimately lead to a better understanding of why the affair occurred and contribute to making needed changes in the relationship. On the other hand, disagreement, dis-approval, and other punishing responses will likely lead to withdrawal and defensiveness.

Additional Strategies for Containing Emotional Expression

These guidelines, approached either from a skills-based or alternative perspec-tive, can help couples to have productive conversations both within and out-side of the sessions. In addition, you can suggest a variety of other strategies to promote constructive interactions between the partners. Given that the expression of strong negative emotions in a dysregulated manner is a signifi-cant risk during these conversations, an overall strategy is to provide increased structure to contain the emotional expression and other dysregulated behav-iors. The following are additional guidelines and strategies that we frequently use to achieve this goal.

Scheduling Couple Conversations Outside of the Therapy Sessions

We noted previously the importance of timing conversations by avoiding situ-ations such as entrances, exits, transitions, and times when either partner is preoccupied. Additionally, it can be helpful for the couple to schedule specific times outside of the therapy sessions when they will have conversations about the infidelity. Of course, this should only happen when the therapist and the couple believe that they have the skills and restraint needed to have these conversations productively. Many unproductive conversations occur when one partner, often the injured partner, pushes for discussion when the other partner is not prepared to talk. Therefore, if both partners know, for example, that they will have a 30-minute discussion Wednesday at 8:00 p.m., focusing on how they will tell others about the affair, then both people can set time aside and be emotionally prepared for the conversation. Limiting the length of these conversations can be helpful. Frequently, couples engage in lengthy conversations about the affair, and as the conversation continues, one or both partners become tired, creating a high-risk situation. If either person experi-ences the conversation as becoming uncontrolled and the couple is unable to refocus the interaction, either partner might request a time-out as described in Chapter 4. Shorter, focused, more frequent conversations are often more productive than wide-ranging, lengthy ones.

Letter Writing as a Prelude to Direct Conversations

When a couple has a conversation about the affair and their emotions are strong, often they begin reacting to each other and to what the other person has said. As a result, the conversation can spiral out of control as the two people experience increasingly heightened emotions in response to each other. To avoid this difficulty, it can be productive to have one partner write a letter to the other partner at various points during the treatment. This approach ensures that the writer is not distracted by the partner's response while writing the letter. In addition, the writer has an opportunity to take his or her time to express ideas precisely, then put the letter aside, and later reread and revise it before sharing it with the partner.

Because the injured partner typically has strong feelings about the affair and the participating partner, during Stage 1 we routinely invite the injured partner to write a letter to the participating partner expressing how the injured partner has experienced the affair and the couple's subsequent interaction. We encourage the injured partner to use effective communication skills as reflected in the guidelines presented previously when sharing thoughts and feelings in the letter. Overall, the goal of the letter is to state how the affair has affected the writer's thoughts and feelings about him- or herself, the other partner, and the relationship. In Table 6.3, we have excerpted the instructions for letter writing from our self-help book for couples who have experienced an affair (Snyder et al., 2007). During the therapy session, you can describe the goal and principles for writing letters and ask the injured partner to write such a letter outside of the session. You also might want to provide some version of Table 6.3 for the injured partner to refer to when writing the letter.

Although either partner periodically might want to write letters or keep a journal just for him- or herself and not intended for sharing, the purpose of the current letter is for the injured partner to write a letter that will subsequently be shared with the participating partner. After the letter is written, you and the couple must decide the next steps of how it can be used productively for a conversation. If you are concerned about how the letter may be written, you might invite the injured partner to allow you to review a draft of it and provide comments before it is finalized. If you do provide feedback, it is important that you encourage a constructive wording of the writer's message and resist inserting your own ideas or perspectives. The participating partner needs to understand that the letter was written by the injured partner and not by the therapist. Once the letter is finalized, its content can be shared with the participating partner in various ways. Eventually, we have the couple discuss the letter in a therapy session. If you believe that the participating partner can read the letter outside of the session without precipitating an unproductive

TABLE 6.3. Instructions for Writing a Letter to the Participating Partner

The guidelines for letter writing are not really different from the guidelines we have already offered for expressing your feelings. The most important point is that you try to write a letter that is balanced, maintains focus, and avoids doing further damage. If you are extremely upset or angry, you have two alternatives: (1) Wait to write the letter until a later time or (2) write an initial letter as a way of "venting" your hurt or frustrations but destroy it later. Be sure you distinguish between a letter intended to be shared with your partner in which you express your feelings more selectively and one written for the purpose of venting and *not* to be shared with your partner. Letters intended for venting that are subsequently "discovered" by your partner can have even more destructive and long-lasting consequences than angry verbal exchanges because they provide a permanent record of your most intense negative feelings.

Begin your letter by identifying your feelings and describing how you are finding it difficult to express those feelings constructively face to face. Acknowledge that your feelings stem from your own perspective and that your partner's perspective might be different. Clarify what you are seeking from your partner at this time: Understanding of your feelings? Clarification of your partner's feelings? Reaching a decision together about how to deal with a situation? Focus your letter by emphasizing one or two primary feelings and the specific situation giving rise to these feelings. *Above all, remember that letters are not intended as a substitute for face-to-face discussions.* Rather, they are a way to express your feelings and thoughts if you think it will be too difficult to talk face to face because you will become upset, your partner will be unable to hear, or an argument is likely to develop.

You also can use letter writing when you are unable to *listen* or respond to your partner's feelings in the way you want. If you and your partner have tried to talk about an issue several times and are unable to do so, consider using letter writing as a way of working through the impasse. Preparing a letter of response that conveys understanding and empathy is different from writing a letter that focuses on your own thoughts and feelings. In writing a letter of understanding, first acknowledge your own difficulty in listening and responding to your partner's views constructively during the prior discussion, if indeed you did experience difficulty. Avoid using the letter to express your own thoughts and feelings. Instead, try to validate your partner's views by expressing your understanding of how your partner could come to think or feel that way, given his or her perspective. Remember: It's not necessary that you agree with your partner, only that you convey your understanding of the thoughts or feelings your partner has expressed. Then request a time to sit down together and invite your partner to clarify any feelings you still find confusing or to amend or correct any misunderstandings that your letter may include.

If subsequent discussions continue to create hurt or to spiral out of control as they did initially, exchange letters again, but this time reverse roles so that you can express your feelings and your partner can communicate his or her understanding of your perspective. Continue to exchange letters, alternating roles as "speaker" and "listener," until each of you feels better understood and able to respond with understanding to the other.

Note. Adapted from Snyder, Baucom, and Gordon (2007). Copyright 2007 by The Guilford Press. Adapted by permission.

interaction for the couple and both people want the letter read before the therapy session, you might suggest that the injured partner give the letter to the participating partner the day before the next therapy session but that they not discuss it before the session. Alternatively, if the couple has great difficulty discussing the affair by themselves, it might be preferable for the participating partner to wait and read the letter during a therapy session.

During the subsequent therapy session, either the injured partner can read the letter to the participating partner if it appears likely that doing so will help to create a constructive emotional atmosphere, or the participating partner can read the letter silently during the session. In either case, once the participating partner knows the content of the letter, the couple discusses it during the therapy session. The primary goal of this discussion is for the participating partner to use the listening skills described previously to demonstrate an understanding and acceptance of how the infidelity has affected the injured partner.

Depending on the couple and the goals at this stage of treatment, you might ask the participating partner to write a letter in response. If you do proceed in this manner, it is important that a letter from the participating partner include an acknowledgment of his or her behavior as well as current thoughts and feelings about him- or herself, the partner, and their relationship.

You might find that letter writing is helpful to the couple at various points during the treatment, providing a mechanism for them to express their thoughts and feelings as they progress through the intervention. It is not intended as a substitute for direct communication, but it can provide a controlled and thoughtful way to express important thoughts and feelings initially before the couple begins discussing them.

Strategies for Enhancing Emotional Experience and Expression

Many partners, particularly injured partners, respond to infidelity with strong, negative, overwhelming emotions and unproductive expressions of those feelings. However, at times, one or both partners might respond in an overly constricted, unemotional, and perhaps intellectualized approach to the affair. Some individuals characteristically deal with strong emotions or difficult situations in this manner. Other persons might adopt a minimizing strategy in response to the enormity of the affair and the emotional numbing that accompanies traumatic experiences. For example, injured partners might respond in this way to avoid becoming overwhelmed by the magnitude of their feelings, or they might minimize expression of emotion to the participating partner in an attempt to avoid further vulnerability, as if to say, "You can't hurt me." Likewise, the participating partner might try to minimize emotional experience as a way to avoid further guilt and minimize the expression of emotion in an effort to counterbalance the strong emotion of the injured partner. Therefore, at times your goal as the therapist might be to enhance the experience or expression of emotion so that the couple does not rush to achieve a superficial resolution of the past painful events. Strategies for enhancing emotional experience and expression within a couple context have been described from a variety of theoretical orientations, and many of these techniques are directly applicable in addressing infidelity. For example, a major emphasis of emotionally focused couple therapy (Johnson & Greenberg, 1995) involves helping partners experience and express emotions that they might be avoiding or minimizing. Epstein and Baucom (2002, pp. 381–392) have incorporated emotionally focused couple therapy in describing a variety of strategies for heightening emotions during a therapy session within a cognitive–behavioral couple therapy framework. To access primary emotions, Epstein and Baucom include strategies such as (1) asking direct questions about what emotions were experienced during a given event; (2) offering reflections of "implied feelings" that were not directly expressed; and (3) having a partner first express thoughts and behaviors that occurred, subsequently linking emotions to more easily accessed cognitions and behavior.

Likewise, to heighten emotional experience during the session, they draw from emotionally focused couple therapy techniques (Johnson, 1996) and discuss the following strategies in detail in their text on general couple therapy (Epstein & Baucom, 2002, p. 387):

- Repeating a phrase at selected moments to heighten the impact of the phrase.
- Using poignant images and metaphors to heighten the experience.
- Altering the therapist's own behavior in a more emotional direction, such as shifting body position or using a volume of speech and inflection that emphasizes the emotional experience.
- Asking individuals to express their internal emotional experience to their partners to transform the internal, subjective experience into an interpersonal experience.
- Maintaining a focus on important emotional experiences or "blocking exits" so that the individual and the couple are not derailed from the emotional experience (Johnson, 1996).

Addressing Long-Term Dysregulation Difficulties

The strategies described thus far in this chapter are intended for use with couples whose difficulty addressing emotions results from either (1) the traumatic nature of infidelity or (2) a mild to moderate level of general difficulty in dealing with emotions for one or both partners. When these circumstances are present, using the strategies that we have discussed can be successful with many couples. However, some couples experiencing infidelity include a partner—and in rare instances, both partners—who suffer from chronic and extreme emotion regulation difficulties. Identifying such individuals can be difficult early in treatment, particularly because most injured partners demonstrate some level of emotion dysregulation in response to the infidelity. In fact, heightened emotions that seem out of control help to define Stage 1 of treatment. However, if emotional dysregulation is extreme and persists, long-term alternative interventions must be considered.

In making this assessment, you should attend to several individual and interpersonal behavior patterns demonstrated by the partner of concern. The following expressions of emotional sensitivity may be present during or outside of the sessions: (1) strong emotional responses to minor or apparently innocuous cues, circumstances, or behaviors from the other partner; (2) strong emotional responses that are out of proportion to the circumstances; and (3) difficulty returning from heightened emotions to normal arousal. Because previously neutral cues or circumstances can trigger strong emotional responses as part of the response to infidelity, it is important to avoid concluding too quickly that an individual has general emotional dysregulation difficulties. Still, certain patterns of behavior might indicate more persistent problems with emotional dysregulation, such as (1) when an individual becomes so upset during therapy sessions that he or she needs to leave the room or terminate the session because of an inability to recover or (2) when a couple describes destructive arguments that sometimes are accompanied by physical aggression or destruction of property. If these behaviors persist for many weeks or even months after a variety of strategies have been attempted to regain equilibrium and contain emotion, then additional intervention modalities might be necessary.

If one partner's emotion dysregulation dominates the session, creates reluctance to raise difficult issues either for the therapist or the other partner, or impedes progress in other significant ways, then some form of individual intervention for the partner might be useful. Otherwise, progress is inhibited or the couple therapy has the tone of individual therapy with the other partner present. Although emotion dysregulation has gained prominence in recent years, primarily within a discussion of borderline personality disorder, difficulties regulating emotion cut across a wide variety of diagnostic categories and individuals with subclinical levels of psychopathology (Snyder, Castellani, & Whisman, 2006). Linehan (1993) has developed a variety of emotion regulation skills for persons with borderline personality disorder that often are taught in a group context and could be of benefit to emotionally dysregulated individuals, even without such a diagnosis.

If a couple needs assistance in addressing emotional dysregulation productively as a unit, several resources are available to the therapist. Kirby and Baucom (2007a, 2007b) have developed a specialized couple-based intervention to address emotion dysregulation that integrates cognitive–behavioral couple therapy and dialectical behavior therapy (DBT). Drawing from DBT, the intervention includes a discussion of the following skills for both partners: (1) introduction to emotion dysregulation, (2) DBT mindfulness skills, (3) DBT emotion regulation skills, (4) DBT distress tolerance skills, and (5) behavioral principles and analysis. Teaching these skills requires a considerable amount of time, and the therapist might elect to focus on those that seem most pertinent to a specific couple. Alternatively, Fruzzetti and Fruzzetti (2003) have developed other strategies for addressing emotion dysregulation in a couple context. In addition, Snyder et al.'s (2006) edited volume on emotion dysregulation in couples can assist therapists in working with such couples. Although detailed discussion of these techniques is beyond the scope of this book, it is important that you consider whether extreme cases of emotion dysregulation can be handled within the context of the couple therapy or whether additional interventions are needed.

Summary

In this chapter, we have discussed addressing emotional responses to infidelity with a direct focus on affective experience and expression. We have described effective communication strategies as well as other structuring strategies such as the use of written letters to help the couple express their thoughts and emotions without becoming overwhelmed or derailed by destructive interactions. Not only can unmodulated, extreme expressions of emotion have obvious destructive consequences, but also, at the other extreme, overcontrolled, unemotional responses can contribute to incomplete processing. Finally, although not common, in some couples one partner has generalized difficulties with emotion regulation, which are accentuated by the trauma of infidelity. Given the considerable pain that often results, such individuals frequently need individual therapy as well.

Overall, Stage 1 of treatment involves dealing with the immediate aftermath of infidelity when emotions are heightened and life feels out of control. Chapters 4, 5, and 6 are intended to work synergistically to help couples through the immediate crisis subsequent to infidelity. When destructive interactions have been minimized, some degree of routine has returned in the couple's life, and the partners are able to talk with each other in a constructive manner, they are ready to move on to the important tasks involved in Stage 2. In the next stage, the couple will seek a more comprehensive, balanced understanding of the factors that contributed to the development of the affair. In the next chapters, we provide an in-depth discussion of how to guide couples through this process.

Resources from *Getting Past the Affair*

Our self-help book for couples, *Getting Past the Affair*, includes information related to the topics discussed in the current chapter. If you are using that book in conjunction with couple therapy, you might find the following sections useful to assign to the couple to read, along with relevant exercises:

Guidelines for sharing thoughts and feelings: Chapter 3 (pp. 58–69) includes a discussion of guidelines for sharing thoughts and feelings.

Writing letters to a partner: Chapter 3 (pp. 76–79) discusses how partners might write letters to each other as a more structured strategy and a prelude to face-to-face conversations. Exercise 3.2 provides the couple with an opportunity to write and exchange such letters.

PART THREE

STAGE 2 OF TREATMENT

Introduction to Stage 2 of Treatment

Coming to a shared, comprehensive understanding of why an affair occurred is simultaneously the most difficult and the most important stage of a couple's recovery from infidelity. It is important primarily because such an understanding can serve as the basis for restoring emotional security for the injured partner, and this security might serve as the foundation for rebuilding trust and intimacy. In other instances, a clear understanding provides the basis for a partner's decision to end the relationship. Although couples working successfully through Stage 1 may begin to restore daily routines and decrease their negativity, failing to use this increased stability as a platform for examining underlying contributing factors to the affair renders them at higher risk for future emotional or physical distance, lingering feelings of mistrust, and increased vulnerability to recurrence of an affair.

GOALS FOR STAGE 2

While the couple works toward a shared formulation of the affair, they also pursue the following secondary goals:

- Restoring predictability regarding fidelity and the long-term future of the relationship.
- Developing a more balanced and realistic view of the partner.

- Expanding an explanatory context that promotes responsibility for one's own contributions and decisions.
- Preparing the groundwork for additional individual and relationship change.

A major threat to a couple's recovery from an affair is the injured partner's continued feelings of insecurity and vulnerability. Neither the participating partner's behaviors nor the long-term future of the relationship may seem predictable. At the base of these feelings may be uncertainty about whether the affair is continuing, could reignite, or could be followed by another affair at some point in the future. Even when injured partners feel reassured about an affair ending and the unlikelihood of another, they may feel insecure about the participating partner's feelings for them because of persistent doubts about one's own attractiveness, desirability, or adequacy. Participating partners often have their own feelings of unpredictability as well. They may attribute the affair in part to characteristics of their relationship or behaviors of the injured partner but may feel unable to discuss these factors, either because they feel guilty or because they anticipate that the partner will be unable or unwilling to address these concerns. Working through these feelings and restoring predictability lie at the heart of recovery.

After an affair, injured partners frequently experience such profound betrayal that they are unable to view the participating partner in any way other than with anger and contempt. When the sole explanation for the affair rests on the faulty character of the participating partner, the ability or willingness to rebuild trust and intimacy with that partner remains thwarted. On the other hand, injured partners occasionally adopt extreme views that absolve the participating partner from any responsibility for his or her involvement in the affair. They may accept blame themselves or assign a disproportionate level of blame to the outside person while minimizing or ignoring the participating partner's role. Participating partners sometimes have their own views of the injured partner that impede efforts toward reestablishing an intimate relationship. They may attribute their own affair primarily to the injured partner's lack of appreciation, caring, understanding, or wish for emotional or physical closeness. During Stage 2, both the injured partner and the participating partner are encouraged to develop a more balanced view of each other.

Promoting partners' balanced views of themselves and each other involves examining (1) diverse domains of potential contributing factors from within and outside the couple's relationship and from each partner separately and (2) ways in which these factors served as predisposing vulnerabilities, precipitating effects, influences that maintained or prolonged the affair, or influences that have rendered recovery more difficult. Couples need assistance in working through these potential sources of contributing factors for the affair. Otherwise, they can become overwhelmed with multiple explanations without a means for organizing them in a way that directs next steps toward recovery; alternatively, they may foreclose on an oversimplified or inaccurate explanation of the affair as a way of ending their confusion. Encouraging the couple to adopt the framework introduced in Chapter 1 promotes a more balanced understanding and guides partners' efforts to address factors in themselves as well as within and outside their relationship.

TREATMENT STRATEGIES FOR STAGE 2

The treatment strategies for pursuing Stage 2 goals generally fall into three classes:

- Establishing a rationale, and creating and maintaining a motivational base for doing Stage 2 work.
- Systematically exploring the contributing factors, which may diverge in content and temporal influence.
- Developing a coherent, shared formulation of contributing factors.

Couples often can work together in Stage 1 interventions aimed at restoring equilibrium and "calming things down." They more frequently experience resistance to Stage 2 interventions that potentially "stir things up." In offering a rationale for pursuing Stage 2 interventions, we emphasize several points. The injured partner needs to learn as much as he or she can about why the affair happened in order to restore the emotional security essential to trust and intimacy. Hence, the participating partner needs to explore why the affair happened in part because it is what the injured partner needs. We also describe anticipated benefits to the participating partner, including gaining the injured partner's trust and restoring intimacy, understanding him- or herself more fully, rebuilding the couple's relationship, and helping the couple make good decisions about the future of their relationship.

Table III.1 lists potential contributing factors to an affair from within and outside the couple's relationship and from each partner. We typically use a guided discovery process to promote couples' exploration of each of these domains. For example, we encourage them to think about such factors before discussing them in the next session, to write down as many of these factors as they can identify, and, depending on the partners' levels of emotion regulation and communication

TABLE III.1. Potential Contributing Factors to Vulnerability to an Affair

Aspects of the couple's relationship

- Frequent arguing or unresolved conflicts.
- Low levels of emotional closeness.
- Too little time devoted to shared fun activities.
- Low levels of physical intimacy.
- Unmet relationship expectations.
- Difficulty balancing both relationship and individual goals.

Influences outside the couple's relationship

- High demands from work or family responsibilities.
- Too much time devoted to activities or persons excluding the partner.
- Stress from illness, financial concerns, extended family, or other sources.
- Too much time spent with individuals who failed to support the couple's relationship.
- Too little time spent with individuals supporting the couple's relationship.
- Frequent exposure to situations providing opportunity for outside emotional or sexual involvement.

Aspects of the participating partner

- Self-doubts and vulnerability to affirmation from an outsider.
- High levels of attractiveness to outsiders.
- Own behaviors that contributed to or maintained relationship difficulties.
- Beliefs about affairs emphasizing positive aspects and minimizing negative consequences.
- Difficulties in honoring long-term commitments.

Aspects of the injured partner

- Self-doubts interfering with emotional or physical intimacy.
- Own behaviors that contributed to or maintained relationship difficulties.
- Difficulties in coping with relationship disappointments or injuries.

skills, to have discussions of these issues between sessions as a way of identifying areas of agreement and disagreement. These efforts may be facilitated by having partners work through our companion book, *Getting Past the Affair*. Within each domain, we encourage partners to consider how potential contributing factors may have exerted their influence across different temporal phases of the affair.

Throughout this exploration process, the therapist needs to structure discussions between partners as they explore and attempt to understand the context of the affair. This approach includes highlighting certain observations, reinterpreting distorted beliefs or cognitions, or drawing inferences from partners' respective histories that they are not able to do themselves. Understanding how past needs and wishes influence an individual's choices in the present may be a critical element to understanding why the individual chose to have an affair or how the injured partner has responded to this event. This exploration process eventually leads to change-directed interventions, which provide important assessment data regarding partners' willingness and ability to implement critical changes essential to reaching an informed decision about how to move on in Stage 3.

After examining potential contributing factors across these different domains, the therapist needs to help the couple integrate the disparate pieces of information they have gleaned into a coherent narrative explaining how the affair came about. The therapist can invite each partner to prepare a verbal formulation that includes contributing factors from each of the domains previously explored in therapy, along with their temporal influences. Alternatively, partners can be asked to write letters in which each person describes what he or she understands to be the relevant factors. Initial formulations and discussion of these in the sessions may be supplemented by the therapist's own understanding and followed by revised formulations to promote more effective integration of all that has been learned during Stage 2 work.

CHALLENGES AND RISKS FOR THE THERAPIST DURING STAGE 2 OF TREATMENT

Several challenges and risks for the therapist can render Stage 2 interventions particularly difficult, including

- Distinguishing *understanding* of contributing factors from *excusing* the participating partner for his or her decisions and involvement in the affair.
- Managing the partners' different time lines and tolerances for continued focus on the affair.
- Managing the partners' dynamics related to their awareness of, and responsiveness to, multiple contributing factors.

As much as injured partners often long for answers to their myriad questions of why the participating partner had the affair, they also often resist explanations that they or their partner might interpret as justifying, rationalizing, or excusing the participating partner's affair. The therapist must help the couple move toward viewing the participating partner from a less negative or contemptuous perspective, while also holding the participating partner responsible for engaging in the affair. Navigating this delicate balance effectively is critical to the successful pursuit of Stage 2 interventions. Hence, it is essential to emphasize from the outset that *understanding* differs from *excusing* the affair. The therapist also needs to emphasize that, although no amount of understanding may lead to the affair's "making sense," failure to recognize and address the full range of potential contributing factors will undermine efforts toward an enduring recovery in the long run.

Injured and participating partners nearly always have different preferences and subjective time lines for moving forward after the affair. Because of the traumatic impact of an affair, injured partners tend to seek a complete understanding of all potential risk factors as a way of eliminating continued uncertainty and potential threat. In contrast, participating partners typically feel an urgency to move on and put the affair behind them. Partners need help in understanding this fundamental difference in perspectives as a means for tolerating it and reducing their respective reactivity to it.

Separate from their respective time lines, additional considerations in partners' dynamics and their relationship may challenge Stage 2 interventions. A critical factor that needs to be addressed early involves either partner's difficulties in regulating his or her own emotions and ability to disrupt intense escalations of negative exchanges. In addition, other features of either partner may interfere with exploring contextual factors, such as lack of introspective skills necessary for recognizing and discussing internal experiences or lack of empathy essential for understanding events from another person's perspective. Partners may also vary in the extent to which they internalize or externalize responsibility for the affair. Dealing with partners' differences in emotional awareness and responsiveness is not unlike therapeutic challenges that accompany couples seeking treatment for difficulties other than infidelity; however, these dynamics are often more pronounced and difficult to contain when driven by the intense feelings and threats to the relationship that follow disclosure of an affair.

CONCLUDING COMMENTS

In the chapters that follow, we address specific strategies and issues essential to helping couples develop a shared formulation for why the affair occurred. Chapter 7 focuses on strategies for articulating a rationale for Stage 2 interventions, helping partners assess their readiness to embark on this next phase of recovery and intervening when partners differ either in their willingness or ability to pursue this work. The ensuing three chapters focus on specific domains of potential contributing factors. Chapter 8 addresses factors from within the couple's relationship, including high levels of conflict, low levels of emotional or physical intimacy, and unmet relationship expectations. Chapter 9 examines factors from outside the couple's relationship, including high demands from work, extensive family responsibilities, and too much time spent with individuals who are unsupportive of the couple's relationship and too little time with supportive individuals. Chapter 10 examines contributing factors from both the participating and injured partner, including developmental experiences potentially compromising relationship functioning as well as more recent dynamics operating within or outside the marriage. In Chapter 11, we examine factors that can render recovery from infidelity particularly complex, including affairs with persons in trusted or influential positions and those complicated by emotional or behavioral problems of one or both partners. Finally, in Chapter 12, we offer specific strategies aimed at helping the couple to integrate their earlier work in articulating a comprehensive shared formulation for why the affair occurred.

CHAPTER 7

Preparing the Couple to Examine Contributing Factors

BRAD: I'm ready to move on, but we seem stuck, going over and over the same old questions. It's not helping us. We need to move forward.

THERAPIST: Moving forward is clearly a valuable goal; explain to me what you mean about feeling stuck.

GAIL: He means he wants me to simply forget about the affair and pretend it never happened.

THERAPIST: Well, you're not likely to do that, but I think that may not be what Brad is asking.

BRAD: I don't expect you to forget about it, Gail. I just want you to stop beating me up about it every day.

GAIL: I'm not trying to beat you up . . .

BRAD: Well, that's what it feels like.

GAIL: I'm just trying to understand.

THERAPIST: Brad, tell me more about what you mean by wanting to move forward.

BRAD: I want us to be able to get back to where we were before. We're not arguing as often or as badly as we were in the beginning, but we're not doing much together either. When I try to reach out to Gail, she pulls back. If I ask her why, she just gets quiet or tells me she's having trouble moving on. And if I ask her why she can't move on, she tells me she still doesn't understand how I could have had an affair with Jill.

GAIL: Well, I *don't* understand, because you just don't want to talk about it and you keep stonewalling me.

BRAD: What do you mean by "stonewalling?" I've answered every one of your questions a hundred times.

THERAPIST: So, Brad, "moving forward" would mean no longer cycling through the same questions?

BRAD: That's right.

THERAPIST: What would it be like to consider different questions instead, questions that might help to move you forward?

BRAD: I don't think there are any different questions left.

GAIL: There are *thousands* of questions left, Brad. You don't know how many questions go through my mind every day, and how many I just keep to myself in order not to upset you.

THERAPIST: But that's not working for you . . .

GAIL: No, it isn't.

THERAPIST: I don't know whether Brad is willing to answer a thousand questions, and it sounds like he's frustrated with answering the same ones multiple times. But, Gail, it also sounds like moving forward without a better sense of how this affair happened isn't going to work for you.

GAIL: That's right. I just can't do that. He wants us to be the way we were. How can we? I used to feel safe. I don't now. I used to trust him, and now I don't. I want to move on too, but I can't just make it happen.

THERAPIST: Well, I agree with both of you that what's going on now isn't working, but I can also reassure you that it's not unusual for couples to get to this point. You've done a really good job of interacting more constructively at home: arguing less, collaborating more, restoring some of your daily routines. But rebuilding trust and restoring intimacy are much more difficult. Let's talk some about why this is so important, and what a more constructive process might look like to help you get unstuck and move forward . . .

We have previously emphasized why exploring and understanding the context for an affair are essential for promoting security. However, couples often become stuck when they enter this stage of recovery. After gaining some initial control over the emotional turmoil that follows an affair, they frequently struggle with where to go next. How do they escape endlessly recycling through the same old questions? How do they move beyond stability and eventually regain intimacy? Developing a shared formulation of why the affair occurred offers the potential to restore a secure and intimate relationship and also provides partners with critical information about how to move forward, either together or separately. Preparing couples to examine contributing factors to the affair involves four steps:

- Establishing a rationale for exploring contributing factors to the affair in a more intensive and comprehensive manner.
- Presenting a conceptual, organizational model.
- Assessing partners' readiness for Stage 2 work and providing them with feedback.
- Preparing partners for anticipated difficulties.

Establishing a Rationale for Exploring Contributing Factors

More often than not, as couples reduce the initial crisis after discovery of an affair, participating partners are ready to move on and place the affair behind them, whereas injured partners may still feel wounded and vulnerable to a possible recurrence of an affair. Injured partners typically need to understand how the affair occurred at a depth and level of detail that are far beyond what participating partners see as reasonable or helpful. Therefore, establishing a rationale for exploring contributing factors often requires interventions aimed primarily toward the participating partner. This rationale involves helping the couple understand how exploring the affair can enable them to accomplish some or all of the following:

- Restore the injured partner's emotional safety as a prerequisite for rebuilding trust and either regaining or preserving emotional and physical intimacy.
- Acquire a more balanced view of the participating partner that promotes understanding of how he or she could undertake such a hurtful action.
- Develop and implement individual or relationship changes to reduce factors that previously undermined the couple's relationship, if applicable.

Furthermore, even if the couple does not ultimately stay together, this process can help the partners gain greater insight into their own and each other's behaviors and potentially help them avoid making similar missteps in future relationships. In addition, the emotional shifts that occur with this deepened understanding can often help injured partners regain emotional peace or experience release from domination by negative feelings.

In the following exchange, Brad and Gail's therapist tried to help Brad understand how examining the factors that contributed to Brad's affair could be helpful to both partners.

THERAPIST: It sounds like this is a difficult time for you, Brad, because, on the one hand, things seem better but, on the other hand, the two of you seem stuck.

BRAD: Right, and I don't know what more to do . . .

THERAPIST: My hunch is that it's probably difficult for Gail too, because she's not sure how to move on either.

GAIL: That's right.

THERAPIST: Brad, I'm convinced that Gail wants to move on as much as you do, but she can't because she still feels shaken by your affair and doesn't feel very secure emotionally. We've talked previously about how an affair is traumatic because it turns upside down everything you ever believed about your marriage, your partner, and even yourself. Nothing seems certain any more.

GAIL: That's pretty much it . . .

THERAPIST: So, until Gail feels like she's looked at this from every angle, she can't feel certain of what else might be lurking somewhere that could threaten your marriage or even lead to another affair.

BRAD: But I've already told her that will never happen, and I'm doing everything I know how to reassure her, even answering the same questions over and over.

THERAPIST: Yes, I know you've been working really hard. But I think part of the problem is that the work you've both done hasn't put Gail's concerns to rest. So she continues to feel uneasy—or unsafe—and then recycles through the same questions or discovers new ones.

BRAD: So what am I supposed to do?

THERAPIST: Well, I'm going to suggest a way that we can explore the various factors that might have made you more vulnerable to an affair. I'll help you focus on what questions and issues might be helpful to you, and we'll approach it in a more systematic, step-by-step way. We'll look first at what was going on in your marriage, then what was going on outside your marriage, and finally what each of you brought into your marriage that potentially placed it at higher risk for an affair.

BRAD: I don't blame Gail for the affair.

THERAPIST: Good for you; I hope none of us blames her. But I also think Gail would feel safer if she could identify ways in which she could contribute to making the marriage feel closer and more satisfying for you both. Just as importantly, Brad, I think this process will help Gail to understand how someone she loves—and who loves her—could have done something that felt so very painful to her. She needs a better way of making sense of that—of putting the pieces of the puzzle together—if she's going to be able to move forward.

BRAD: I need that too—a way of making sense of it—because right now even when we're getting along, I never know when the other shoe is going to drop.

THERAPIST: That's right. But the point of doing this isn't just to figure out how the affair happened. It's also to figure out what each of you can do to make sure that it won't happen again. Brad, I think it is great that you've already pledged to Gail that it will never happen again. But that probably isn't going to be enough unless she's convinced that you both understand how this happened and have eliminated whatever risk factors are under your control.

BRAD: If that's what it takes, I guess I'm willing to try . . .

Participating partners may be reluctant to explore contributing factors to the affair for a variety of reasons. Many want to move beyond the injured partner's current distress and anticipate that such exploration may maintain or intensify their partner's turmoil. Others have difficulty tolerating their own guilt or shame, which may be heightened by such discussions. Some fear driving their partner further away by exploring difficulties in the relationship or highlighting aspects of the injured partner that were unsatisfying before the affair. Still other participating partners may struggle against disclosing their resentments toward the injured partner for past hurts or betrayals. Before pursuing Stage 2 work, it is essential to explore these potential sources of reluctance to examining contributing factors and discuss ways of reducing feared outcomes of such an exploration.

Sometimes, although less often, the injured partner may also need to be convinced of the need to systematically explore contributing factors to the affair. The injured partner may be experiencing a fragile sense of stability in the relationship and fear that discussing the affair will threaten that stability. Or an injured partner may have already settled on a set of explanations for the affair and prefer to avoid the disruption that could result from further exploration of contributing factors. The dialogue below demonstrates a therapist's efforts to engage a wife in the Stage 2 process after her husband's affair.

THERAPIST: Sue, as I was explaining why I believe this next phase of our work is important, I sensed from your appearance that you're unconvinced or confused or something. What are you thinking and feeling?

SUE: I just don't see the point of it. We know why Philip's affair occurred. Our marriage was fine, he's said so himself. It was a stupid mistake—selfish—caving in to temptation that presented itself at work. That's it. I don't like it, but there's nothing really I can do about it.

THERAPIST: Right, you can't undo it, but it still seems to gnaw on you.

PHILIP: She's as angry as she was 3 months ago when she found out.

THERAPIST: Sue, you've told me that you want your marriage to continue, and I believe you. But I'm concerned about how you're going to make sense of this in a way that lets you move on.

SUE: I just have to put it behind me.

THERAPIST: I agree you need to work at putting it behind you, but I can see that you're finding that difficult to do. I think one major reason it is still so upsetting is that it's hard for you to make sense of how Philip did this. Recognizing it as a stupid or selfish doesn't really explain how Philip came to make such a mistake.

SUE: There isn't any explanation . . .

THERAPIST: Well, there's probably no explanation that would allow Philip's affair to make sense. And even if there were, no explanation would ever serve as justification. But right now, there's so much about his affair that remains unknown that it sits between the two of you like a big boulder.

SUE: That's right . . .

THERAPIST: And it's pretty hard to get close to someone when there's a boulder between you.

SUE: Yes, well, a boulder might keep us at a distance, but it also might keep me safe. Having a boulder between us makes it pretty hard to get hurt too.

THERAPIST: Yes, and eventually you may decide that safe distance is more important to you than vulnerable closeness. But I think there are more choices available to you between those two extremes. I'd like to help you understand Philip's affair better. And as you're gaining a better understanding of what happened and why, you can always decide to back off if that's what you decide is important to you. But at least you'll have a choice of staying distant or possibly taking some risks of moving closer. Would you be willing to do that?

SUE: I guess I could give it a try . . .

Presenting a Model for Organizing Risk Factors

We have noted previously that couples need a road map for recovery from infidelity. Exploration of factors contributing to an affair needs to be based on an understanding of what to examine, in roughly what order, and how to synthesize the information that has been gathered into an overall picture that makes sense. In Chapter 1, we presented an organizational model for working with affair couples that integrates factors from four domains that potentially contribute to an affair—from within the marriage, outside the marriage, and from both of the partners. We noted that the work should proceed within a temporal framework, and that it is essential to distinguish among predisposing or precipitating factors and factors that serve either to maintain the affair or to make recovery more difficult. At this point in therapy, we recommend that you present this organizational model to the couple. In doing so, it is important that you

- Identify the four domains to be considered and the order in which they will be examined.
- Encourage a systematic step-by-step approach to maximize understanding.
- Discourage premature foreclosure on an incomplete formulation.
- Clarify what topics will likely be unproductive to discuss and will, therefore, be avoided.

An effective way of introducing the four domains is to provide the couple with the summary table of potential contributing factors, previously described in the Introduction to Stage 2. It can be useful to read through these four domains during the session, not as a way of eliciting new information about any one area but as a way of providing an overview and possibly noting some factors that have already been identified either in the initial assessment or during Stage 1 work. In the initial description of these domains, it is also useful to begin distinguishing among different temporal aspects of contributing factors: those that exerted an influence primarily before the affair (either as predisposing or precipitating factors) and those that exerted an influence primarily during the affair (maintaining the outside relationship or preventing discovery or disclosure) or following the affair (making recovery easier or more difficult). It is helpful to emphasize to the couple the importance of examining the entire spectrum of potential factors step by step before drawing any final conclusions. This approach helps to ensure that factors that are less obvious or more difficult to discuss are not neglected, and it helps prevent either partner from settling on incomplete explanations.

Just as critical as outlining important domains to be considered is identifying topics of discussion that are not likely to be constructive. Specifically, as discussed in Chapter 4, you should discourage the couple from discussing the "gory, explicit details" of what sexual behaviors did or did not take place. Rarely do such discussions contribute to increased understanding of why the affair occurred or to a lessening of the traumatic impact. Instead, they serve only to enhance or intensify vivid images that can haunt the injured partner and make recovery more difficult.

Moreover, you should discourage focusing on qualities of the outside-affair person that the injured partner does not have or that the couple's relationship currently lacks. Comparisons of a marriage or committed partner with an affair partner are unfair because affair relationships differ so dramatically from a marriage or committed relationship. Two people involved in an affair devote their limited time and full attention to pleasing each other with relatively few outside distractions and burdens. We share with our couples research findings indicating that the majority of marriages that begin as affair relationships eventually end in divorce. Moreover, holding an injured partner solely responsible for whatever was lacking in a marriage or committed relationship is usually unrealistic because it ignores contributions from the participating partner. Finally, it is not constructive for partners to criticize one another for characteristics or situations that are beyond that person's control, such as aging, health problems, or the demands of rearing children. Instead, for example, if inadequate self-care or failure to set limits on intrusions from children interfered with quality time between partners, it is important to identify what both partners can do to address these matters.

Assessing Both Partners' Readiness for Stage 2

To undertake Stage 2 work successfully, both persons first need to be able to express their thoughts and feelings about the affair as well as to listen to the same from the other partner. Moreover, they need to be able to manage their feelings when their discussions become overheated and are no longer constructive. It is neither essential nor realistic to anticipate that couples will be able to follow these guidelines perfectly. However, expecting couples to undertake this difficult work on their own outside of the sessions likely sets up the couple for failure if they have not yet been able to express negative feelings with some control or show the ability to listen to the other's perspective. As a general rule, the more difficulty that either partner has in articulating his or her thoughts and feelings, hearing the other's perspective, or managing intense feelings, the more important it is to preserve much of this work for within the sessions when you, as therapist, can guide and safeguard the process.

It is not unusual for one partner to be less eager than the other to explore the context for the affair. When we perceive that one or both partners are reluctant to pursue this next stage of recovery, we encourage them to talk about their feelings of reluctance within the session. If they fear getting into difficult issues without feeling prepared to weather the emotional pain that might ensue, we reassure them that we will not go faster than we believe they can handle, and we will do the most difficult work within the sessions. If they fear that the process of exploration will go on forever, we remind them that we are also committed to moving forward steadily. We encourage the partner who is more ready to undertake Stage 2 work to discuss his or her concerns about what might happen if the couple did *not* examine how the affair came about, for example, failure to restore a sense of intimacy or inability to resolve problems in the relationship that potentially contributed to unhappiness for either partner.

As therapist, you need to discuss the potential advantages of Stage 2 work for both partners. Table 7.1 summarizes potential benefits to both partners from developing a shared understanding of how the affair came about. Most importantly, express your confidence in the couple's ability to undertake these efforts, noting what progress they demonstrated previously in reducing their emotional distress, reestablishing daily routines, or establishing more effective boundaries with individuals outside their marriage. Negotiate an initial, small step that both partners find agreeable, for example, having each person list important strengths that were in their marriage previously but that began to

TABLE 7.1. Understanding the Context of the Affair

The goal of this next phase of treatment is to help partners develop a shared understanding of the context in which the affair occurred. Potential contributing factors to consider include
- What was happening in the relationship.
- Outside factors in the environment, such as stress from work, children, or extended family.
- The participating partner's own behaviors, history, and personality.
- The injured partner's own behaviors, history, and personality.

The process of examining the full range of potential contributing factors, and developing a shared understanding of how the affair came about, has several benefits. For example, this process can
- Help both partners expand or modify some of their initial explanations of why the affair occurred.
- Help the injured partner understand more fully the participating partner's motivations in having the affair. For example, the participating partner may not have intended to hurt the injured partner, despite making bad decisions that brought about considerable pain.
- Help the injured partner understand various factors that contributed to the affair and how these factors can be addressed so that affairs are less likely to occur in the future.
- Promote greater compassion for each partner as an individual by increasing understanding of each person's flaws and vulnerabilities and of how they evolved.
- Help both partners recognize areas of vulnerability in their relationship that might be strengthened, reducing the likelihood that this type of event will recur.
- Help partners identify hurtful behaviors that make recovery more difficult now.
- Help partners to reach good, informed decisions about moving forward—either together or separately—based on a deeper understanding of factors that placed their relationship at risk for an affair and current efforts to reduce or eliminate those risks.

diminish either before or after the affair. Have them bring those lists to the next session to discuss as a first step toward strengthening their relationship and reducing its future vulnerability.

Preparing the Partners for the Challenges of Stage 2 Work

Couples are more likely to benefit from Stage 2 interventions when they understand what is going to be involved and can anticipate some of the issues that can make this work particularly challenging. Presenting the organizational model for examining potential contributing factors, as well as articulating a clear rationale for doing so, helps move couples toward the initial decision to begin examining the context of the affair. However, even when both partners commit to this next phase of treatment, their efforts can be derailed if they are not prepared for some of the unique challenges of Stage 2 work.

Differences in Subjective Time Lines for Recovery

Compared with injured partners, participating partners typically believe that the couple can move faster toward recovering from an affair. We find it useful to acknowledge partners' different expectations for recovery in an empathic way that highlights implications for how both partners deal with this dilemma. Specifically, we emphasize with participating partners that injured partners nearly always need more recovery time because of the traumatic nature of the relationship injury. We suggest that a time frame of 6 to 12 months is typical for many couples to recover, with considerable variability extending outside this window. However, with injured partners, we also emphasize that recovery requires moving forward, and we identify some possible discrete markers of progress to work toward, such as reduced frequency, intensity, and duration of flashbacks; decreased preoccupation with the affair; and suspension or diminished repetition of questions once they have been answered.

Differences in Emotional and Cognitive Style

Partners' differences in emotional and cognitive style can become intensified and antagonistic after an affair. When one partner seeks to reduce conflict or promote closeness by talking about relationship issues, and the other tries to protect the relationship by avoiding difficult discussions, each partner's efforts can evoke behaviors in the opposite direction by the other. A well-established "demand → withdraw" pattern is often seen in distressed couples, in which one partner's pursuit of relationship discussions triggers retreat by the other and vice versa. This pattern frequently becomes intensified among couples struggling to recover from an affair. We help partners to anticipate that such differences may continue or increase during difficult discussions in Stage 2 work. We attempt to avoid this dynamic by encouraging each partner to contribute to more constructive exchanges by moving a bit toward the center. Doing so often means that injured partners need to control the intensity of their emotional expression, step back from discussions that are not constructive, and engage in self-soothing strategies so that the partners can subsequently reengage more constructively. Similarly, participating partners need to work on increasing their tolerance for uncomfortable discussions, distinguishing discussions that are unpleasant from those that are unproductive, and making judicious use of time-outs to keep discussions at a constructive level of emotional intensity. When appropriate, we review techniques for damage control, previously described in Chapter 4.

Distinguishing Understanding from Excusing

Injured partners may experience resistance to Stage 2 interventions if they, or the participating partner, confuse understanding the context for the affair with excusing the participating partner from his or her responsibility for participating in the affair. It is important to reiterate throughout Stage 2, particularly when examining contributing factors that involve the injured partner, that no one *causes* his or her partner to have an affair. Regardless of what stressors the participating partner was experiencing or how the injured partner was behaving, the participating partner did not have to respond by having an affair.

Continued Flashbacks or Emotional Disequilibrium

Despite their efforts to draw upon the strategies emphasized during Stage 1, partners may continue to be vulnerable to flashbacks or periodic episodes of anger, despair, or intensely negative exchanges between the two of them. It is important to protect the couple from feeling hopeless at such times, noting that such lapses are an inevitable part of recovery. Injured partners should be reminded of strategies for managing flashbacks, as described in Chapter 5: recognizing and acknowledging flashbacks when they occur and clearly expressing to the partner whether, at that moment, the injured partner needs reassurance and closeness or separate time alone. Both partners should be reminded of strategies described in Chapter 4 for recognizing when their feelings may be getting out of control, using constructive time-outs to interrupt intense negative exchanges, and then using specific techniques for bringing their feelings to a more moderate level.

Difficulties in Developing Empathy

In examining the context for the affair from a broad perspective, a primary goal is helping the injured partner to develop a more balanced view of the participating partner and what happened, a goal that Jacobson and Christensen (Jacobson & Christensen, 1996a) refer to as "empathic joining" around a common concern. A balanced view requires developing an explanatory framework that extends beyond extreme, negative attributions about the participating partner's underlying character or motives, such as being selfish, unloving, or intentionally hurtful, to consider how the decision to have an affair could have arisen from a broad host of contributing factors, perhaps including many outside the participating partner. To the degree appropriate, helping the injured partner view the participating partner as a flawed human being who has vulnerabilities and shortcomings along with a number of strengths and positive qualities can help move the process along. Again, noting either partner's vulnerabilities and exploring how these qualities developed throughout life in no way excuses responsibility from the decisions that person made.

Specific questions the therapist can pose to promote empathic perspective taking in both partners include the following:

- "Have you ever known a good, loving person who made a bad decision that hurt someone? If so, how did you make sense of it?"
- "Have you ever struggled with doing the "right thing" yourself in the past? Have you ever failed? If not, what might have happened if your personal history had been more difficult or less supportive; might you have been less successful in always making the 'right choices?'"
- "Have you ever been disappointed by someone in the past? What was required from you to be able to reach an understanding of how that person came to disappoint you? How did you feel once you reached that understanding?"
- "Have you ever disappointed someone in the past? What was required from the other person to be able to reach an understanding of how you came to disappoint him or her? How did you feel once the other person reached that understanding?"
- "As best you can, imagine right now that you are your partner. Try to experience inside yourself what your partner is thinking and feeling right now. What is it like for you as you do this exercise?"

Both Pam and Tom, a couple we have followed in earlier chapters, experienced concerns about pursuing Stage 2 interventions. Pam worried about opening herself up to renewed interrogations from Tom about her involvement with her coworker Mark. Tom worried that Pam would exploit the process and look at factors outside of herself as a way to minimize her own responsibility. The following exchange reveals how Pam and Tom's therapist worked to help Tom be more receptive to examining contributing factors to Pam's affair as a means for promoting empathic understanding.

THERAPIST: Tom, earlier Pam was describing her concerns about beginning this next phase of our work together, but my sense is that you have some reservations as well.

TOM: I guess so.

THERAPIST: Help me understand those.

TOM: It's just that sometimes she still doesn't seem to acknowledge what she's done . . .

PAM: (interrupting) I know what I did . . .

TOM: . . . and take responsibility for it. So I guess I'm reluctant to give her more reasons for placing responsibility elsewhere.

THERAPIST: Could we agree that, no matter what broad set of factors we identify that could have contributed to Pam's involvement with Mark, ultimately she takes responsibility for her affair? No matter what was going on, nothing or no one forced Pam to have an affair; that was her decision.

TOM: Sure.

THERAPIST: And, Pam, do you agree to that too?

PAM: Of course.

THERAPIST: Good. Tom, I can understand that starting these discussions is hard for you. On the one hand, it's really important to you that Pam not minimize her own responsibility for her affair, is that right?

TOM: Yes.

THERAPIST: But, on the other hand, somehow you have to figure out how to make sense of how someone you love, and you believe loves you, could have done such a thing, and that's really hard.

TOM: It is hard and at times seems impossible.

THERAPIST: What would happen if you don't figure out how to do that?

TOM: Well, I guess eventually if I can't get past this, we'll never be close again.

THERAPIST: You'd like that—to be close again . . .

TOM: Of course.

THERAPIST: And for that to happen, you're going to have to figure out how a good person—someone you love and depend on to love you—could have done such a hurtful thing.

TOM: I guess that's right. I know it won't help if I just keep replaying in my mind what she did and how unfair and hurtful it was.

THERAPIST: Well, it was unfair and it was extremely hurtful, but ultimately it won't help you get close to Pam again if you can only focus on her personal shortcomings or thoughts of her not caring for you, and not be able to even consider other things going on with her and in your life together that may have contributed to her decision to have an affair.

TOM: I guess so. There has to be some kind of explanation. It just doesn't make sense.

THERAPIST: No, it probably will never make complete sense, but particularly not if you're unable to consider what else may have been going on. Could we talk about that for a few minutes: what it might take to consider how a good person could make a really bad decision?

TOM: Okay, sure.

THERAPIST: I'm wondering if you've ever struggled that way—not like having an affair—but really struggled with doing the right thing and maybe ever fell short . . .

TOM: Well, sure, I think probably everyone has fallen short at some point . . .

THERAPIST: Yes, I think you're probably right. If you would, tell me about a time when you struggled with that sort of thing, a time when you perhaps fell short, and how you eventually came to make peace with yourself . . .

In the short discussion that followed, Tom described a time as an adolescent when he had stayed out late with his friends, been persuaded to try marijuana, and then had an accident with his parents' car. His parents had been furious and grounded him for most of the summer. But eventually they forgave him, and Tom recognized that he had not been confident enough of himself to resist his friends' taunts and do what he had known was right. Although he continued to have mixed feelings about going through the Stage 2 process, the discussion was useful in increasing Tom's willingness to consider a broader range of influences potentially contributing to Pam's affair.

Summary

Before exploring the factors that contributed to the context for the affair in a more intensive and comprehensive manner, couples need a clear rationale describing why this work is essential to restoring security as well as reaching an informed decision about how to move forward. They also need to know what factors they will discuss and how the discussions will proceed. Such understanding can provide couples with the structure and motivation needed to engage in this very demanding and difficult process. Going back to discuss and reexperience the feelings involved in any trauma is extremely upsetting for most people. You, the therapist, can greatly facilitate the process by letting the couple know that you understand their reluctance and at the same time expressing your confidence in them as a couple and yourself as a knowledgeable guide to help them through the process.

Resources from *Getting Past the Affair*

In our companion self-help book for couples, *Chapter 6*, "Why Stir Everything Up?," addresses reasons for exploring the broader context of the affair and introduces partners to specific domains to examine. The chapter also describes information that is *not* likely to be useful for understanding the affair. A separate section (pp. 150–153) helps partners examine their own readiness for this next phase of work and learn how to encourage the other to participate. The chapter concludes with exercises designed to help partners identify what they hope to gain from the process and to devise coping strategies for challenges they may encounter along the way.

CHAPTER 8

Examining Relationship Factors

THERAPIST: In our last session, I suggested that we begin to consider factors that potentially put your marriage at risk for an affair, and we agreed to begin by talking about what was going on in your marriage. Tell me about the discussions you've had along those lines this past week.

VICKI: It's been hard for us to talk about it. I know that we were going through a tough time before Bill's affair. The business has really been stressful the past couple of years. And then after my Dad died—and the awful way it happened—I think I just went into my shell and wasn't very available to Bill.

THERAPIST: In what ways were your discussions this past week difficult?

VICKI: I just don't like thinking about it. I still feel angry at Bill for cheating on me when I needed him the most and angry at myself for driving him further away when we were already struggling.

BILL: It wasn't your fault, Vicki. I keep trying to tell you that . . .

VICKI: Yeah, you tell me that. But whenever I ask how you could have betrayed me, it comes back to the same thing: We were in a bad place; you felt rejected by me; then I didn't respond to your efforts to be supportive, so you sought the advice of another woman, and then it led to something more . . .

BILL: What do you want me to say?

VICKI: I just don't know any more.

THERAPIST: You want to understand how this happened . . .

VICKI: I *need* to understand . . .

THERAPIST: But it's hard, because some of the contributing factors may include what was happening in your marriage and in some ways that also involves what was going on with you. And then you don't know whether to feel angry or guilty.

VICKI: Sometimes I feel both . . .

THERAPIST: And there are probably other feelings as well, like feeling anxious or uncertain about whether it could happen again.

VICKI: I always worry about that . . .

BILL: That's not going to happen—ever.

THERAPIST: Your commitment to that is important, Bill. But it's also important that you understand that Vicki continues to feel vulnerable because the affair still seems so confusing. For her to feel secure again, you're going to have to reach a fuller understanding of how the affair happened in a way that makes better sense to both of you. And part of that will require examining what was going on in your marriage.

BILL: I don't want Vicki to feel like the affair was her fault, or for her to think I feel that way.

THERAPIST: Yes, you know that, regardless of what was going on in the marriage, the decision to have an affair was still yours alone.

BILL: Right. Believe me, I know that. But I'd also like for Vicki to understand what was going on from my perspective, not to excuse what I did, but maybe so that she wouldn't see me as a complete jerk who totally stopped caring about her or about us. And if we're going to make this work, we've got to deal with our marriage and make it stronger than it was. Vicki, I'm not blaming you in any way for my affair. I promise I'll never do that. It's about wanting us to be able to make our marriage work again. I'm desperate for that, but I can't do it alone and I need your help. Please . . .

A bad relationship doesn't cause an affair, any more than a good relationship prevents one. About half of men and one third of women who have had an affair report having been happily married at the time (Glass & Wright, 1985). And many relationships go through difficult times or suffer from chronic challenges that do not result in an affair. Still, many times an affair occurs in a relationship that has become vulnerable because of either high levels of relationship stress or conflict or low levels of emotional or physical closeness. It is important that couples struggling from infidelity examine their relationship both before and after the affair, – not only to better understand how the affair came about but also to plan more effectively for how to move forward.

Managing the Therapeutic Context and Process

Helping a couple to examine potential contributing factors to the affair from their relationship requires two sets of therapeutic skills. The first set involves general skills for maintaining a collaborative alliance and protecting the process from hazards described in Chapter 7 (e.g., dealing with partners' differences in subjective time lines and their tendency to confuse the notion of *understanding* with *excusing*). The second set of therapeutic skills required in Stage 2 work is helping partners to explore known risk factors identified from previous clinical and research studies.

This chapter focuses on specific factors within couples' relationships that, from a normative perspective, are known to increase a relationship's vulnerability to an extramarital affair. It is unlikely that all these factors are contributing sources of an affair for any given couple or that any single factor bears exclusive responsibility. However, as the therapist, you can guide both partners in exploring each of these factors for their potential role in placing the couple's relationship at increased risk. Common contributing factors to an affair from the couple's relationship are summarized in Table 8.1 and frequently involve one or more of the following:

- Difficulties in resolving differences or managing conflict.
- Deficits in emotional intimacy.
- Deficits in physical intimacy.

Examining relationship factors can be a useful first step toward exploring the broader context for the affair because it does not single out either individual but rather has a joint couple focus. It is especially important to promote a constructive tone early in the process as a way of encouraging participation by both partners and preparing them for the subsequent, more difficult Stage 2 work. Techniques for promoting a constructive tone include inquiring about positive relationship qualities as well as negative ones and reframing negative qualities from a more positive perspective when possible. For example, partners' previous reluctance to discuss relationship problems might be framed as reflecting well-intentioned but misguided efforts to protect their relationship

TABLE 8.1. Potential Contributing Factors from the Couple's Relationship

Frequent or intense conflict

- Frequent conflicts, nit-picking, or unresolved tensions.
- Escalation of minor differences into major arguments.
- Disagreements or tensions lasting for long periods of time without resolution.

Common sources of relationship conflict

- Specific areas of interaction (e.g., finances, children, the sexual relationship, use of leisure time, household tasks).
- Relationship and family boundaries (e.g., how much time to spend alone, with each other, or with children, extended family, friends).
- Shared resources (e.g., how to share material possessions or space).
- Opportunities and responsibilities (e.g., work in and outside the home).
- Differences in preferences or values (e.g., preferences for planning vs. spontaneity, differences in spiritual beliefs).
- Differences in personal style (e.g., level of emotional expressiveness, comfort with taking charge).

Ineffective strategies for managing conflict

- Under- or overcontrol of feelings (e.g., excessive anger or emotional detachment).
- "Demand → withdraw" patterns in which one partner repeatedly pursues and the other persistently avoids discussion of important relationship issues.
- Differences in emotional and cognitive style (e.g., inability to balance "talking about feelings" with "finding solutions").
- Differences in timing (e.g., rushing in too soon or waiting too long after an argument to pursue resolution).
- Efforts to win; insisting on being "right" or "winning" an argument.

Feeling emotionally disconnected

- Difficulty in sharing emotional experiences or feeling understood.
- Not working together as a team to accomplish common tasks.
- Not sharing visions or dreams for the future.
- Not setting aside enough time to play together.

Feeling physically disconnected

- Insufficient touches, hugs, or other nonsexual forms of physical closeness.
- Differences in levels of sexual desire.
- Low frequency of lovemaking.
- Dissatisfaction with the quality of sexual intimacy.
- Difficulties in talking about sex.
- Barriers to sexual intimacy (e.g., differences in work schedules, physical health problems, specific sexual difficulties).

(continued)

TABLE 8.1. (continued)

Dissatisfaction with respective roles

- Unhappiness with responsibilities related to work outside the home.
- Dissatisfaction with roles in the home as a partner (e.g., responsibilities involving housework, meals, yardwork).
- Unhappiness with roles as a parent (e.g., opportunities to play with the children, responsibilities for child care or discipline).

from hurtful conflict. It is sometimes helpful to restate partners' descriptions of negative qualities using softer or less pejorative language or to acknowledge legitimate differences in partners' perspectives. Relationship problems often result not from either partner's behaviors independently but rather from the interactive effects of both persons' behaviors.

An affair often impacts how partners view their relationship history. Participating partners sometimes emphasize negative aspects of the relationship as factors that led to or maintained the affair. Injured partners sometimes minimize these negative influences or emphasize more positive features earlier in the relationship that they believe should have protected the relationship from an affair. Differences in partners' emphasis on different time periods in their relationship and on strengths versus weaknesses can foster polarization in their views. As the therapist, you need to help them achieve a balanced perspective that incorporates both strengths and deficits across the broad time span of their relationship.

While exploring relationship factors that potentially increased vulnerability to an affair, there are two concurrent goals. One is to identify relationship contributions as a way of contextualizing the affair within a broad, comprehensive framework; thus, the focus is on the *past* and how the affair developed. Second, this same information serves as a potential means of reducing risk factors, strengthening the relationship, and providing the couple with new data about their ability and commitment to change in the *future*. Balancing these two goals—identifying contributing factors versus attempting to change them—assumes special importance when examining factors from the couple's relationship. On the one hand, it is important to avoid disrupting the exploration process by focusing on change efforts prematurely; in some instances, one or both partners may not yet be ready to engage change efforts productively. However, discussing ways to strengthen the relationship can provide an important motivational basis for the more difficult challenges of examining individual factors later in Stage 2. Information regarding the motivation of both partners to make important relationship changes, either independently or collaboratively, also will be critical in Stage 3 as partners reach an informed decision about how to move forward, either together or separately.

Difficulties in Resolving Differences

Relationships become at risk for a broad range of adverse outcomes, including an affair, when they are characterized by an excess of negatives and a scarcity of positives. A stable but emotionally disengaged relationship can be just as vulnerable to an affair as an emotionally intense but chaotic one. Some research suggests that happily married couples engage in at least five positive communication exchanges for every negative one (Gottman, 1994). Other research indicates that, once couples reach a level of significant or chronic distress, they become highly sensitized to negative exchanges—responding with disproportionate anger or frustration to even mildly negative relationship events—and fail to recognize or underrespond to positive events (cf. Epstein & Baucom, 2002).

In considering relationship factors potentially contributing to the affair, couples should consider the frequency and levels of conflict, their strategies for managing conflict, and the multiple sources of the differences between them. While discussing these issues and how they might have provided the context for the affair, couples also might become invested in changing these patterns as they are highlighted. Working with them to make changes can be appropriate, but at this point the major emphasis is on clarifying the relationship factors that contributed to the context for the affair.

Levels of Conflict and Strategies for Managing Differences

There is considerable variation in the frequency of couples' arguments, the length and intensity of their conflicts, and the subjective impact of these disagreements. For example, Mayra and Antonio both acknowledged having "fiery" temperaments: Each reacted quickly and strongly when they disliked something the other had said. But they also cooled down quickly, sometimes laughing or even giving the other a playful hug, and neither of them took these exchanges seriously. In contrast, Gayle and Michael rarely argued, but each knew when the other was upset because the partner would withdraw into cold silence or one-word-response exchanges that could last an entire day. Neither one liked this pattern, but their discomfort with open conflict kept them from discussing or resolving differences. Gayle sometimes confronted Michael with hurt feelings from something he had said or done weeks earlier;

he frequently had little recollection of the event and resented Gayle's hanging onto her hurt.

Couples sometimes struggle with unresolved differences because of basic deficits in expressing or responding to difficult feelings or in examining differences constructively and reaching decisions together. For these couples, it will be beneficial to help them communicate more effectively, for example, by promoting basic communication skills based on the guidelines presented in Chapters 5 and 6. At other times, couples may struggle with unresolved conflict because of individual or relationship dynamics that interfere with implementing the communication abilities that both partners possess. For example, partners may differ in their preference for exploring feelings versus seeking action-oriented solutions; when conflicts intensify, these differences can become polarized so that neither partner feels understood or valued by the other.

Some couples struggle because the partners have different internal clocks for stepping back, gaining perspective, and reengaging in discussion. It is not uncommon for one person to persist in efforts to resolve a disagreement beyond their partner's ability to continue constructively in the moment, with the result that one partner increases his or her demands for engagement and resolution while the other withdraws further as a strategy for decreasing the negativity. Other couples struggle because both partners seem determined to "win" by asserting greater legitimacy for their own perspective and insisting on their own preferred solution. One of your roles as the therapist is to help couples distinguish between basic communication deficits versus other dynamics that interfere with implementing their communication skills. For example, you might say, "Talk with me about the times when you communicate well, and how those differ from the times you struggle more. What seems to help you communicate better, and what seems to get in the way?" As you elicit this information, encourage each partner to emphasize what he or she could do differently rather than focusing on changes desired from the other.

Sources of Conflict

Some couples argue over seemingly infinite situations without an apparent common theme, whereas others appear to struggle predominantly in one area while managing differences in other areas more effectively. For example, some couples struggle primarily around issues of finances, parenting strategies, allocation of their leisure time, or interactions with friends or extended family. Differentiating among generalized versus more focused conflicts can help couples distinguish between the need to develop basic communication and decision-making skills versus the benefit of seeking information or guidance for more specific recurring struggles in a particular area. After an affair, couples' styles of managing conflict frequently become more exaggerated. Couples characterized by frequent disagreements before the affair may exhibit even more frequent or intense arguments; those who previously avoided conflict may now retreat even further into silence or isolation to avoid further hurt. The therapist's task is to help couples examine how high levels of conflict or unresolved differences before the affair placed their relationship at risk and how difficulties in managing differences may be interfering with recovery and moving forward now.

When specific sources of recurring conflict have been identified, the therapist can help the couple by promoting alternative agreements in moving the couple past a roadblock or adopting a new perspective. For example, you might say, "It sounds like the two of you have struggled with different views about parenting for quite some time, and that these differences have created some distance between you. My hunch is that this is a complicated area that will require some time to work through. But in the past month since this affair was revealed, your teamwork as parents has ground to a halt, especially around your children's bedtime, and right now that's making things even worse. Let's see if we could come to an interim agreement as a way of making this work better for now."

As another example, Vicki and Bill came to realize that their discomfort with conflict, acquired in part from frequent and intense arguments that dominated their first marriages, prevented them from addressing minor disagreements both at work and home. These disagreements subsequently festered and left each of them more resentful. Clarifying this pattern of avoidance as one factor that contributed to their relationship deterioration was important in understanding Bill's affair. In addition, their therapist decided to promote a brief decision-making conversation around this issue to help them build confidence in their ability to move forward after Bill's affair.

VICKI: I don't like the way we deal with differences at work. You seem upset with some of the decisions I make, but instead of talking with me you just withdraw or sulk. That gets old really quick, and then I don't feel like pursuing the issue with you any further. And it makes me uneasy because that pattern got especially bad during your affair.

BILL: I know it's a problem. I'm just not sure what to do about it. It's not like we could just stop dealing with the business during the day to discuss things between us when clients were calling or coming into the office.

VICKI: Then why didn't we deal with them when we got home?

BILL: Vicki, I was exhausted by the time we got home. Besides, we agreed a long time ago to try to keep work and home life separate so that conflicts we have from either one didn't spill over into the other.

VICKI: But it didn't work then, and it certainly isn't working now!

THERAPIST: It's not unusual for couples who work together to have difficulty separating work from home life, especially when they own a business together. What I think is important to understand is that in attempting to separate work and home life, it meant in reality you ignored problems at work, and that created difficulties for your marriage, is that right?

VICKI: Exactly, it drove us apart. When things happened at work, we didn't deal with them, and then we were distant at home. We didn't separate work and home; we maintained the avoidance at both places.

THERAPIST: Bill, do you agree that this is what happened?

BILL: Yes, but it really wasn't just to avoid problems. Working together can be great, but it also is hard. I wanted our home life to be separated from the business, but I guess that really isn't possible if we're having troubles in one of those areas.

THERAPIST: That's right. The goal of reducing spillover of tension from one setting to the other is a good one, but that will probably require creating times in each setting to address issues that arise. So I think we've realized that not dealing with business problems when you work together is a major factor that got you in trouble as a couple. And that will be critical when we think about how you want to move forward in the future and what would need to change if you stay together. We don't need to resolve how to integrate home and business life right now because it probably is pretty complex, and our focus for now is trying to understand how the affair developed. But we could spend a bit of time thinking about how to handle the one aspect of it that you just mentioned: how to address work problems in a way that doesn't interfere with your marriage. Can you think of some better ways of doing that?

BILL: Well, Vicki and I usually go to lunch together, and we could use that time to raise any concerns that have come up . . .

VICKI: Or if they come up in the afternoon, maybe we could take 20 minutes or so there at the office before leaving for home.

BILL: But we're not always going to resolve them in 20 or 30 minutes, Vicki.

VICKI: I know that, Bill. But think about it. When we have problems at home that haven't been resolved, we do pretty well in avoiding those topics at work. We just wait until we get back home to deal with them. Why couldn't we do the same thing with problems from work: leave them there if we need to until we go back the next day, even if we have to go in early?

BILL: (*after a long pause*) . . . I'm just not sure it will work.

THERAPIST: Try describing your concerns to Vicki . . .

BILL: We just don't do that well, Vicki. We go home with some issue between us and the cloud hangs over us the entire night. I try to get you into a better mood, but you stay stuck. You won't laugh or play. You might watch TV with me, but there's no discussion . . . and there's certainly no closeness.

THERAPIST: You'd like to leave the uncomfortable feelings as well as the conflict at work.

BILL: That's right.

THERAPIST: Ask Vicki what makes it hard for her to do that . . .

BILL: Could you leave the bad feelings at work instead of bringing them home? I just hate when we do that.

VICKI: It *is* hard for me to do that, Bill. You're better at setting your feelings aside than I am. I used to resent that because it seemed not genuine, and I felt like you were ignoring my feelings. Plus, I never trusted that we were going to get back to the issue or resolve it, so I became discouraged and resentful.

BILL: I admit that I avoided going back to the same issue when we returned to work the next day, but that's partly because I figured it was just going to renew the cycle of bickering and withdrawal all over again.

THERAPIST: Describe what you could do differently . . .

BILL: Well, for my own part, I can commit to addressing work-related issues at the office, either by our going in half an hour early, discussing them over lunch, or even staying half an hour late.

VICKI: And I'm willing to do a better job of separating my feelings from work from our time at home. I think I can do a better job of that if I know we're both committed to setting aside time at work to deal with the issues that come up there. Just try to be patient with me and if I seem stuck in a bad mood, point it out gently and give me some time to work my way out of it, okay?

BILL: I can try . . .

In this example, the therapist first wanted to isolate the couple's pattern for integrating work and personal life that contributed to relationship difficulties. This clarification was critical for understanding the context for the affair and the changes needed in the future if the partners remain together. In many situations, this topic would continue to be the sole focus of the session: isolating possible relationship factors that help to explain one partner's decision to have an affair. In this instance, the therapist believed that the couple could address one aspect of their problem at this point without losing their focus on understanding how the affair came about. In fact, the therapist needed only to provide brief prompts or redirections, because Vicki and Bill had good communication skills and shared concerns over a common frustration.

Deficits in Emotional Intimacy

Two people often decide to marry or form a committed relationship because each feels emotionally close to the other. Each may describe the other as easy to talk to, fun to be around, caring, or compassionate. Sometimes partners describe being drawn to one another by common interests and values or by shared dreams for the future.

Couples in which partners have lost feelings of emotional closeness are particularly difficult to treat. Lack of emotional connectedness is frequently cited as a contributing factor to affairs by partners of both genders, but particularly by women. Whether or not deficits in emotional intimacy contributed to the affair, once an affair has occurred, a dramatic disruption in emotional connection between partners typically follows. Hence, when helping couples to examine risk factors and work toward recovery from an affair, it is not enough to address deficits in managing and resolving conflict. Instead, it is also vital to explore how the couple potentially failed to develop or maintain a strong emotional bond as well as how they are currently struggling with emotional intimacy.

How does emotional intimacy between partners develop? Pathways to "falling in love" vary but frequently include one or more of the following:

- Spending time together in mutually enjoyable activities.
- Working together as a team to accomplish common goals.
- Engaging in discussions in which deep or vulnerable feelings are

expressed by one person and are understood and accepted by the other.

- Sharing in activities reflecting deeply held values or beliefs.
- Creating shared visions or dreams for the future.

For some couples, a strong emotional connection is lacking from the outset. It is important that, as the therapist, you distinguish between couples who previously demonstrated strong emotional bonds and those who did not. For example, you might ask, "Were there periods in the past when you felt closer? If so, when did that feeling start to change? Can you remember what was going on at that time?" Couples who had strong emotional bonds in the past can often be helped to resurrect patterns of interaction that previously felt close but subsequently faded or were disrupted by other factors. Couples who never developed strong emotional connections may require more intensive interventions aimed at increasing positive emotional experiences and shared activities. In addition, helping couples to recognize these relationship patterns as contributing to the potential for an affair is central to the work of Stage 2.

A common problem for couples after an affair is that interactions that used to feel satisfying and natural now feel uncomfortable or forced. Mealtimes may be spent in silence rather than sharing the day's experiences. Being together with friends or family might feel awkward. Talking about the future may seem artificial because the future seems so uncertain. Participating partners sometimes sit back and fail to initiate emotional exchanges because they do not know what the injured partner will accept. Injured partners often fail to initiate emotional closeness because they are waiting for intimate feelings to return on their own or because they are looking for initiatives from the participating partner as evidence of commitment to the relationship.

As the therapist, you need to confront the contributing sources for the couple's lack of emotional connectedness, both past and present, and explore how those factors contributed to the context for the affair. We emphasize to couples that, after an affair, feelings of closeness are often the last element of relationship health to return. It is easier to change behaviors, or even to change thinking patterns, than it is to change feelings. Therefore, it is important to develop or restore patterns of behavior that increase the likelihood of feeling close at some point in the future, recognizing that these patterns may feel unnatural or awkward in the short term. In promoting these exchanges, it is also important that you recognize the limits of what each partner can tolerate, pressing at the boundaries but not pushing the couple into activities that either partner might find overwhelming or aversive.

For example, you might confront a situation of enduring distance as follows: "I understand that it's been a long time since the two of you have felt very close, and now, after this affair, it's even harder to be close when you may want or need it the most. Those feelings of closeness may not develop quickly, but it's important that we try to identify ways you can interact that at least provide some opportunity for feelings of closeness to grow. What kinds of activities have helped you to feel closer or less distant in the past?"

Deficits in Physical Intimacy

For many couples, physical and emotional intimacy are closely intertwined. For some partners, emotional closeness is an important precondition for physical closeness, whereas others describe physical connection as a vital pathway to feeling emotionally close. Although gender differences in this regard are common, with women more frequently citing emotional intimacy as a prerequisite for physical intimacy, it is important not to assume that this trend holds for any particular couple.

Physical closeness extends beyond sexual exchanges. It involves touching in caring but nonsexual ways throughout the day: reassuring hugs, holding hands, casual touches when passing in the hallway or working together in the kitchen, snuggling on the couch or in bed. In working with couples after an affair, it is important to inquire about ways in which nonsexual physical exchanges previously felt uncomfortable or lacking for either partner, along with ways in which such exchanges have been disrupted by the affair. Equally important is exploring the sources of deficits in this area. For example, deficits in physical connection before the affair may be linked to family or other socialization experiences that failed to encourage physical expressions of closeness. Or physical closeness expressed by hugs, kisses, or caresses may have been viewed exclusively as a forerunner to sexual intimacy, potentially limiting their expression. The therapist should inquire about early learning experiences: "How was physical closeness shown in your family growing up? Were your parents openly affectionate with each other? How about with you?"

After an affair, previous patterns of physical closeness may be disrupted by anxiety, hurt, or resentment. As part of a more generalized retreat and self-protection, the injured partner may withdraw from any physical exchanges that previously were linked to emotional or sexual intimacy but now feel unsafe. Or withholding of physical exchanges, even of a nonsexual nature, may be used to convey continued hurt or anger. Participating partners may be equally apprehensive about initiating physical closeness, sensing their injured partner's distress and wishing to avoid forcing an unwanted exchange that may increase the tension or discomfort between them. We sometimes ask partners, "How does it feel more difficult now to be affectionate, either in initiating hugs or kisses or responding to your partner's overtures?"

Deficits in sexual intimacy often stem from factors similar to those underlying deficiencies in nonsexual closeness, but they can result from other sources as well. Partners may describe long-standing differences in their levels of sexual desire or the extent to which sexuality is an important part of their overall identity. One or both partners may be uncomfortable with initiating or responding to sexual overtures or with pursuing greater variety in the nature of sexual exchanges. Beyond differences in levels of sexual desire, either partner may struggle with individual difficulties in becoming sexually aroused or reaching orgasm. An inability to discuss differences in sexual desires or expectations or to resolve differences in this regard can easily lead to chronic dissatisfaction or a progressive decline in sexual intimacy.

The primary goal of addressing difficulties with physical intimacy at this point in treatment is to clarify whether it was a relationship factor that increased the likelihood of the affair. If this area has been problematic, then you will want to discuss how the couple could work to improve physical closeness at this point if they wish to do so, along with noting it as a future intervention goal if they decide to stay together. Help partners discuss their visions of what a physically intimate relationship would look like, emphasizing nonsexual as well as sexual exchanges. What steps would each partner be willing to take, either currently or in the future, in working toward these visions? If the partners differ in their wants or expectations, what compromises can they work toward in moving forward toward a better physical relationship for them both?

Taking the Long-Term Perspective: Relationship Strengths and Challenges

When couples explore relationship issues that potentially increase vulnerability to an affair, two common factors may contribute to selective or distorted recall. First, partners may focus primarily on more recent times in their relationship leading up to the affair, ignoring earlier times that were potentially quite different. Frequently, they highlight more recent relationship problems and overlook earlier relationship strengths. Second, partners may focus on different aspects of the relationship: one focusing primarily on the negatives, the other on the positives. Two patterns in this regard are particularly common.

In the first, the participating partner emphasizes problems in the relationship as a major factor leading to the affair, sometimes portraying the affair as a nearly inevitable consequence of these problems. However, the injured partner defensively counters that the problems were not that significant or should have been offset by positive exchanges or commitments they shared. In the second pattern, the participating partner adopts the opposite stance, emphasizing the positive aspects of the relationship, including the participating partner's professed commitment, as reasons for the injured partner remaining in the relationship and moving on together rather than ending the relationship. In either case, these perspectives can easily become polarized; as one partner emphasizes the positive aspects of the relationship, the other one highlights the shortcomings.

Focusing on either the positive or negative elements or viewing the relationship only from more recent events rather than from a longer term perspective does not allow either partner to achieve a balanced view that is likely to result in the best informed decision about how to move forward. In exploring potential vulnerability factors from the relationship, you, as the therapist, need to actively and explicitly resist each of these tendencies by promoting a long-term view that integrates both the strengths and the challenges of the couple's relationship. This goal can be addressed by posing one or more of the questions listed in Table 8.2, for example, asking partners to discuss what initially attracted them to each other, what they regard as their best achievements as a couple, or some of the challenges they have overcome together in the past.

Brad and Gail struggled with this task. Brad viewed Gail as questioning everything about their relationship from the very beginning after his affair with his student, Jill. He feared that in doing so Gail would conclude that their relationship had been a mistake from the beginning and hence was not worth trying to salvage now. The more he tried to convince her that their relationship had been a healthy one, the more she emphasized parallels between how they had begun their relationship and Brad's affair with Jill. The following portion from one of their sessions demonstrates their therapist's efforts to promote a more balanced perspective from both partners.

BRAD: Why can't you see that we were good together, and that we could be good together again?

GAIL: I'm not saying we were never good together.

BRAD: Yes, you are. Whenever I talk about how we used to admire and encour-

TABLE 8.2. Encouraging a View of the Relationship from a Larger Perspective

What were your reasons for becoming a couple?

- What initially attracted you to each other?
- Why did you marry or make a long-term commitment to this relationship?

How have you grown individually and as a couple?

- How have you both helped each other grow as individuals?
- How have you brought out the best or the worst in each other?
- How has your relationship grown to accommodate new or difficult challenges?

What have you done well?

- What are your best achievements as a couple?
- What would you miss most if you ended your relationship?

What challenges have you overcome together?

- What have been the most difficult times you've faced together in the past?
- How did you manage to get through those times?
- In what ways did previous challenges make you stronger as a couple? In what ways did they leave you feeling hurt, disappointed, or more vulnerable?
- How have you reconnected in the past after feeling particularly hurt?

How does the current crisis fit into the big picture?

- Has your partner been truthful in the past before this affair?
- Did this affair occur at a time when your relationship was particularly vulnerable?
- Looking back at the time before the affair, was there more good in this relationship than bad?

---

age each other, you just look away as though it never happened. You used to look up to me and respect me, and I admired your enthusiasm and determination to take everything in . . .

GAIL: That's just it, Brad. You liked being on a pedestal and my being naive and easily impressed. We weren't equals. You needed to be superior.

BRAD: I didn't need to be superior. I just liked being helpful and maybe feeling appreciated sometimes.

THERAPIST: Brad, what are you feeling right now?

BRAD: I get so frustrated, like she can't see a single good thing about me or the marriage. That everything was a fake or unhealthy from the beginning.

THERAPIST: So you feel dismissed?

BRAD: No, not dismissed. It's just that I need her to see there were good things in our marriage that are worth trying to get back.

THERAPIST: So it's more like feeling anxious or worried that if she can't see that, there's not much chance of working together now?

BRAD: Yeah, I guess so, more like anxious.

THERAPIST: Anxious she could end it . . .

BRAD: Yeah.

THERAPIST: (*after a pause*) Ask Gail what she's feeling.

BRAD: Well, what *are* you feeling?

GAIL: Well, actually, *dismissed* fits it pretty well. Whenever I try to point out what wasn't working and why I'm not willing to just "get over" the affair and go back to the way things were, you ignore what I've said and keeping telling me we just have to make it work like it used to.

THERAPIST: So maybe dismissed, but what other feeling?

GAIL: Scared, actually.

THERAPIST: About what?

GAIL: Scared that we *will* go back to the way it was – with Brad being in charge and expecting me to look up to him all the time, and my feeling uncertain of myself and unwilling to challenge him or fearing that if I try to meet him head-on as an equal he'll just go out and find some other little doe-eyed coed to worship at his feet . . .

BRAD: That's not fair . . .

THERAPIST: Gail, can you say that in another way that Brad might be more able or willing to hear?

GAIL: Brad . . . okay . . . look, maybe that wasn't fair. But you just can't expect it to go back to the way it was in the beginning. I was still an undergrad, and you were finishing your PhD and were brilliant and charming . . .

BRAD: So you can still remember that . . .

GAIL: Yes, and there were lots of good things about those times, I'll admit. You were a role model for me, and you also reminded me of my brother in a way . . . protective toward me. I liked that.

BRAD: I wanted to be more than a big brother . . . still do . . .

GAIL: But that's just it. I'm not sure you were ever ready for me to become an equal partner – not professionally and not in our marriage.

BRAD: Gail, that's not fair. I don't think I ever tried to hold you back . . .

GAIL: It's not that . . . (*long silence*)

THERAPIST: Try to put your feelings into words. You're doing a good job, Gail.

Try to express your fears without invalidating the past, and see how that
works.

GAIL: Okay . . . Brad, I know that in many ways you're genuinely happy for me
when I'm successful professionally. You pressed the department hard to
give me a position. You help me prepare for my classes. I appreciate that.
But if I ever challenge you—whether it's related to work or to things at
home—you just dismiss me as though I'm that naive little 22-year-old
who still needs your protection but just doesn't know it, and I resent
that.

BRAD: I'm willing to work on that . . .

GAIL: But here's what frightens me the most, and I'm not sure you can change
this. I think you *need* someone to look up to you, to have you on some
kind of pedestal. It's not just that it feels good to you—I like it too when
someone's looking up to me—but I think you won't be happy or feel content if you don't have a wife who does that, and I just can't do it any more.
Of course I can respect you, but not in a way that puts you above me.

THERAPIST: Talk more about that . . .

GAIL: It's just not healthy for me. Brad, I can't keep you on a pedestal because
always looking up to you makes me feel like you're looking down on me. I
realize now that after the first few years and moving beyond hero worship,
I started to resent the lack of equality between us and I started pulling
away from you.

BRAD: I could feel you pulling away . . .

GAIL: So you know it wasn't all sunshine and roses between us.

BRAD: Well, not after the first few years maybe.

GAIL: That's all I need you to see—that how we started out worked well
because of where we were in our lives, but that we changed—I grew up—
and we can't try to recreate that now and expect it to work.

THERAPIST: Brad, what is Gail most needing for you to hear?

BRAD: I guess she wants me to know that we can't go back to the way it was in
the beginning, no matter how good that might have been then.

THERAPIST: Good for you. And what are you most needing for Gail to hear
from you?

BRAD: That it wasn't always bad or wasn't that we never had a good thing
going.

GAIL: I know that, Brad.

THERAPIST: What else?

BRAD: I guess I want her to know that I'm willing to try to do it differently. I know I screwed up big time, Gail. I just don't want you to give up on us. I want us to make it work.

THERAPIST: You'd like to see if you could create a new way of relating . . .

BRAD: That's right . . . So can we?

GAIL: I don't know, Brad. That's the million-dollar question. I haven't given up yet, or I wouldn't be here. But we're not who we were back then. I'm willing to try, so long as I know we're working on a new way of relating, not returning to the old one.

THERAPIST: Absolutely, that will be a major task for you to consider when you decide how to move forward in your relationship. And for now, it seems critical to realize that the relationship that developed initially with Brad in the "professor/expert" role might have worked for a while, but over time it no longer fit who you were as a couple and contributed to your drifting apart. Is that right?

Implications for Change: Next Steps in the Relationship

As the couple discusses relationship factors that put them at risk for an affair, understandably they will venture into discussions of whether their relationship can change in the near and distant future. As we noted earlier in this chapter, the primary goal at this point in treatment is to identify factors that contributed to the affair, while also promoting initial efforts to make changes in these domains. Partners should be reassured that commitments to make relationship changes in the short term do not obligate them to any particular path in the longer term. Changing on behalf of the relationship now does not commit them to remaining in the relationship. Instead, these initial change efforts provide critical information about whether they are able to implement and sustain changes in their relationship, whether these changes make a difference in the short run, and whether they are sufficient for maintaining the relationship in the long run.

Summary

To restore emotional security after an affair, couples first need to understand what factors potentially contributed to their vulnerability to unfaithful behavior. Common contributing factors from within the relationship include frequent or intense conflict, an accumulation of unresolved differences, lack of emotional closeness, and deficits in physical intimacy. Developing a balanced understanding of relationship factors requires examining both strengths and challenges, not only in the months leading up to the affair but also from a long-term perspective. Couples can become stuck when either partner settles too quickly on a formulation that incorporates only a few factors to the exclusion of others, emphasizes only deficits to the neglect of strengths, or selectively focuses on one part of the couple's history and ignores other parts. As the therapist, your role is to promote a process of guided discovery that encourages systematic appraisal of the relationship across a broad set of domains and temporal perspective. Identifying potential contributing factors should be coupled with exploring intermediate steps to reduce or eliminate these factors, as a means not only of strengthening the relationship but also of garnering important information about partners' ability to change, which is essential for reaching informed relationship decisions later in the therapy process.

Resources from *Getting Past the Affair*

In our companion self-help book for couples, *Chapter 7*, "Was My Marriage to Blame?," includes information related to the topics discussed in the current chapter. The first portion of that chapter (pp. 161–175) helps couples examine what their relationship was like before the affair, including how well they dealt with differences, their level of emotional connection, and their level of physical intimacy. The latter portion of the chapter (pp. 175–182) helps them to examine the ways in which their relationship was healthy or unhealthy from its outset and what would be required to build a strong relationship now. The chapter concludes with three exercises. Exercise 7.1 encourages partners to identify major sources of conflict in their relationship and describe what they can do, either individually or as a couple, to address these conflicts more effectively. Exercise 7.2 helps couples identify ways of promoting greater emotional and physical intimacy. Exercise 7.3 asks partners to identify what strengths they have had as a couple in the past and how they can build on those strengths to help them through this difficult time and work toward a better future.

CHAPTER 9

Examining Outside Factors

TOM: I don't see how you can expect me not to worry as long as you're still working there with Mark day after day.

PAM: It's my *job*, Tom. I've worked for years to get where I am in the firm, and I'm not about to throw it all away.

TOM: But you're ready to throw our marriage away?

PAM: I didn't say that.

THERAPIST: Tom, try to stay focused on your concerns and describe the uneasy feelings you're having in a way that you think Pam might be more able or willing to hear . . .

TOM: Well, you told us last time that we should use this past week to think about what was going on around us that maybe put our marriage at higher risk for an affair. And it just seems to me that Pam works with a lot of guys and very few women in her office, so she gets a lot of attention and that makes me feel uneasy.

PAM: There are plenty of other women where I work . . .

TOM: (*interrupting*) . . . But not at your level . . .

PAM: That's not my fault.

THERAPIST: Tom, I'm wondering if there may be more to it than simply the fact that there are more men than women in the office where Pam works. What specifically concerns you?

TOM: Pam, you're the kind of woman that men are going to notice. You're good-looking, you dress well, you're really good at what you do, you have a great personality . . .

PAM: (*a bit sarcastically*) Sorry if that's a problem for you . . .

TOM: No, I know those are good things. But given those qualities, men are going to be on you like flies on honey. I don't expect them not to notice you, and I don't blame you when they do. But what that means is that you have to go out of your way to let them know that you're married and not available.

PAM: You don't think they know that?

TOM: Well, they probably know you're married—you do wear your wedding ring.

PAM: Just what do you expect, then?

THERAPIST: Pam, that's a really important question. Right now it seems that you may be feeling like you're on the hot seat, and that's not particularly comfortable. But figuring out how your situation at work may have some built-in risks could be pretty important, not only in terms of developing some safeguards but also in letting Tom know that you view the situation seriously and are open to changing parts of it if necessary. So would you be willing to spend some time on this today, thinking about what some of those risk factors might be and then at some point perhaps considering whether there's anything you could do differently at work to make things seem more secure?

PAM: I guess so, as long as Tom isn't insisting that I quit my job.

TOM: That's not what I'm asking.

Even strong relationships can become more vulnerable to an affair when exposed to chronic or severe outside demands or stressors, particularly if they are not offset by outside resources that support or strengthen the relationship. Sometimes such vulnerability develops slowly over years, such as when partners allow themselves to become increasingly involved in work or responsibilities of rearing children to the neglect of their own relationship. At other times, vulnerability is precipitated by more discrete changes, such as a move to a new community and loss of social supports or pursuit of one partner by someone outside the relationship. Whether the causes are gradual and insidious or more sudden and dramatic, understanding the potential role of outside factors in contributing to the relationship's vulnerability to an affair is critical.

Managing Therapeutic Context and Process

In examining outside influences, the emphasis should remain on identifying potential contributing factors, being careful not to move too quickly toward change-based interventions that can interrupt or stall the exploration process. However, occasionally when examining outside contributing factors, one discovers "lightning rod" issues or concerns that, until addressed, may disrupt further Stage 2 work. This situation occurs most frequently when ongoing outside influences are perceived by the injured partner as significantly increasing the risks of a continued or repeated affair, for example, persistent pursuit by an outside person or continued engagement of the participating partner in outside activities that were previously associated with unfaithful behavior, such as going to singles bars after work with friends. In those cases, some intermediate problem solving may be necessary to defuse or contain these outside influences to permit further Stage 2 work to continue.

Outside influences commonly contributing to vulnerability to an affair are summarized in Table 9.1 and are the focus of this chapter. They include

- Typical demands and stressors encountered in the ordinary course of daily living.
- Less common stressors distinguished by their chronicity or severity.
- Exposure to individuals or circumstances undermining relationship values of fidelity.
- Inadequate resources or outside support for the couple's relationship.

Common Intrusions and Distractions

Few if any relationships escape exposure to common demands, stressors, or mere hassles that characterize daily living. We think of these factors as *intrusions* and *distractions*, external pressures that intrude into the relationship by increasing negativity, impatience, or general stress levels of one or both partners and putting demands on partners' time that distract them from caring for themselves and each other. Although these outside influences can arise from virtually anywhere, common sources include strains from work, involvement

TABLE 9.1. Potential Contributing Factors from Outside the Relationship

Intrusions and distractions

- Work outside the home.
- Outside commitments (e.g., children's schools, religious groups, or community service organizations).
- Responsibilities of raising children.
- Responsibilities of extended family (e.g., expectations of spending time with relatives or caring for an aging parent).
- Household tasks.
- Hobbies and other interests.

Excessive stress

- Chronic financial strains or similar relationship stressors.
- Difficult life transitions (e.g., becoming parents or "empty nesters," moving to a different community, starting a new job).
- Chronic health problems.
- Ongoing conflicts with others (e.g., extended family, neighbors, coworkers).

Undermining of relationship values

- Temptations and opportunity (e.g., work settings that involve extended time alone with someone of the opposite gender).
- Pursuit by someone outside the relationship.
- Friends and acquaintances who devalue fidelity.
- Cultural stereotypes of marriage and affairs (e.g., repeated exposure to books or movies that portray affairs in unrealistic, romanticized ways).

Lack of social support for faithful relationships

- Absence of couple friends to support your marriage.
- Lack of involvement in couple-based social groups or activities.
- Failure to cultivate friendships intended to support your accountability to a faithful relationship.

in the community, rearing children or commitments to extended family, routine household tasks, and hobbies or similar interests.

Work and Other Commitments Outside the Home

For almost all couples, one or both partners work outside the home. Any work situation, regardless of its nature or status, has the potential to generate negative spillover into the relationship when it involves high levels of stress, low levels of satisfaction, or excessive time demands. In our experience, negative influences of work arise from both participating partners and injured partners. Participating partners sometimes cite excessive work involvement and neglect by the other partner as a reason for seeking attention from an outside person. We have also known participating partners who have become vulnerable to an affair in part from their own work-related stresses or demands, sometimes citing lack of appreciation and their own emotional isolation as key factors.

In exploring work-related factors as a potential source of vulnerability to an affair, it is important to distinguish between the intrinsic demands from work versus self-generated stresses resulting from misplaced priorities or poor decisions. For some people, high needs for achievement and a determination to "get ahead" take precedence over relaxing at home with one's partner to nurture the relationship. For others, success at work becomes a highly valued source of affirmation and a predominant part of one's identity, particularly in the face of conflict at home or feelings of inadequacy as a partner or parent. In challenging assumptions or enduring patterns of work-related behavior potentially compromising the couple's relationship, we emphasize two principles: (1) *balance*, acknowledging objective realities regarding the need or desire to work while balancing equally important but sometimes less apparent needs of the couple's relationship for time together, nurturing, or play; and (2) *value-based decisions*, confronting partners with discrepancies between expressed priorities (e.g., placing one's family first) and actual behaviors (e.g., devoting excessive time in the evenings or on weekends to work-related activities rather than to the couple or family).

Not all work outside the home comes in the form of employment. For many individuals, volunteer service to children's schools, religious organizations, and various civic groups can be equally vital and draining. Community organizations rely extensively on volunteers and seem to have a knack for identifying individuals whose values regarding service make it difficult for them to say "no." Such service can be immensely rewarding, become deeply intertwined with one's sense of identity or worth, and be difficult to decrease once commitments are accepted for fear of letting others down. Challenging overinvolvement in volunteer activities outside the home can be therapeutically difficult if these pursuits have already been labeled by the other partner as less important or less worthy because they are unpaid, particularly if the other partner justifies his or her devotion to work on the basis of the income generated.

We generally strive to affirm the healthy values of service and giving to others while emphasizing the same principles we highlight when challenging intrusions from paid work, that is, the importance of maintaining balance and allocating time and energy consistent with one's explicit priorities. For example, "Carol, you've told me previously that you decided early in your marriage not to work outside the home so that you could devote more time to your children. Your contributions as a volunteer at their schools and as a leader in the PTA seem consistent with that decision and with the importance you place on your children. But I'm concerned about whether the evenings and weekends devoted to these activities might sometimes actually pull you away from your family. Could you talk about how you struggle with that balance?"

Children and Extended Family

Most couples with children describe them as a major source of joy as well as a source of demands on time and energy. Literature regarding the family life cycle shows typical declines in overall relationship satisfaction after the arrival of children, with continued declines being common as children progress through toddlerhood and adolescence; relationship satisfaction often does not return to earlier levels until the last child leaves home. The transition to parenthood brings disruptions in sleep, intrusions into partners' time and energy previously devoted to each other, potential declines in frequency of lovemaking, and sometimes financial concerns, particularly if one partner terminates employment outside the home. Each successive stage of children's development brings its own unique challenges, for example, managing time devoted to children's extracurricular activities in evenings and on weekends or contending with adolescents' sometimes stormy progression toward independence.

Partners frequently can identify the general stresses of rearing children but might have less insight into how specific stresses have impacted each partner or the relationship. For example, one partner may feel resentful about demands from parenting but feel too guilty to express it to the other. Or either partner may wrestle with feeling ineffective as a parent or not enjoying the children as much as he or she had anticipated. Differences in attitudes or values around children's privileges, responsibilities, or discipline strategies can contribute to parental conflict. So too can feelings of being burdened with a disproportionate share of parenting tasks. Some couples report little conflict over children, but they describe a pattern of consistently placing needs of their own relationship below the preferences or perceived needs of their children (e.g., rarely going out as a couple because it makes one of their children unhappy). With those couples, we emphasize the need to care for their own relationship as a means of protecting one of their children's most important assets, namely the integrity and quality of their parents' marriage.

In exploring interactions regarding children as potential intrusions or distractions on the couple's relationship, we discuss normal challenges of parenting but strive to identify how specific components affect each partner and the relationship. We also distinguish between common challenges experienced by most couples and special circumstances that may pose additional hardships on parents, such as children with physical health problems or those with emotional or behavioral difficulties. We examine specific strategies the couple has used to manage the demands of parenting and ways the strategies have been helpful or have fallen short.

Separate from strains related to parenting, couples often struggle with demands from extended family. These demands may be as simple as family members' expectations that the couple should spend discretionary time (e.g., weekends or holidays) with them rather than having separate time alone. Or they may be more complicated and involve significant conflict between one partner and either extended family members or in-laws. Increasingly, it is common for couples to experience demands of caring for aging parents, often just as their own children are leaving the home. In some cases, couples struggle with caring for a family member with special needs involving physical or psychological impairments. Again, although partners can often identify such concerns as sources of stress, they frequently have little understanding of how these stresses specifically impact each partner or the relationship. Hence, the therapeutic task involves going beyond identifying such stressors at a general level and instead articulating the impact of specific aspects of the situation on partners' respective experiences.

For example, "You've both talked some about the challenges of caring for Dave's parents since his dad's stroke, but I'm curious about how that's impacted each of you. What I'm especially interested in knowing isn't so much the details of what you each do because we've already talked some about that, but more about what these changes have meant to each of you. Nancy, could we begin with you? What has this been like for you, and what's your understanding of what it's been like for Dave? Start first with the parts about you, okay?"

Household Responsibilities and Discretionary Activities

Once couples move beyond a dating relationship and share a common residence, they have to negotiate how to manage routine tasks such as meals, finances, laundry, housecleaning, home maintenance, yard care, vehicle maintenance, and so forth. Common difficulties in managing these tasks include

- Failing to divide responsibilities between partners in ways that feel equitable to both.

- Differences in partners' expectations about how to manage specific tasks or how to prioritize responsibilities in the home versus leisure time as a couple or separately as individuals.

- Having inordinate levels of household or related responsibilities sometimes brought on by the couple themselves (e.g., moving to a large home requiring additional upkeep).

- Specific skill deficits (e.g., inexperience in constructing a budget or managing finances).

It is useful to distinguish between situations that are intrinsically stressful (e.g., an aging home that requires frequent repairs) versus those that arise because of issues in the couple's own relationship (e.g., preferences for restoring an older home vs. the convenience of purchasing a newer one). Partners can more easily unify as a team around a shared outside stressor, but differences in attitudes or values may lead to polarized positions and increased resentments.

In Chapter 8 we noted that couples become connected emotionally in part by working together as a team to accomplish common goals and by spending time together in mutually enjoyable activities. Partners sometimes struggle to balance this "we" part of their relationship with the separate "me" parts that reflect individual hobbies and related interests. It is unreasonable to expect partners to share the exact same interests or relinquish all outside activities when they become a couple. Moreover, separate hobbies or interests can reduce stress and enhance each partner's emotional and physical well-being. However, relationships become vulnerable when either partner devotes excessive time or energy to outside interests or when partners have not negotiated how to manage differences in respective needs for time alone. Research indicates that satisfied couples allocate their leisure time to a healthy blend of shared as well as separate activities; in contrast, distressed couples frequently consist of partners who spend a large percentage of discretionary time alone or with others rather than with each other.

Excessive Stress

Separate from the ordinary demands of everyday life, couples sometimes struggle with stressors distinguished by their chronicity or severity. Losing a job or changing jobs, moving to a new community, the onset of physical health problems, or the death of a parent are common events shared by many couples. Nevertheless, these or similar situations can compromise a relationship when either partner becomes overwhelmed and less emotionally available to the other. When exploring outside factors that can increase vulnerability to an affair, couples often can identify such stressors because they stand out among routine daily challenges. However, despite recognizing their importance, partners often find it difficult to discuss these situations effectively because of their emotional complexity.

It is important to consider how stressors contribute to vulnerability to an affair. Earlier, we noted that common stressors may exert an influence by increasing partners' negativity or by placing additional demands on partners' time that distract them from caring for themselves and each other. However, in addition to these indirect effects, chronic or severe stress may increase partners' vulnerability more directly. For example, when under acute stress, individuals may not think clearly and are more susceptible to impaired judgment and poor decisions. Sometimes the inability to manage or resolve acute stress contributes to feelings of inadequacy, and affirmation from an outside person assumes greater potency. Similarly, chronic or severe stress can produce such high levels of negativity that an individual becomes vulnerable to seeking relief or comfort through an affair.

Clearly, not all individuals exposed to intense or enduring stress succumb to having an affair. Explanations such as "I was just unhappy" or "The stress finally got to me" will not be sufficient for understanding how an affair occurred. Hence, it is important to inquire about the subjective experience and meaning of such stressors for both partners and how these stressors interacted with other individual or relationship vulnerabilities in contributing to the affair.

For example, the profound grief that accompanies the death of a child may initially bring partners together but subsequently become too difficult to talk about, particularly if one partner eventually is able to move on emotionally but the other remains overcome by the loss. Partners may find it difficult to express their frustrations or resentments about the other one's physical health problems that limit activities they once enjoyed together—hiking, playing tennis, lovemaking—because these resentments are comingled with genuine empathy and sadness on the partner's behalf. Similarly, emotional difficulties of either partner (e.g., depression, anxiety, or alcohol abuse) may pose unique challenges to the couple and lie outside their ability to communicate effectively.

In such situations, the therapeutic challenge involves going beyond identifying the overt stressor to uncovering the complex feelings that frequently lie underneath and clarifying how the stressor increased the couple's vulner-ability to an affair. After first asking, "Separate from the affair, what have you found most difficult to deal with individually or as a couple over the past year?," we then proceed to ask, "Talk about how this has been difficult, not so much in terms of what has happened but more in terms of the feelings that go along with it." The ensuing process is similar to what might unfold in indi-vidual therapy, except that each partner is encouraged in turn to be a "par-ticipant observer" to gain a better understanding of the other's experience. In this manner, feelings of hurt versus anger, guilt versus resentment, or needs for closeness versus despair can often be clarified in ways that enable both part-ners' reactions to the situation to be more understandable to the other.

Exposure to Negative Influences

In addition to intrusions from outside stressors or distractions, relationships also can become vulnerable when either partner is exposed to negative influ-ences that undermine or devalue relationship commitment and fidelity. Such influences are rampant throughout popular culture, including television, movies, and books that portray affairs as common, exciting escapes from the drudgery of long-term relationships, with few negative consequences. These depictions of affairs, used to arouse the viewer or reader, disregard surveys finding that 70–80% of Americans state that extramarital sex is always wrong and that most others express at least some disapproval (Smith, 1994). Such cultural portrayals also ignore consistent findings regarding the negative con-sequences of infidelity for participants, their relationships, and frequently for other family members as well (Allen et al., 2005).

   Challenges to relationship values of commitment and fidelity can occur on a more personal level, particularly when either partner spends time with persons who acclaim the benefits of a single life and make jokes or other derogatory comments about being "tied down" to one partner. Sometimes friends who are unhappy in their own relationships are all too willing to par-ticipate in "partner bashing," in which each person describes the shortcom-ings of his or her partner and the other listens sympathetically without chal-lenging the speaker. At times, individuals in committed relationships might be invited by their single friends to social gatherings without their partner where flirtatious interactions among both single and married persons may be widespread. Friends or acquaintances may disclose their own affairs, empha-sizing the exciting aspects and either overlooking or discounting the adverse impact and risks.

Other challenges to fidelity include repeated exposure to temptations or opportunities for intimate involvement with someone outside the relationship. Common examples include work settings that involve extended time alone with someone who is appealing, for example, traveling together or working extended hours together on a project when few others are present. Some situations inherently provide shared emotional experiences that can promote feelings of closeness, for example, celebrating a project's success after months of effort or worry or working side by side in particularly difficult settings in which mutual emotional support may lead to a sense of intimate connection. Such circumstances are not restricted to employment settings and can occur in volunteer activities through schools, churches, synagogues, or other civic organizations. In such circumstances, the two people can convince themselves that being together is for a "noble" or worthy cause and ignore the risky behaviors that might follow.

Pursuit by an Outsider

A particularly salient threat to fidelity arises when someone in a committed relationship is pursued by an outside third person. Discussions about the outside person are likely to be among the most difficult and emotionally intense issues to address when examining outside factors during Stage 2 interventions. These discussions will be even more difficult if the participating partner has maintained contact with the outside person and particularly if the affair is ongoing. As we noted in Chapter 4, whether or not the affair has ended will, in part, determine the kinds of discussions that the couple will need to have about the outside-affair person. In encouraging partners to critically evaluate the status of problematic outside relationships, we explore a variety of potential indicators suggesting that the outside person has assumed special significance, including the following:

- Is the partner willing to give up the outside friendship for the sake of his or her committed relationship?
- Is the partner willing to confront the outside person about "mixed signals" he or she is receiving about the boundaries of their relationship?
- Are there *any* aspects of interactions with the outside party that the person would be reluctant to disclose fully with his or her partner?

When appropriate, you may need to address problematic or inadequate boundaries with outside persons following guidelines presented in Chapter 4.

Even when all contact with the outside-affair person has ended, discussions about this person's role in the affair may be extraordinarily difficult. As a general rule, we encourage the participating partner to discuss his or her understanding of the outside person's contributions to initiating or maintaining the affair as fully as possible before inviting the injured partner's comments. This sequence is intended to reduce the participating partner's defensiveness and elicit more information than might otherwise be disclosed. Nevertheless, differences in partners' perspectives may still be problematic.

For example, if the participating partner attributes the affair primarily to the outside person's pursuit and accepts little personal responsibility, the injured partner will likely respond negatively and focus more strongly on the participating partner's role. Alternatively, if the participating partner focuses on his or her own role and characterizes the outside person in an overly positive or virtuous manner, the injured partner will likely respond negatively because the outside person is usually perceived by the injured party as a coconspirator in the betrayal. If the injured partner describes the outside person in demonic or intensely negative ways, the participating partner may feel provoked to defend the outside person, which inevitably leads to further turmoil between the participating and injured partner. Finally, either partner may be reluctant to address specific characteristics or behaviors of the outside person for fear of provoking increased emotional turbulence at a time when the couple's relationship still feels fragile.

No single therapeutic strategy will address the myriad dynamics that can make discussions of the outside person more constructive. Instead, the therapist can only strive to be aware of these multiple influences and address them as they emerge, containing negative escalations, addressing partners' respective apprehensions and working to provide a safe therapeutic context, and promoting balance in exploring contributions from the outside person while recognizing that other factors and persons also played important roles.

Some outside relationships begin innocently, for example, when participants do not intend for an emotional or physical relationship to develop but ignore risk factors or "warning signs" along the way and then find themselves dealing with strong feelings of attraction or susceptibility to more intimate involvement. Sometimes the outside person has significant emotional issues or needs that increase the likelihood of seeking involvement with someone else, whether that person is already in a committed relationship or not. In such situations, efforts by the person in a committed relationship to slow down, de-escalate, or completely suspend further involvement may be met with considerable resistance in the form of pleading, persistent intrusions, or threats to retaliate unless the desired relationship is maintained. Persons in committed relationships may also find themselves being pursued by outside persons who are exploitive or predatory in nature, with a history of seeking intense but short-lived involvements with others for personal satisfaction. In other circumstances, the outside person may be well adjusted psychologically but did not maintain appropriate boundaries, fell in love, and pursued the other person.

In evaluating how exposure to outside negative influences placed a couple's relationship at higher risk for an affair, two additional issues warrant consideration. The first is the extent to which the participating partner actively discouraged pursuit by others. Interests expressed by an outside person can be flattering, affirming, and exciting. Explicitly resisting or opposing flirtatious or intimate interactions can be just as important as not promoting them. Such efforts go beyond token behaviors such as wearing a wedding ring; rather, they extend to behaviors such as including one's partner in social gatherings whenever possible, actively referring in a positive manner to the other partner when he or she is absent, avoiding or leaving situations in which flirtatious or inappropriate exchanges arise, and being explicit and conspicuous about one's commitment to a faithful relationship. Some partners might avoid saying directly to the pursing individual that a behavior is inappropriate for fear of being offensive or having misinterpreted that person's intentions; however, it is rarely offensive to speak positively about one's partner and committed relationship.

The second issue meriting close examination is the extent to which the participating partner ignored, denied, or did not recognize early indicators of an outside relationship that was progressing along a "slippery slope" toward emotional or physical closeness. It is not uncommon for outside-affair relationships to begin as healthy friendships that then assume a special or intimate nature. Discussions move to a deeper level; casual touches or friendly hugs linger; interactions that previously occurred in a group context now exclude others and take place in more private settings.

As the exchange between Tom and Pam at the beginning of this chapter suggests, Pam's work situation caused Tom to worry about her susceptibility to attentions from her male coworkers. The fact that Pam and her colleague, Mark, continued to work together bothered Tom, but his concerns extended more generally to Pam's failure to discourage men's solicitous and occasionally flirtatious behavior. Later in that same session, the therapist explored how Pam's situation at work may have increased her risk of inappropriate interactions with colleagues.

THERAPIST: Pam, you talked earlier about how you never intended to have an affair with Mark, but that your relationship with him developed over a long time, and eventually you found yourself much more involved than you had anticipated. Can you talk more about how that happened?

PAM: Well, that's right, I never imagined that I would be one of those women who cheated on her husband. That's not like me.

THERAPIST: But somehow the affair occurred nevertheless, and now it's really important to examine more closely how that happened. What safeguards were absent, or what early warning signs did you miss?

TOM: You've always had guys chasing you, Pam, even back in college when we first met. You were never without a boyfriend. As soon as one relationship ended, there were other guys waiting in the wings eager to take up the chase. And I think you sometimes let them know somehow along the way that you might be interested in something more at some point.

PAM: I admit, I never liked staying at home while other girls were out on dates, so I tried to make sure that never happened to me.

TOM: I always worried back then that maybe that would happen to us, that you'd get bored or grow tired of me and let some other guy come in and sweep you off your feet.

PAM: But that never happened. I knew I wanted something different in my life and someone I could count on. That's why I married *you* . . .

TOM: But it *has* happened now, Pam. You *did* let it happen, just like I worried it could . . . (*long pause*) . . .

PAM: I know, Tom—and I am so incredibly sorry—I swear I will never let that happen again. Mark and I have no interactions any more except what's absolutely necessary. And I've agreed that I wouldn't ever meet with him in either of our offices without the door being open, and no more working together at night even if there are others around.

THERAPIST: Pam, you've done a good job of setting clearer boundaries with Mark, and I think that's been really helpful to you and Tom as you try to get a foothold and begin moving forward. But I hear Tom expressing a more general concern about subtle messages that he thinks you may be sending that convey an openness to having men flirt with you, or maybe about your not sending explicit messages that you're *not* open to that kind of flirtation. I'm wondering if *you* think that sometimes happens.

TOM: (*interrupting*) That's right, Pam. I mean—you have pictures of our daughters in your office, but none of me.

PAM: Tom, you don't *like* any pictures I have of you . . .

TOM: Well, I've changed my views on that now. I want you to have pictures of me in your office so that other men are reminded of who I am—and who you and I are.

PAM: I'm glad to do that . . .

TOM: And I want to start attending those office parties and picnics with you instead of staying at home with the girls.

PAM: Tom, I've invited you in the past . . .

TOM: Sometimes, but not always. You invite me to the Christmas party and the summer picnic, but not to those Friday happy hours you go to once a month. If you're going to go, I want to go with you, and I think other husbands and wives should be invited, too. I think it should be as a couple; otherwise, it's just asking for trouble.

PAM: What about the girls after school?

TOM: If we're going to change things in our marriage, we'll have to figure out how to manage that. Maybe they could go to your sister's home on those Friday evenings, and we could take her kids some other week so she and Toby could get a night out together.

PAM: (*Looks down at the floor, no longer responding.*)

THERAPIST: What are you thinking, Pam?

PAM: I don't know. I mean, I know that Tom hates my going to those Friday happy hours now. They just remind him of everything that's happened recently.

THERAPIST: Are you reluctant to give those up . . . or to include Tom?

PAM: It's not that I'm reluctant to include Tom . . . and, yes, I'm reluctant to give them up. A lot of business actually gets done at those happy hours—I mean, connections are made, strategies are hatched—and if you're not there you get left on the sidelines.

THERAPIST: And you don't think you could do that if Tom were there?

PAM: I think I could. Actually, there *are* other spouses who come to the happy hours, mostly wives I guess. It's just that, Tom, whenever you've come to social events related to my work, you're so gloomy in how you look and act that it makes me feel really uncomfortable.

TOM: I don't particularly like the people you work with, especially some of the guys.

PAM: Well, you can't expect me to want you to come to these things and then behave in a way that makes me and everyone else uncomfortable because it's clear how miserable you are being there.

TOM: (*Looks away.*)

THERAPIST: (*to Tom*) Doing that differently might be especially hard for you now . . .

TOM: I don't know, not really. I mean, I really despise Mark and everything he stands for. But lately I've decided not to let guys like him intimidate me any more. There actually are some people whom Pam works with I like . . . and I could focus on them. And as far as the others go, I can fake it as well as anybody. I can be pleasant and cheerful if that's what it takes. If I don't let Pam go to any of these things, she's going to be resentful . . .

PAM: (*interrupting*) I don't have to go to all of them, Tom . . .

TOM: Okay, but that's not the point. What I'm saying is that I want to be visible in your life. I want others to see me and to know that you and I are a couple. There have been too many ways that I've been behind the scenes—maybe because you put me there, maybe because I chose to be there—but that has to change. I'm willing to work at being more inter-active and fun when I'm with your coworkers and friends, but you need to include me more and also make our marriage more obvious to others even when I'm not around.

PAM: I can do that . . .

Inadequate Support for the Relationship

Virtually any relationship can become compromised if exposed to unrelent-ing demands, overwhelming stress, or factors eroding commitment to faith-ful behavior. Partners can strengthen their relationship by seeking support from other individuals or couples who actively encourage their relationship and commitment to fidelity. Hence, in examining outside factors potentially contributing to vulnerability to an affair, it is important not only to identify negative influences but also to explore the partners' failure to seek out protec-tive positive influences.

There are at least three common ways in which partners receive sup-port for their relationship. The first is by participating in social groups that explicitly support and encourage couple and family activities. Many couples experience this kind of support through their involvement in religious orga-nizations, and others find it in community activities that emphasize family life, such as couples' involvement in their children's school or extracurricular events, or couple-based activities, such as cooking groups or cycling clubs. Other couples find support for their relationship by socializing with other couples who demonstrate commitment to a faithful relationship and consistently exhibit respectful, caring exchanges between partners. Couples can also find support for their relationship by identifying a close friend who is willing to help them be accountable in their relationship, not by soliciting or encouraging complaints about the other partner but instead by challenging the person to examine his or her own contributions to the problem or responsibility for taking steps to make the relationship better.

In examining how Bill's affair with a member of their church had developed, he and Vicki identified several ways in which they had become isolated from individuals and couples who had supported them in the past.

VICKI: Somewhere along the way, I think we just got lost.

THERAPIST: Talk with Bill about what you mean by that, about how you both got lost.

VICKI: Well, I know that I certainly felt lost. After Dad died, my interest in lots of things just vanished. It was all I could do to return to our business and keep things running at home. I had no interest in going out or dealing with others. I didn't want to go to church. I felt resentful when others tried to tell me that my dad was in a "better place" and then I felt guilty for feeling that way. I realize now that I became really depressed . . .

BILL: And I didn't know how to help you with that. I tried staying home with you but that didn't seem to work.

THERAPIST: Who was in your lives whom you could turn to for support?

VICKI: I think that's part of the problem. Bill and I used to have couples in the church with whom we occasionally socialized, but we had already cut back on that when we were struggling in our business and then I became even less comfortable with those couples.

THERAPIST: Did you have any friends of your own you could draw on?

VICKI: Not really. Probably my closest friend is my sister, but I couldn't really talk with her about Dad.

THERAPIST: Why is that?

VICKI: We had different ways of seeing the situation. I had a really complicated relationship with my dad, sometimes feeling really close to him but then feeling disappointed when he would drink, and then trying to rescue him. My sister was just generally angry at my dad and unsympathetic. After he died, I couldn't talk with her about my grief.

THERAPIST: Could you and Bill talk?

BILL: That was part of the problem. I wanted to be supportive, but the advice I tried to give Vicki about moving on never helped . . .

VICKI: I didn't want your advice . . .

THERAPIST: (to Bill) And when you were confused about how to help, was there someone you turned to?

BILL: I thought about going to our minister, but Vicki was already in conflict with him so that didn't feel like an option to me.

THERAPIST: And that's when you turned to a woman in your Sunday school class . . .

BILL: I thought she could provide a woman's perspective that would be helpful, and initially it was.

THERAPIST: But then it became something else . . .

BILL: Yeah, pretty stupid as I think about it.

THERAPIST: Not stupid, perhaps even understandable, but clearly a problem. (pause) Did you have any guy friends to turn to?

BILL: That's just it. When Vicki and I married, we pretty much gave up our individual friends. We just didn't have time for them any more, and a lot of them were single anyway. Between the business and our children, we barely had time for each other let alone for other friends.

THERAPIST: Early on, one of the ways of committing to each other was to put limits on time you spent apart with others. And with each of you already having children from your first marriage, there wasn't much opportunity to spend time with others. But I'm concerned that in shutting others out you also cut off important sources of support for yourselves and your marriage.

VICKI: I can see that now . . .

BILL: Me too.

THERAPIST: So in moving forward, at some point it's going to be important to consider how to restore a healthier balance: continuing to make sure you give first priority to your marriage and your family but also making sure that you build in time with people who can support and help you when you're going through difficult times.

Summary

Relationships can become more vulnerable to an affair when subjected to overwhelming stressors or simply the routine demands of everyday life that make it more difficult for partners to care for each other and their relationship. Such risks are magnified when outside negative influences either implicitly erode commitment to a faithful relationship or more actively encourage emotional or physical involvement with another person. Discussions about influences of the outside-affair person present special therapeutic challenges. Couples need to examine not only how they were exposed to negative risk factors but also how they failed to seek out or maintain protective positive influences encouraging faithful behavior and supporting their relationship.

Resources from *Getting Past the Affair*

In our companion self-help book for couples, *Chapter 8*, "Was It the World Around Us?," includes information related to the topics discussed in the current chapter. The first portion of that chapter (pp. 189–194) explores outside intrusions and stressors, followed by an examination of how outsiders may have actively or covertly undermined the couple's relationship. Consideration is also given to how partners can draw appropriately on others for support and encouragement. The chapter concludes with two complementary exercises. Exercise 8.1 encourages partners to identify negative influences outside their marriage, including distractions, significant stressors, or interactions with persons devaluing commitment and faithfulness in relationships, along with identifying strategies to reduce these influences. Exercise 8.2 helps partners identify and draw on outside resources and people who can help support and strengthen their relationship.

CHAPTER 10

Examining Individual Partner Factors

GAIL: I never saw it coming. I mean, I'd heard the rumors, but I didn't want to believe them. And when I asked whether you were sleeping with Jill, you said "No," and I wanted so much to believe you. I can't believe how stupid I was, how everyone must have looked at me with pity or maybe just laughed at me behind my back. I am *so* angry, Brad. How could you have done it?

BRAD: I know, Gail. And I'm as sorry as you are angry. I *really* am. I don't know what came over me, how I screwed up so badly. I just know I'll never let anything like that ever happen again.

GAIL: That's not good enough, Brad . . . I know you mean it, but it's just not enough.

THERAPIST: Gail, talk more about what you mean by that. What's not enough?

GAIL: There has to be more to it. I know we've talked about how Brad and I drifted apart, what with his being wrapped up in his work and not feeling like he could share it with me and my frustrations with my own work. And I know how tempting it must have been for Brad, having Jill look up to him and all that. I mean—it's not like I forget what it was like for Brad and me when he was teaching and I was still a student. But it doesn't add up. It's still no excuse . . .

BRAD: (*interrupting*) I'm not looking to be excused . . .

GAIL: It's not enough to explain it, Brad. Look, lots of couples go through bad times and drift apart for a while. And there are always going to be "temptations" out there. But if that's all it takes for you to get involved with someone else, then I'm never going to feel safe again.

THERAPIST: What would be "enough"? What would you need to feel safe again?

GAIL: I need Brad to figure out what it was about him that let him step over the line. He says he doesn't know what "came over" him. Well, I need for him to figure that out! I'm not okay with it remaining some kind of "mystery" that we'll never solve. That may be convenient for Brad, but it's *horrible* for me.

THERAPIST: Try talking with Brad about what you need in a way that you think he'll be able to hear.

GAIL: (*long pause*) Brad . . . please, listen. You have to understand. I can't just put your affair behind me and go on, no matter how much I'd like to. What happened is something I never believed could happen to us. Maybe you didn't mean to hurt me, but you did . . .

BRAD: Gail, you're asking for answers I just don't have . . .

THERAPIST: Brad, I don't think Gail is expecting you to give her the answers, at least not right now. But I do think she's asking you to commit to a process of finding them, of spending time in here together to figure out how it is you did something that's not consistent with what you believe in. That's part of why it's scary for her, because it just doesn't make sense.

BRAD: I understand . . .

THERAPIST: So what Gail needs to know is whether you're willing to take the next step, to go beyond looking at what was happening around you to look at what was going on *inside* of you. I understand that could feel uncomfortable for you, because there might have been things going on with you that you're not particularly proud of . . .

BRAD: Well, I'm certainly not proud of what I did . . .

THERAPIST: So would you be willing to take some time in here to figure that out together—perhaps mostly for Gail but also partly for you—to figure out what was going on with you and what it would take to address that, so you can know with more certainty that you're no longer vulnerable in those same ways? I know that's vital for Gail, but I believe that would be helpful for you as well.

BRAD: I'm not sure what that would take, but I guess I'm willing to try . . .

THERAPIST: Good for you. Let's talk about what that would involve . . .

As reflected in this exchange, after contributing factors from within and outside the couple's relationship have been examined, crucial questions about how the affair happened still persist. It is rare that injured partners restore enduring security by exploring only their relationship and outside factors without also examining risk factors from within the partners themselves that made them more vulnerable. Even if they find initial relief without exploring individual contributing factors, these feelings rarely last. Participating partners may also remain unsettled if individual contributing factors are not addressed, particularly if they perceive important features of the injured partner that jeopardized the relationship and have not yet been discussed.

Examining potential contributions from both the participating and the injured partner can be the most difficult part of Stage 2 interventions. Partners may genuinely lack insight into their own thoughts and feelings. Some may have good awareness of thoughts and feelings around the time the affair developed or following its revelation, but have little understanding of how these factors relate to important experiences earlier in their lives that potentially left them more vulnerable. Others may lack even a rudimentary language for labeling or describing feelings. The more that partners struggle to identify their own inner experiences, the more important it is for the therapist to engage them in a guided discovery process to bring the factors into awareness so that they can then be discussed and understood by both partners.

With other couples, exploring individual contributing factors is made difficult not by lack of insight but from defensiveness in one or both partners or reluctance to be open and disclosing. Exploring one's own potential contributions to an affair requires facing difficult thoughts and feelings in oneself—those that potentially create anxiety, guilt, or embarrassment—and being vulnerable by disclosing them to a partner with whom there may still be considerable conflict or mistrust. Participating partners who already fear being vilified by the injured partner are understandably reluctant to reveal additional aspects of themselves that place them in a negative light. Injured partners may be similarly reluctant to explore their behaviors before or after the affair if they fear that their participating partner will seize upon such factors as an excuse for their own actions.

Difficulties in accessing inner experiences and the anxiety attached to such exploration can lead to heightened negativity in one or both partners. Couples who previously have made substantial gains in containing initial turmoil and examining relationship and outside factors may now show a resurgence of hurt feelings, anger, or retreat. Hence, the role of the therapist becomes more complicated and even more crucial during this phase of Stage

2 interventions, both encouraging the disclosure and discussion of individual contributions to the affair but also managing the anxiety or negativity that sometimes accompanies this process.

In this chapter, we pay particular attention to these considerations, not only identifying common sources of vulnerability to an affair related to participating and injured partners but also describing specific therapeutic strategies for examining these factors.

Potential Contributions from the Participating Partner

Setting the Context

As therapist, you need to ensure that the participating partner understands the importance of exploring his or her own thoughts and feelings leading up to, during, and after revelation of the affair. In Chapter 7, we introduced initial points to emphasize when providing a rationale for pursuing Stage 2 work, namely to (1) restore emotional security for the injured partner, (2) achieve a more balanced view of the participating partner, and (3) lay the foundation for individual or relationship change. It is often necessary to revisit those points when preparing to explore individual contributions to the affair.

We remind the participating partner of the importance of restoring predictability and security for the injured partner by developing a comprehensive and credible formulation for the affair. The message we emphasize is essentially "If for no other reason, we encourage you to do this work because it's what your partner needs." For some participating partners, this message is enough. However, there are additional reasons that more directly involve the participating partner. First, we want to reduce the participating partner's confusion about his or her own involvement in the affair because of risks accompanying such confusion. Participating partners who fail to gain a full understanding of their own thoughts and feelings related to the affair often experience continued guilt or shame that detracts from, rather than promotes, relationship intimacy. Some interpret the affair as evidence that they must not really love the injured partner and, hence, need to end the relationship with the injured partner as a way of restoring "internal balance" or self-respect. And, of course, participating partners who fail to address aspects of themselves that contributed to the affair remain more vulnerable to similar behaviors in the future, whether in the current relationship or a different one.

We want participating partners to examine not only what aspects of themselves potentially contributed to the onset of the affair but also what contributed to its continuation. For example, participating partners may fail to recognize feelings of guilt or responsibility for the outside person that hindered—or *still* hinder—ending the affair. Or they may find it difficult to disclose feelings of loneliness that accompany ending the affair while trying to recommit to a primary relationship dominated by antagonism or emotional distance.

An additional important part of setting the context for this work involves ensuring the injured partner's involvement in a constructive manner. Because of its "guided discovery" nature, this phase of Stage 2 may be more similar at times to individual therapy than couple-based treatments. When working primarily with one partner, we encourage the other partner to adopt the role of "participant-observer," listening intently to understand the partner in an "expanded" way but at times allowing the therapist and other partner to work more intensively one on one within the conjoint session. Hence, when working to explore individual contributing factors from the participating partner, the therapist must also carefully monitor and balance the injured partner's involvement.

For example, if the injured partner appears to be tuning out or not attending, we might promote more engagement by saying "Barb, I'm wondering what thoughts or feelings you're having as you're listening to Nathan talk about what he was experiencing when his interactions with Sara began to move beyond friendship." In contrast, if the injured partner becomes overly intrusive, attacking, or inclined to adopt a "cotherapist" role, we may discourage such behaviors by (1) selectively ignoring the injured partner, (2) gently asking the injured partner to hold these thoughts for a few minutes until the participating partner's exploration of a particular feeling or situation comes to a resting point, or (3) reframing the injured partner's comments in a more benign or constructive manner. For example, "Barb, as you were commenting on the similarity of Nathan's affair to his father's affairs, I sensed both hurt and perhaps hopelessness in your voice. I'm wondering whether you worry about what attitudes Nathan may have unintentionally picked up from his father, or whether you have some ideas about a different set of values that might better guide your relationship."

Ensuring a constructive framework for exploring individual factors also requires attending to subtle differences in language and tone. Consider differences between these two comments: (1) "Nathan, the way you cheated on me is just like the way your dad cheated on your mom" versus (2) "Nathan, I'm not sure you had much opportunity to learn how a couple gets through difficult times together, given what happened in your parents' marriage." In both statements, the injured partner makes a connection between events in the couple's own relationship and events in the participating partner's past that potentially increased vulnerability to an affair. However, the former is more critical and less empathic than the latter. Moreover, if the injured partner states the first, even if this observation is correct, it makes it more difficult for the therapist to pursue the connection unless the injured partner's interpretation is first softened by restating or reframing it in a more empathic or encouraging manner. Partners will differ in their abilities or motivation to phrase their observations and insights about the other person appropriately, so often you need to talk with them directly in the session to shape their comments in a way that will be helpful rather than cause alienation.

Conducting the Process

In addition to setting the context, it is especially important to direct or conduct the process when exploring individual factors. By "conducting the process," we mean directing who speaks first, when the other partner is invited to comment, which material is examined first and at what level, and when connections between the present and the past are explored. For example, when initially exploring contributing factors from the participating partner, we want the participating partner to take the lead rather than the injured partner. Understandably, partners are more willing to consider and explore feelings, needs, or shortcomings they first identify themselves. Once the factors are disclosed and framed by the therapist in an empathic manner, the other partner can be invited to share his or her own reactions or insights. One way of facilitating this process is to encourage the participating partner to talk directly with the therapist, as in this example: "Nathan, talk with me about what was going on with you back then, back when you first became aware of looking forward to interactions with Sara. What kinds of thoughts and feelings were you having, for example, about yourself or your marriage or maybe about life in general?"

When examining individual factors contributing to an affair, a general principle is to examine first those factors that arouse lower levels of anxiety or defensiveness before turning to those that potentially are more difficult either to understand or to express. Ways of implementing this general principle include the following:

- Considering more recent events before discussing those that occurred in the more distant past.
- Attending to conscious thoughts and feelings before exploring those that lie outside immediate awareness.

- Examining explicit beliefs and attitudes before underlying feelings, needs, or fears.
- Emphasizing strengths and resources before considering vulnerabilities or deficits.

Even when similarities or connections to the past seem obvious to you as the therapist, you may elect to defer commenting on that connection or offering an interpretation until you are confident that (1) the person to whom you are addressing the comment is emotionally prepared to receive it, and (2) the other partner will not misuse your observation as additional ammunition to criticize or attack the partner at a deeper level. When examining individual contributing factors from either partner, we encourage the person to become "intently curious" about what was going on with him or her and how it came about. For example, during the session we might ask whether a given feeling is familiar and, if so, whether the person can recall previous times of experiencing or struggling with that feeling, for example, "Nathan, you've said that when you first started having feelings about Sara, you were feeling pretty discouraged about things. Work wasn't going well; you and Barb were stressed out with the new baby, and life wasn't going the way you had imagined it to be. Can you talk with me about previous times in your life when you've felt discouraged? I'm especially interested in times when you were feeling somewhat ineffective."

Or we might give an assignment to reflect on such feelings during the week, as in this example: "Nathan, during the coming week, I want you to think about some of the feelings you've described today, for example, discouraged, frustrated, or alone. And then for each of those feelings, I'd like you to list any times you've had similar feelings in the past. Try to remember the earliest times you had those feelings, before you and Barb even met. And try to remember times you felt them in your relationship with Barb before you and Sara ever became involved. What were those feelings like at those times, and how did you try to cope with them? Jot down some thoughts, bring those back next time, and share with me what you've remembered and any additional thoughts you have. We're trying to see whether there are any patterns in what you've experienced over time that might help us understand your affair."

As the therapist, you also need to attend carefully to issues of when and how to invite involvement in the exploration process by the other partner. Overall, you are attempting to create a collaborative mind-set between the two partners in which they work together to understand the participating partner. This dynamic is similar to Jacobson and Christensen's (1996b) notion of "unified detachment," in which the couple steps back from the problem and takes a descriptive rather than evaluative stance, for example, by working together to identify situations that led to feelings of rejection for the participating partner, an important factor in the development of the affair. To make it safe for the participating partner to self-disclose, it is important to put that person in the lead in shaping the direction of the factors that are discussed. For example, when examining individual contributions from the participating partner, we typically delay inviting comments from the injured partner on any potential factor until first eliciting disclosure and exploration by the participating partner. That is, we encourage the injured partner to comment on material already at hand before introducing new material, in essence "staying with" factors the participating partner has disclosed. We also encourage the injured partner to reflect what the participating partner has disclosed from the participating partner's perspective before the injured partner offers complementary or contradictory perspectives. In other words, we teach the injured partner an important skill often used by therapists: "Reflect and validate before offering a new or extended perspective." It is not essential that the injured partner agree with the participating partner's account, particularly when the participating partner has expressed thoughts and feelings regarding the injured partner. However, as the therapist, you need to promote a process of generating and considering as many potential contributing influences as possible, not in order to excuse the affair but to make the participating partner's involvement less bewildering and the partner less "unidimensional" in a negative way.

For example, we might say, "Barb, you've been listening intently to Nathan describing what was going on with him as his interactions with Sara started to become more intense. He's described feeling lost. As best you can, without excusing how Nathan ultimately handled those feelings, can you describe *from Nathan's perspective* what that must have been like for him when he started feeling lost?" If the injured partner struggles with this task of experiencing empathy for the participating partner, we might first elicit similar feelings or experiences in the injured partner's life: "Barb, try to recall times when you've felt lost yourself. You may have felt that way when you first learned about Nathan's affair, but maybe there have been times earlier in your life when you've had similar feelings of being lost, perhaps in a less intense way. Can you describe what those experiences were like for you—how you struggled, and how you managed to move forward?" After the injured partner gets in touch with similar feelings from his or her own life, often it is easier for him or her to reflect and express empathy for the participating partner's experience, although not for the purpose of excusing the affair.

In the sections that follow, we consider aspects of the participating partner that potentially increased his or her attraction or vulnerability to an outside emotional or sexual relationship, positive qualities enhancing the participating partner's attractiveness to an outsider, and aspects of the participating partner that make terminating or recovering from the affair more difficult. These potential contributing factors are also summarized in Table 10.1.

Factors Contributing to Attraction to an Outside Person

People can become more vulnerable to an affair when they experience discontent with themselves, their relationship, or life in general. Other persons may be drawn to an affair not by something lacking in their life but by special positive qualities of the outside person or relationship. Hence, it is important when exploring attraction to an outside person to distinguish between attraction based on negative "deficit" factors versus positive "enhancement" factors. The former may have implications for change efforts in remediating deficiencies, whereas the latter may have implications for interventions aimed at accepting limits inherent in any committed relationship.

Beyond the initial promise of excitement or pleasure, an affair relationship can provide comfort and retreat from the ordinary stressors of everyday life, affirmation of an individual's attractiveness or worth, or unconditional acceptance, so long as the outside relationship remains buffered from expectations or challenges that eventually befall any long-term committed relationship. The primary functions of individuals in an affair are to please, affirm, comfort, support, and delight one another. These qualities are valued in most close relationships; however, when these qualities occur within affairs, they are either misplaced and should be enhanced in the primary relationship or are carried out in a manner that threatens the primary relationship. Hence, in examining thoughts or feelings in participating partners rendering them more vulnerable to an affair, it is important to examine ways in which these experiences either were lacking or were not restricted to appropriate relationships. For example, in what ways did the participating partner struggle with doubts about his or her own attractiveness? What other self-doubts were present related to roles in or outside the home? In what ways was the participating partner seeking a deeper emotional or physical connection, or was the anticipated benefit simply escape, distance, or relief? Involvement in an outside relationship can also evolve in part from feelings of anger or resentment, perhaps from feeling insufficiently appreciated or admired or possibly from a sense of entitlement after perceived abandonment.

TABLE 10.1. Potential Contributing Factors from the Participating Partner

Attraction to an outside person based on needs or concerns of the participating partner

- Affirmation of self-worth.
- Affirmation of sexual attractiveness and adequacy.
- Desire for emotional connection and intimacy.
- Pursuit of someone to fulfill unrealistic relationship expectations.

Qualities of the participating partner that promote attraction from others

- Positive qualities such as emotional sensitivity and warmth, physical attractiveness, and social status.
- Failure to convey clear boundaries and a commitment to one's marriage or primary relationship.

Factors lowering resistance to an outside emotional or sexual relationship

- Inability or unwillingness to commit to an exclusive relationship with one person.
- Lapses in judgment.
- Reluctance to confront marital/committed relationship difficulties.
- Engaging in the affair as a way to express discontent in the marriage/committed relationship.

Aspects of the participating partner that contribute to continuing an affair

- Emotional attachment or feelings of responsibility or commitment to the outside person.
- Positive aspects of the outside relationship.
- Pessimism about the outcome of the marriage/committed relationship.
- Feelings of entitlement or lack of concern about "getting caught."
- "Compartmentalization": mentally isolating the marriage/committed relationship from the outside relationship, as if they are unrelated experiences, and not thinking of the other while engaging in either one.

Aspects of the participating partner that interfere with work toward restoring the marriage

- Difficulty tolerating intense feelings expressed by the injured partner.
- Frustration or impatience with the difficult, slow process of recovering from the affair.
- Confusion about, or difficulty in expressing, his or her own thoughts and feelings.
- Difficulty in moving beyond his or her own feelings of guilt or shame.
- Difficulty in envisioning how the marriage/committed relationship can become secure and satisfying for both partners.

In exploring underlying needs or feelings of the participating partner potentially contributing to the affair, we typically use language that denotes a low level of intensity in order to reduce reactivity of either partner; often partners will reject strong statements or comments about themselves that suggest major weaknesses or shortcomings. For example, rather than referring to feeling "abandoned," we describe feeling "distant" or "alone." Similarly, instead of implying feelings of "inadequacy," we refer to feelings of "uncertainty" about oneself. We initially accept such feelings, desires, or needs uncritically, without evaluating their reasonableness or justification and without generalization to some pervasive trait or character deficit. It is first important simply to explore in as many ways as possible *what* the participating partner was experiencing and then *how* those thoughts or feelings increased susceptibility to an affair. Consideration of *why* the participating partner was thinking or feeling as he or she was, and what the implications of that may be for reducing vulnerability in the future, is deferred until those experiences are understood in their own right.

For example, earlier we described how a therapist might encourage a participating partner, Nathan, to focus initially on identifying the feelings he was experiencing about himself when he first became involved outside of his marriage. After these feelings were identified in session, Nathan was encouraged to reflect during the week on previous times he had experienced feeling discouraged or ineffective. In the next session as he began to disclose these earlier experiences, his therapist began to explore events in his marriage and at work around the time of his affair that had reactivated these long-standing self-doubts.

Sometimes participating partners' feelings and needs that contributed to an affair seem easily understood by both partners in light of circumstances at the time. For example, a participating partner might say, "I was really overwhelmed at work. The workload was unbearable, and when that happens for a long time, I know I don't think well and I need some comfort to get through it. I start consuming huge amounts of food, I drink too much, and I look for a quick fix to help me get through a horrible time." At other times, the participating partner's needs and feelings may seem distorted or disproportionate to what was going on within or outside the relationship as the affair was evolving. For example, a different participating partner might comment, "I had just gotten a great annual evaluation at work and shared it with Marie, but she didn't seem as excited for me as I had expected. I know it doesn't make sense, but it was the final straw that just sent me over the edge."

Some wants or needs go unmet even in a good relationship because of unrealistic expectations of the relationship or the other partner. At other times, underlying feelings increasing vulnerability to an affair stem not as much from current circumstances but rather from enduring dispositions to think or feel a particular way. For example, feeling neglected by one's partner when he or she becomes absorbed in other responsibilities may tap into long-standing concerns of being insufficiently valued by significant others. In such situations, as the therapist, you can help partners distinguish between enduring dispositions or vulnerabilities to feel a particular way versus current events that trigger that underlying tendency.

The following exchange reflects Brad's examination of individual factors that contributed to his affair with his graduate student, Jill. Although Brad showed some insight into his needs for admiration and implicit beliefs about how men elicit such admiration, his efforts to convince Gail that he was no longer vulnerable to such feelings were somewhat typical of initial exploration at this stage.

BRAD: Gail seems to think that I'm insecure and I'll never be happy unless women are fawning all over me.

GAIL: I never said that, Brad. I said that I think you really like having younger women admire you.

THERAPIST: Brad, I'm curious about whether you could respond to Gail's statement at that level . . .

BRAD: Of course it feels good to be admired. Who wouldn't like that?

THERAPIST: It does feel good to be admired. So what do you think Gail is concerned about in that regard?

BRAD: Well, she probably thinks I like it too much, or that I'm drawn to women who show me attention.

THERAPIST: And what do *you* think about that?

BRAD: I don't know. It's possible I guess, maybe to some degree.

THERAPIST: Could we explore that a little bit?

BRAD: Sure.

THERAPIST: What I'm interested in exploring with you is whether some of that liking to be admired ever takes on a kind of intensity to it, either in terms of being really drawn to someone who provides it or perhaps feeling a bit frustrated when someone doesn't.

BRAD: You mean like with Gail?

THERAPIST: I'm not sure—possibly. Tell me more what you're thinking about.

BRAD: Well, we've talked earlier about how Gail and I first got involved, when she was a student in one of my classes. I think she did admire me back then . . .

GAIL: I did—for good reasons . . .

BRAD: And I really liked that. It wasn't the only reason I was attracted to you, Gail, but you made me feel good about myself.

THERAPIST: Good in ways that maybe were sometimes hard to feel on your own . . .

BRAD: Probably. I know I came across as sure of myself and all that, but I really wasn't.

THERAPIST: Can you tell me more what you mean by that?

BRAD: It goes way back. Is that what you're looking for?

THERAPIST: Sure, if it applies . . .

BRAD: Well, it probably does, at least to some extent.

THERAPIST: In what way?

BRAD: Well, you remember that my folks divorced when I was 7, and my dad moved across the country a couple of years later.

THERAPIST: I remember you told me that you didn't have much contact with him after that.

BRAD: That's right, practically no contact at all. He remarried and I didn't fit into his new life.

THERAPIST: So that mostly left just you and your mom . . .

BRAD: Yeah, and her boyfriends.

THERAPIST: What does that mean?

BRAD: It just means that eventually my mom figured it was time to get on with her life and find someone to replace my dad.

THERAPIST: And how did those relationships work out?

BRAD: You mean with my mom? Well, eventually I guess they didn't work out all that well. Either my mom became disillusioned with them, or she didn't provide them with what they needed. Anyway, she never did remarry.

THERAPIST: And where was she in your life during those times, especially when she was in the middle of a new romance?

BRAD: She was a good mom . . .

THERAPIST: Yes . . .

BRAD: And she made sure I was okay or taken care of. But I guess as I grew up and reached adolescence, she pretty much figured I could take care of myself.

THERAPIST: Were there ever times you felt left out or ignored by her? I'm not suggesting that she wasn't a good mom, but it does sound like she was struggling to find her own place in life, and I do wonder how that may have impacted her time with you.

BRAD: Well, there were times when I was pretty much on my own, and I didn't particularly like that.

THERAPIST: And how did you learn to cope with that in terms of being alone?

BRAD: You mean, how did I get girls to notice me?

THERAPIST: Okay . . .

BRAD: I learned how to be helpful, to recognize when I had something I could offer them that they needed. I guess Gail's right about that in some ways. I'm certainly not wealthy like the guys my mom chased, but I'm smart and I've learned a lot and that gets me noticed. I learned how to share what I knew and be helpful. So I'd tutor the girls, you know, or help them with their papers, and they loved it. And I do like being looked up to or appreciated . . .

THERAPIST: Being looked up to is important for you. It helps get you connected . . . less alone. Could we talk about what it was like for you when it felt like Gail's admiration was slipping somehow . . . ?

At that point, the session transitioned to discussing how their relationship changed as Gail became busy, pursuing her own graduate studies and later taking a teaching position in the same department. After a fuller discussion of this more recent time in Brad and Gail's relationship, the therapist asked Brad to identify any parallels he might see between what he did when he felt lonely while growing up and how he responded when Gail became more distant.

Qualities of the Participating Partner
That Attract an Outside Person

Affairs develop not only because participating partners may seek something they are lacking but also because they may possess something found desirable by others. That is, persons can become vulnerable to an affair by virtue of their strengths and resources as well as their needs or deficits. For example, the participating partner may be physically attractive, emotionally sensitive, and easy to talk with or particularly vivacious and engaging. He or she may have a high-status position that others seek to benefit from by developing a "special" relationship. Individuals having such positive attributes can become more vulnerable to an affair if they fail to (1) appreciate the attributes that make them attractive to others, (2) acknowledge their own behaviors that may inadvertently encourage others to pursue emotional or physical involvement, or (3) recognize behaviors of others that cross appropriate boundaries and actively resist or discourage them.

For example, Tom was uncomfortable with the way Pam's male coworkers flirted with her: telling sexually suggestive jokes in her presence, touching her arm when they talked, or teasing her in playful ways that suggested a level of familiarity that went beyond a business relationship. Pam dismissed Tom's concerns, asserting that it was "harmless" and simply served to promote "high energy" and "strong collaborations" within the firm. After her affair with Mark, Pam was forced to acknowledge that, although such playfulness or flirtation might be innocent from her perspective, some of her male coworkers potentially interpreted it as her openness to more serious engagement, as Mark clearly had. Hence, she needed to monitor more closely the ambiguous signals she was giving. It was not enough to know her own boundaries; she needed to be more proactive in communicating those boundaries clearly to others.

In some situations, participating partners might not be able or willing to minimize their positive qualities. For example, one participating partner declared, "I can't help it if I'm outgoing and physically attractive. Do you want me to try to be boring and look ugly?" It is not helpful for participating partners to reject responsibility for how their positive qualities contributed to the context for the affair. Rather, it is crucial that they recognize how they use those qualities or how others might respond to them.

Factors Lowering Resistance to an Outside Relationship

Few individuals enter a committed relationship expecting to be unfaithful to their partner. Nevertheless, whether in response to their own feelings or pursuit from an outside person, many individuals eventually engage in an affair. Hence, it is important to examine the factors that lowered the participating partner's resistance to an affair. Some of these factors may reflect enduring characteristics of the partner, for example, unwillingness or inability to commit to an exclusive relationship with one person; long-standing patterns of impulsivity, high-risk behaviors, or lapses in judgment; or a self-centered perspective that fails to consider adverse consequences for others. In other cases, the participating partner's reluctance to confront relationship difficulties lowers resistance to an affair offering an alternative escape. In some instances, the affair can be a means of expressing discontent with the relationship, sometimes an expression of anger or other times a last-chance ploy to call attention to the participating partner's unhappiness and provoke changes by the other partner. Occasionally, resistance to an affair is lowered by more transient or situational factors, for example, impaired judgment from alcohol or other substance use combined with opportunity or intense feelings accompanying recent trauma or loss. One way of exploring resistance-lowering factors is to inquire about what circumstances led to transitioning from "the slippery slope" (e.g., contemplation of an affair or risky behaviors) to actual involvement in the affair.

Failure to set appropriate boundaries with other individuals is a notable factor that lowers resistance to affairs. In some situations, poor boundaries result from participating partners' resistance to having limits placed on their behaviors. Those partners may benefit from clarifying relationship values (e.g., fidelity) that at times conflict with personal preferences (e.g., deep emotional conversations with a coworker). Other participating partners recognize the importance of boundaries but fail to recognize where those boundaries need to be drawn, for example, engaging in flirtatious behavior without anticipating how others might respond in pursuing more intimate exchanges. Some participating partners recognize the need for boundaries but struggle to adhere to them. For those partners, interventions may need to focus on strengthening internal resources (e.g., recognizing initial feelings of attraction and setting firm limits before the feelings become too strong) or drawing on outside resources (e.g., attending certain social events only with one's partner or a trusted friend in order to raise awareness and accountability to appropriate boundaries.

In some instances, significant psychopathology plays an important role in the participating partner's affair and makes treatment more difficult as well. Although there are no empirical data on this issue, the prognosis for a couple seems less positive if the participating partner engaged in affairs because he or she has antisocial or narcissistic traits and believes that he or she is above social norms and mores. This belief suggests that the participating partner is at risk for additional affairs, particularly if he or she is not remorseful or is inordinately defensive about the current affair. In this instance, an important goal of treatment may be to ensure that the injured partner becomes fully aware of this pattern of behavior and is able to make a good decision about whether to continue the relationship.

In a similar vein, a participating partner's dependence on alcohol or other substances can be a complicating factor. In these cases, the substance often has played a major role in the decision to become involved in the affair and if the participating partner continues to use, the injured partner will likely continue to feel vulnerable to an affair's recurrence. In addition, the emotional upheaval that is often engendered by engaging in couple treatment for the affair and the painful exploration involved during treatment can trigger greater substance use and endanger the sobriety of the newly abstinent. Effective couple-based interventions have been described for helping a dependent partner develop and maintain sobriety (see e.g., a summary by Fals-Stewart, Birchler, & O'Farrell, 2003). Only when this person has developed stable skills to combat the urges to use substances should the focus of treatment turn to the affair. Injured partners are often highly supportive of this focus, given that the alcohol is often causing relational disruption in addition to the affair. Overall, it is important to resist supporting the myth that if someone has an affair, he or she must be "psychologically disturbed." It is also important to acknowledge that, in some instances, psychopathology does play a significant role in the development of the affair as well as in its treatment. Both members of the couple must become fully aware when psychopathology is a factor, so that they can make reasonable predictions about future behavior and the magnitude of change needed to create a healthy, happy relationship together.

Factors Potentially Maintaining an Affair

Some affairs are short lived, as in a one-night stand. Although most affairs end within 6 months, a significant percentage (25%) continue up to 18 months and some (roughly 5%) may persist for years without becoming known to anyone except the two participants (Marshall, 2005). Injured partners sometimes exclaim not only, "How could you do this?" but also, "Why didn't you stop?" The second question becomes particularly important when the affair was discovered by the injured partner rather than disclosed by the participating partner, because the former begs the question of whether the affair would still be ongoing if it had not been exposed.

By far, the most common reason why affairs continue are feelings of emotional attachment to the outside person. In some cases, the affair relationship has provided opportunities for extended intimate discussions combined with physical closeness, acceptance, and understanding not challenged by competing expectations or demands, and special times or experiences together such as romantic dinners or weekend trips to enchanted places. When affairs continue for an extended time, these experiences may feel similar to the best parts of an intense courtship or sustained honeymoon. The feelings of love and attachment that can accompany such experiences are genuine and often powerful. They result in part from an outside relationship that has been carefully nurtured by one or both participants and sheltered from many of the stressors that marriages or other long-term committed relationships inevitably confront. The participants maintain the affair in part to avoid the emotional loss that would occur otherwise. In some instances, the participating partner and the outside person might have made long-term commitments to each other. If strong positive feelings for the outside person persist, the participating partner might experience ending the affair as a betrayal of that person. Affair couples sometimes discuss the fact that difficult times might lie ahead for their relationship, but insist that they will be there for each other even when times are rough.

Addressing feelings of love and attachment to the outside person can be quite challenging in conjoint sessions. The participating partner may be reluctant to disclose such feelings to the injured partner, who may feel deeply wounded or threatened in listening to the participating partner's feelings for a third person. However, failure to address these feelings at some level potentially leaves the injured partner unaware of an important factor in the affair's continuation or the participating partner poorly equipped to deal with feelings of loss. We use an understated language that refers to "missing" the other person or the closeness of that relationship. When appropriate, we also relate such feelings to the participating partner's tendency to associate emotional and physical closeness to each other, an attitude that potentially serves the primary relationship quite well, as reflected in the following exchange involving Pam and Tom:

THERAPIST: Pam, it sounds like once you and Mark became intimate, it became more than just a physical relationship.

PAM: Yes, even from the beginning.

THERAPIST: You're not the kind of person who's likely to be sexual with someone you don't also care about on a personal level . . .

PAM: No . . .

THERAPIST: And on one hand that's a good thing—preferring to combine emotional with physical closeness—but it also possibly makes that relationship more difficult to stop as well as more hurtful to Tom.

TOM: I try not to think of that . . .

THERAPIST: It's difficult, I know. We've talked before about how affair relationships are different from a marriage—protected from daily hassles and
stresses—and how that tends to allow positive feelings to continue or
become more intense. This understanding is important partly as a way
of making sense of how Pam's affair could have continued but also in
understanding some of the feelings that accompanied your decision to
end that relationship, Pam.

PAM: I needed to make a decision, and I chose my marriage. I want this to
work, Tom.

TOM: Then why do you sometimes still pull back from me?

PAM: Because sometimes things still aren't right between us. You get upset
with me or we're arguing about the kids or about my need to work while
at home or whatever . . . You can't expect me to feel close to you at those
times.

THERAPIST: It's hard sometimes, because you've made a decision based on your
values and what you want in the long run, but in the meantime you've
chosen—for good reasons—to end one relationship that was devoted
exclusively to positive experiences in order to recommit and work on
your relationship with Tom.

PAM: That's right . . .

THERAPIST: And, right now, you and Tom are really struggling . . .

PAM: Yes, sometimes. But I try to remind myself of our better times in the past
and my hope that we can recover those kinds of feelings.

TOM: I'm hoping for that too, Pam.

As Pam's comments suggest, an affair can be more difficult to end when
the positive aspects of that relationship are accompanied by deep pessimism
about the primary relationship's potential to improve. Moreover, separate
from positive feelings for the outside person, the participating partner sometimes feels responsible for the outsider's well-being. Participating partners prepared to end an affair can still fail to do so if the outside person persists in
expressing deep desires or needs for the relationship, emotional fragility, or,
in more extreme cases, threats of self-harm. In some cases, threats by the
outside person are not about self-harm but instead about retaliation against
the participating partner (e.g., by threatening to make the affair public). And,
of course, some affairs are maintained not from a sense of responsibility but

rather from a sense of entitlement and limited concerns about the affair being discovered.

Injured partners also struggle with understanding *how* the participating partner simultaneously maintained the affair and their own relationship, particularly if the primary relationship remained generally positive and there were few indications of involvement with an outside person. It is not unusual for an injured partner to exclaim, "How could you go on that way, making love with her and then coming home for dinner and making love with me as though nothing was going on?" In addressing such concerns, it is useful to talk with both partners about the process of *compartmentalization*, which potentially permitted the participating partner to mentally isolate thoughts and feelings from the two conflicting relationships.

We help partners understand the process of compartmentalization by first describing common examples from everyday life, such as trying to shut out conflict from home when focusing on challenges at work. For example, few passengers would want an airplane pilot to think about a recent argument with his or her partner while piloting the airplane. Thus, compartmentalization can be an adaptive cognitive–emotional process, but when it is applied to two simultaneous romantic relationships, its use is misdirected. For most participating partners, engaging in an affair *does* create inner conflict at some level, whether clearly experienced or not. Some participating partners minimize their internal conflict, sometimes quite successfully, by compartmentalizing or keeping the two relationships separate in how they experience the world. Many participating partners in one way or another explain, "When I was with you and the kids, I was engaged and not focusing on my other relationship. When I was with her, I managed to shut you out and just enjoyed that relationship. It may sound terrible, but that is what I did."

Understandably, injured partners struggle with such an explanation because it portrays a rather extreme "mental gymnastic" to be able to separate major parts of life in this way. Completely shutting out thoughts of one intense relationship when involved in a different one goes beyond typical daily experiences of compartmentalization. Furthermore, if such an explanation is accepted, it can be frightening because it suggests that having a good relationship is not enough to ensure against an affair. Moreover, the participating partner's ability to compartmentalize and demonstrate happiness in the primary relationship means the injured partner might not recognize that another relationship exists. When compartmentalization is a significant factor in developing or maintaining an affair, helping the participating partner to live life in an integrated manner can be a significant challenge.

Qualities of the Participating Partner
That Interfere with Recovery

When examining individual aspects of the participating partner, it is important to consider not only those factors that contributed to the onset of the affair but also those qualities that may make recovery more difficult. For example, the participating partner may have limited tolerance for continued negative responses from the injured partner or may feel frustrated with the slow, difficult process of recovery. If so, reviewing issues discussed earlier in the therapy (e.g., the traumatic impact of the affair for the injured partner, the likelihood of continued occasional flashbacks, and differences in subjective time lines) may help to increase the participating partner's tolerance and patience.

Occasionally, participating partners remain mired in their own guilt and shame about the affair. Sometimes that guilt serves to reassure the injured partner of the participating partner's remorse and decrease the injured partner's insecurity or punishing behaviors. At other times, the participating partner's guilt persists despite genuine entreaties from the injured partner to let go of the guilt as a way of moving forward together. In those situations, we may talk about the adverse impact of sustained or exaggerated guilt and discuss ways of challenging those feelings. In essence, the participating partner might have difficulty forgiving him- or herself, a topic that we address more fully in Chapter 13.

The participating partner may also have difficulty fully engaging in the recovery process if he or she remains ambivalent about the decision to end the outside relationship or feels doubtful or pessimistic about the long-term outcome of the primary relationship. Such ambivalence, although understandable, eventually takes an emotional toll on both partners and becomes a self-fulfilling prophecy. We emphasize with participating partners that holding back and not working to strengthen this relationship to the fullest extent possible greatly increases the likelihood that it will not succeed. Similarly, holding onto the outside relationship, either in fantasy or by continuing to interact emotionally or physically with the outside person, virtually guarantees that the relationship with the injured partner will remain compromised. Consciously or not, some participating partners "allow" their committed relationship to dwindle and end by failing to make a full effort to improve it. For some participating partners, this "slow death" is easier than directly confronting the decision to end the committed relationship, either to be alone or to pursue the relationship with the outside person. If you sense that such a process might be happening, it is important to raise this concern directly.

Potential Contributions from the Injured Partner

Managing Context and Process

Similar to examining individual factors from the participating partner, when exploring potential contributions from the injured partner, it is important first to establish a context for this work and then actively direct the therapeutic process. The most critical context involves reemphasizing that, *regardless of his or her contributions to vulnerability in the couple's relationship, the injured partner is not responsible for the participating partner's decision to engage in an affair.* We restate the goals of examining the injured partner's contributions to the primary relationship, namely to gain a more balanced view of the participating partner and to lay the foundation for subsequent efforts toward relationship change. Moreover, in addition to exploring the injured partner's potential role in relationship vulnerability contributing to the onset of the affair, it is important to examine aspects of the injured partner adversely influencing the recovery process.

By and large, as the therapist, you want the injured partner to take the lead in this exploration process rather than allowing the participating partner to point out shortcomings of the injured partner. Typically, participating partners have already shared enough information in discussing relationship factors or their own feelings related to the affair that injured partners have ample basis for considering their own contributions to the relationship problems. For example, you might begin with, "Ian, you've been listening over the past few sessions to Hannah's description of what it was like for her in the relationship before her affair as well as her efforts to recommit to her relationship with you now. Can you talk some about how that's been helpful to you in thinking about your own roles in your relationship?"

However, there may be times when the participating partner needs to be more than simply a participant-observer in the injured partner's exploration, because the participating partner has a unique perspective on how the injured partner potentially contributed to susceptibility to an affair. Moreover, injured partners who are still hurt and confused about how the participating partner could have become involved in an affair may actively seek more explanations from the participating partner during examination of their own roles: "I really want to know: What did I do or not do that contributed to this?" As the therapist, you need to titrate the participating partner's involvement in the therapeutic process at this stage carefully, sometimes facilitating engagement but also ensuring that the injured partner retains the primary lead in order to minimize defensiveness or reactivity.

Similar to the process for examining contributions from the participating partner, we generally advocate beginning with more recent experiences, such as those in the relationship before or after revelation of the affair, before exploring earlier developmental experiences outside of the current relationship. Exploring childhood or adolescent experiences too early runs the risk of provoking defensive resistance to examining more enduring or unresolved issues. Hence, we begin with thoughts and feelings more readily accessible to the injured partner before exploring those lying outside of immediate awareness.

When possible in order to reduce defensiveness or blame, we reframe aspects of the injured partner potentially contributing to the affair as having positive elements as well. We may promote a discussion of how the injured partner might have had positive intentions or motivations, but the way that those motivations were carried out in the relationship actually might have helped create the context for the affair. For example, "Ryan, you've heard and acknowledged Donna's frustrations with your tendency to avoid discussions of your relationship that, in some ways, led her to feel more desperate. But I'm wondering whether your not wanting to get into such discussions sometimes reflected your wish to protect the relationship from what felt like destructive arguments. Can you talk about how you struggled with that balance?"

In the following sections, we consider aspects of the injured partner that potentially increased the vulnerability of the relationship to an affair as well as the injured partner's reactions to the affair that might make recovery more difficult now. A summary of these possible influences from the injured partner is provided in Table 10.2.

Factors Contributing to Vulnerability in the Relationship

Initial cues regarding contributions of the injured partner to vulnerability in the relationship may come from prior discussions of the relationship or from the participating partner's descriptions of thoughts, feelings, or needs that contributed to the affair. In this regard, helping the injured partner to explore his or her role in risk factors considered previously in Chapters 8 and 9 may be productive. For example, in what ways did the injured partner contribute to negative exchanges in the relationship: by initiating or escalating arguments or by being demanding or critical? Did the injured partner show low tolerance for differences in opinions or preferences, insisting on agreement or confusing preferences with core values? Some partners contribute to a cold or antagonistic atmosphere not by escalating in negative ways but instead by holding onto hurts and being slow to forgive or reengage in efforts to resolve differences.

TABLE 10.2. Potential Contributing Factors from the Injured Partner

Aspects of the injured partner that contribute to vulnerability of the relationship before the affair

- Difficulty in meeting a partner's needs (e.g., for emotional or physical intimacy or for personal growth and fulfillment).
- Unrealistic expectations or demands placed on the participating partner.
- Negative behaviors that were too frequent or intense (e.g., excessive criticism or unwillingness to work toward compromise).
- Difficulty in recovering from relationship disappointments or conflicts.
- Difficulty in recognizing or dealing with differences in relationship patterns or styles of thinking and feeling.
- Reluctance to acknowledge or work on own contributions to relationship difficulties.

Factors leading to delay in detecting or responding to signs of vulnerability to a potential affair

- Ignoring signs of the participating partner's increasing emotional or physical withdrawal.
- Minimizing the participating partner's concerns about the marriage/committed relationship or requests to consider couple counseling.
- Overlooking behaviors reflecting possible problems with boundaries (e.g., excessive flirtation or time alone with an outside person or secrecy about interactions with another person).

Qualities of the injured partner that make recovery more difficult for him- or herself

- Reluctance or inability to engage in self-care behaviors.
- Fear of vulnerability leading to unwillingness to risk closeness again.
- Moral convictions that block efforts to reconcile with an offending partner.
- Personal pride or influence from others discouraging efforts to work on the marriage/committed relationship.

Qualities of the injured partner that make recovery more difficult for the participating partner

- Difficulty in containing intense negative emotions such as anger, anxiety, or grief, which make positive interactions or constructive discussions more challenging.
- Efforts to undermine the participating partner's relationships with important others such as children, extended family, or friends who support the marriage/committed relationship.
- Persistent pursuit of additional details that do not contribute to a better understanding of the affair or repeatedly going over details that are already known.

Injured partners also sometimes contribute to their relationship's vulnerability by their emotional distance. They may be detached and unresponsive, or they may simply lack relationship awareness, leaving the participating partner without opportunities for sharing deep feelings. Other injured partners may lack the capacity or the desire to engage in discussions about inner thoughts and feelings. Sometimes a partner's low levels of emotional responsiveness or enthusiasm may be seen by the other as detracting from opportunities for sharing excitement, passion, play, or joy.

Lack of physical closeness can also place a relationship at risk. To what extent did the injured partner find it uncomfortable or simply lack interest in pursuing closeness through hugs, hand-holding, kisses, or sexual intimacy before the affair? It is useful to distinguish between discomfort or disinterest in physical closeness that predates the couple's relationship versus similar feelings that emerged in response to other relationship difficulties. Problems of sexual desire or arousal and specific sexual dysfunctions, or, conversely, high demands regarding frequency or content of sexual exchanges may all serve to disrupt the couple's physical intimacy and promote consideration of sexual involvement with an outside person.

The couple's relationship may have incurred increased risk by the injured partner's overinvolvement in activities or responsibilities either within or outside the home. It is not enough simply to identify examples of overinvolvement; rather, as the therapist, you should explore the underlying reasons for such behaviors. For example, exaggerated involvement in children's activities may relate to the injured partner's own experience of disinterested or uninvolved parents as a child and a determination to parent in a different way. Also, some men have affairs shortly after the birth of a child in response to feeling displaced or unimportant as the wife places a major focus on the newborn. In these instances, although the high demands of parenting an infant might be an important factor in the context for the affair, the couple still needs to explore whether the ways that one or both partners responded to this demand could have been handled better. Another form of overinvolvement—excessive devotion to work—may stem from underlying worries about being an adequate provider or enduring self-doubts from previous failures. Regardless of the specific content of these risk factors, the goals of exploring and reframing underlying vulnerabilities of the injured partner are twofold: (1) to enhance self-understanding in order to make these dispositions more amenable to change and (2) to promote empathic awareness by the participating partner of those underlying causes contributing to the injured partner's behaviors.

Delay in Detecting or Responding to Risk Indicators

Although there is ample evidence suggesting a higher risk of infidelity among individuals experiencing marital distress (see Allen et al., 2005, for a review), other findings suggest that as many as one half of married men and one third of married women reporting involvement in extramarital sex describe their marriage as "happy" or "very happy" before the affair (Glass & Wright, 1985). Hence, it is not reasonable to presume that the injured partner should have been able to detect the partner's unhappiness or vulnerability to an affair before its occurrence. Nor do we suggest that, even if the injured partner had responded to such indicators, the affair would not have happened. Rather, we approach these issues recognizing that, for a significant percentage of couples, there are a variety of ways in which an injured partner's failure to recognize or respond to clear "warning signs" may have contributed to the risk of an affair developing or continuing.

One such path involves overlooking or ignoring signs of relationship difficulties, including the partner's emotional or physical withdrawal. This pattern may relate to the injured partner's pervasive trust in the participating partner, an inability to conceive of unfaithfulness by someone in a caring, committed relationship, or a tolerance for periods of relationship distress and optimism that relationship problems will resolve on their own in due time. Sometimes an injured partner's failure to respond to relationship difficulties involves denial or avoidance of uncomfortable discussions, leaving the participating partner pessimistic regarding the potential for constructive change. A heightened form of such avoidance involves continued resistance to repeated requests for couple counseling.

Another way in which injured partners may contribute to the risk of infidelity is by overlooking the participating partner's clear violations of implicit or explicit relationship boundaries. There is a distinction between pathological jealousy and appropriate questioning of a partner's excessive flirting or secrecy about interactions with others. Similarly, there is a difference between pathological possessiveness and establishment of clear boundaries that differentiate what behaviors should occur solely between committed partners and those that can occur in other relationships. Failure to recognize and respond to inappropriate behaviors may reflect a poor understanding of healthy relationship boundaries, or it may indicate self-doubts and reluctance to provoke the other person's negative reactions when restrictions on that person's behaviors are requested or imposed. As the therapist, you need to distinguish between the need to educate partners about appropriate boundaries versus the need to strengthen partners in asserting and adhering to relationship boundaries that they already comprehend.

Qualities Interfering with Recovery for Self or Partner

Just as important as factors contributing to a partner's affair are those influencing recovery. Injured partners can make recovery more difficult for themselves by failing to engage in adequate self-care or by engaging in behaviors that are harmful to themselves either emotionally or physically. We noted the importance of self-care earlier in Chapter 5 when describing strategies for restoring emotional and physical equilibrium. Being physically or mentally exhausted precludes the energy required for difficult relationship discussions or repair and leaves the individual more emotionally fragile and reactive. Failing to pursue appropriate outside social support reduces resilience to ongoing frustrations in the couple's relationship. The heightened emotional reactivity that accompanies inadequate self-care, including intense anger, anxiety, or grief, can also make recovery for the participating partner more difficult. Recurrent emotional volatility of either partner eventually wears the relationship down, leaves both partners discouraged or exhausted, and robs partners of the opportunity to restore secure attachment or build hope for the future. As the therapist, you may need to reexamine issues of self-care in either partner, not only as a means for restoring equilibrium but also as an essential step in the ongoing recovery process.

Recovery may also be hindered by an injured partner's persistent insecurity or reluctance to take steps toward rebuilding emotional and physical closeness. Apprehensions about becoming emotionally vulnerable or being hurt again are a normal response to an affair, and these concerns are not likely to disappear either quickly or completely. As the therapist, you need to facilitate a balance between recognizing and responding empathically to understandable anxiety or "holding back" and, at the same time, promoting informed risk taking and moving forward to rebuild intimacy and trust. We talk further about rebuilding trust in Chapter 14. During Stage 2, a more immediate concern may be the need to address the injured partner's persistent pursuit of further explanations or details of the affair that do not contribute to a better understanding of why it occurred. Such questioning typically is aimed at reducing feelings of vulnerability based on a belief or hope that if every possible aspect of the affair could become known, the affair might be more understandable or at least less likely to recur in the future. Of course, Stage 2 is based on the premise that reaching a shared understanding of contributing factors is essential to recovery. However, also important to recovery is the injured partner's becoming reconciled to the realization that the participating partner's affair may never make "complete" sense and that the possibility of a recurrence can be significantly reduced but never entirely eliminated.

Injured partners also need to be confronted with any negative behaviors toward the participating partner that are blocking recovery. Persistent anger can seep into daily interactions in countless ways, for example, reminding the participating partner continuously of his or her offense, undermining relationships with children or extended family, insisting on unreasonable constraints such as having no social interactions except those monitored by the injured partner, and so on. Sometimes such behaviors are driven primarily by the wish to retaliate and punish the participating partner. In other cases, injured partners may be following misguided advice from family or friends to "tighten the leash" or show the participating partner that he or she "can't just get away with this." Injured partners may also persist in endless questioning or other negative behaviors from an underlying fear that if they relinquish these behaviors, the participating partner might forget what has happened and be more susceptible to violating boundaries again. In essence, some of the ways that injured partners behave negatively toward participating partners described in Chapter 4 can persist and make recovery much more difficult. Exploring specific factors underlying continued negative behaviors hindering recovery is a prerequisite to engaging effectively in interventions to address those influences.

In the session described next, the therapist helped Vicki explore ways in which her own feelings were making recovery from Bill's affair more difficult. Vicki and Bill had already explored Bill's feelings of helplessness during Vicki's depression after her father's death. However, Vicki's continuing regrets and feelings of guilt about her depression were making it more difficult for her to embrace opportunities for closeness between the two partners currently.

VICKI: I still feel responsible somehow . . .

BILL: Vicki, we've been over and over that. You're not responsible. The affair was my decision—I'm not proud of that, but I own it. I wish you could just move on . . .

THERAPIST: There's a tone of frustration in that . . .

BILL: Yes. I feel horrible for Vicki, not only for what I put her through but now for what she continues to put herself through. And ultimately I feel like . . . (long pause)

THERAPIST: You feel like . . . (waiting)

BILL: . . . Like it keeps us stuck. And then I feel awful even saying that because it sounds like I'm blaming Vicki for our struggles when I'm the one who had the affair.

VICKI: Well, I feel awful too, Bill, because I know that even though it was your decision to have the affair, I contributed to making things worse for you.

THERAPIST: Vicki, I appreciate your openness to looking at how your own role in the marriage and ways in which you weren't at your best possibly contributed to the difficulties you and Bill were having before his affair. But what's important is being able to use that information to figure out how to avoid similar risks in the future. What I'm hearing from Bill is his concern that, rather than using the understanding to strengthen your marriage, right now it's making you feel even worse. And that's getting in the way of moving forward . . .

VICKI: I'm not sure what to do about it. I mean, I can see how it's getting in the way . . .

THERAPIST: But seeing how it's getting in the way hasn't helped you get beyond it . . .

VICKI: No.

THERAPIST: Could we look at how blaming yourself—as bad as that feels—is maybe serving some kind of protective role for you?

VICKI: What do you mean?

THERAPIST: Well, I'm not exactly sure. But, for example, it does keep you and Bill from becoming more intimate and maybe that feels safer right now. Or maybe when you blame yourself, it makes the affair feel more under your control somehow and less scary than if it were in Bill's hands. As you hear me say this, does any of it seem possible or likely to you?

VICKI: I don't want to stay distant . . .

THERAPIST: No, I don't think you like the distance either. But when you think about getting really close again—both emotionally and physically—and trusting in that really deep way we've talked about, what feelings go along with those thoughts?

VICKI: Well, sometimes it feels really good and I start feeling hopeful again.

THERAPIST: And other times?

VICKI: (long pause) . . . Sometimes I feel absolute panic. I know I shouldn't, but I do – and I don't have any way of talking with Bill about that without hurting his feelings or pushing him further away.

BILL: Vicki, you're not going to push me away by talking with me. What does make me feel pushed away is when you refuse to talk about your feelings and pull back into your shell and blame yourself. That's what is pushing me away.

THERAPIST: Vicki, let me try to help you talk with Bill about that panic in ways that I think he can hear and can help you feel less frightened . . . less frightened about having the feelings and less scared about what will happen if you share them with Bill . . .

After this exchange, Vicki was able to examine how her continued guilt related to a long-standing disposition to blame herself for hurtful or disappointing events in her life and how this tendency placed her at higher risk for depression. As she began to view her own contributions from a more balanced perspective, Bill was able to examine his roles in the marriage and behaviors culminating in the affair in a more complete and balanced manner as well. For example, he was able to express empathy for Vicki's struggle with depression while also describing his frustrations with the distance it created between them.

Summary

Examining individual factors that increase vulnerability to an affair is an important extension from considering what was going on *around* partners to exploring what was going on *inside* them. This expansion in focus often elicits heightened defensiveness and reactivity between partners. The work may also be more difficult if partners have limited capacity for articulating their own thoughts and feelings or responding empathically to those of each other.

Establishing the context for this work and carefully managing the therapeutic process are critical to this phase of Stage 2 interventions. The relevance of more distal experiences in partners' lives varies considerably across couples and individual partners. The more remote, emotionally difficult, or inaccessible these experiences are, the more likely you will need to emphasize more individually focused interventions within conjoint sessions to address them. As a general rule, we advise pursuing a process that moves from more recent to more distant events and from more conscious thoughts and feelings to those that lie outside immediate awareness. It is important to emphasize individual strengths as well as needs or deficits that potentially contributed to increased vulnerability to an affair.

Despite successfully examining influences from within and outside the relationship and exploring potential individual risk factors from each partner, some couples continue to struggle because of particularly complicated affairs, such as those in which the outside person holds a special position of trust or power. We consider these special circumstances further in the next chapter.

Resources from *Getting Past the Affair*

In our companion self-help book for couples, *Chapter 9*, "How Could My Partner Have Done This?," emphasizes factors from the participating partner that may have contributed to the affair. These factors include influences that potentially led to initial involvement in an affair as well as those that contributed to the affair's continuation. For couples for whom the affair is still ongoing, this chapter addresses factors that may have a role in this as well. Chapter 9 in the self-help book also considers reasons the participating partner may be finding it difficult to move on emotionally, even after the affair has ended. Exercise 9.1 encourages partners to examine aspects of the participating partner that may have initially contributed to the affair, whereas Exercise 9.2 addresses features of the participating partner that may either help or hinder recovery.

Chapter 10, "What Was My Role?," follows a similar path, initially examining features of the injured partner that may have potentially rendered the couple's relationship more vulnerable to an affair as well as aspects of the injured partner that may be either helping or hindering recovery. That chapter also encourages the injured partner to consider whether he or she missed potential warning signs along the way that would have indicated vulnerability to an affair and whether the injured partner can take steps currently to reduce the likelihood of an affair's recurrence in the future. Exercise 10.1 encourages partners to examine aspects of the injured partner that may have initially contributed to vulnerability in the couple's relationship, and Exercise 10.2 addresses features of the injured partner that may be facilitating or hindering recovery.

CHAPTER 11

Complex Affairs

A s noted throughout this book, infidelity involves a complicated set of phenomena for couples to address and for a therapist to manage clinically. Any time there is a significant violation of trust in a couple's relationship, the effects are likely to be damaging, if not devastating. Although we have provided a wide range of clinical examples that demonstrate the "many faces of infidelity," most affairs include two consenting adults who are "equals" in most regards. However, some affairs involve relationships in which this sense of equality between the two persons involved in the affair is not present (e.g., when the outside person is a supervisor or pastor). In these cases, making sense of the affair becomes more complicated. When a sense of inequity exists between the two persons having an affair, it is likely to change how the couple attributes responsibility to the participating partner. In addition, assumptions about other individuals and even institutions can be shattered. Therefore, it is important to give consideration to infidelity that occurs within the context of such "special relationships."

Moreover, once an outside person becomes a part of the participating partner's life, the participating partner might give lower priority to the injured partner or in some way begin relating differently. Even so, during an affair, most participating partners continue to live with their spouses or committed partners, along with their children. That is, even while an affair is ongoing, the basic family unit of functioning continues in some fashion, even if it is compromised. However, there are instances in which the injured partner learns that the participating partner has been leading a "double life" that goes far beyond emotional or sexual involvement with another individual. In such circumstances, the injured partner must deal not only with deception and violations of exclusivity but also with a newfound uncertainty about the meaning of the relationship and, more broadly, the injured person's entire adult life. Thus, some affairs take on such magnitude and scope that the psychological meaning or interpretation of life as a committed couple and experiences over many years come into question.

These atypical or increasingly complex affairs demonstrate many of the same characteristics that we have discussed thus far, and the overall treatment strategy is the same. Therefore, in the current chapter, we do not introduce different or unique intervention strategies. However, these particularly complex situations require that, as the therapist, you remain attentive to specific factors that will need to be emphasized in helping couples come to grips with these potentially overwhelming life circumstances.

Affairs with Persons in Trusted Positions

Trusted Professional Relationships

At times, an affair develops between one partner and another individual who had been placed in a particularly trusted position in the life of the participating partner or the couple. For example, one partner might become involved with a pastor, priest, or other religious leader; a therapist; or a physician. Persons in these and similar positions are generally regarded as playing unique and important roles in people's lives. In seeking services from professionals in such roles, individuals sometimes lower the boundaries that they typically observe in mutual, reciprocal relationships. For example, individuals disrobe and present their bodies for detailed scrutiny to their physicians. In doing so, individuals assume that the relationship is confined to these particular interactions within the physician's professional role. Furthermore, the focus is expected to be on the patient's needs without reciprocal concerns for the needs or desires of the physician, beyond the scope of the physician's professional responsibility.

Similarly, an individual might tell a religious leader about transgressions, temptations, or a variety of religious and spiritual concerns that would not be disclosed to other persons. Underlying such self-disclosures is the assumption that the religious leader's interest is focused on the spiritual, moral, and religious well-being of the individual making the disclosure and that the disclosed information and related vulnerability will be honored and handled appropriately. Within many organized religions, it is considered appropriate for religious leaders to visit people in their homes or in hospitals and to be available at times of grief, during illnesses, and in other situations that involve personal vulnerability. Likewise, many religious institutions consider it appropriate for a religious leader to take a person's hand or offer a hug to someone at a time of distress. These lowered boundaries are viewed as acceptable and are based on the understanding that the relationships formed at such times will not advance into personal, romantic ones.

In secular contexts, individuals often seek therapists for similar reasons: to address distress, to try to understand themselves more fully, or to seek advice or direction for troublesome aspects of their lives. In doing so, clients lower their boundaries and disclose feelings and thoughts that are rarely discussed in other settings. There is an assumed trust and expectation that the therapist will maintain appropriate personal boundaries, will use the information only to meet the client's needs, and will not become involved romantically with the client.

In all of these examples, one partner lowers a personal boundary, typically with an increased sense of vulnerability, but does so because the other individual is in a position that society deems safe and is distinguished by different norms, rules, and expectations to protect the well-being of the more vulnerable individual. When a partner has an affair with an individual in one of these positions of trust, the response of both the injured partner and the participating partner can be increasingly distressed and confused. For the injured partner, often there is a disruption not only regarding the trustworthiness of the participating partner but also in the relationship with the outside person in the trusted position as well as for the institution that the outside person represents. Such an experience typically leads to further distress and confusion if the injured partner also had a relationship with the trusted outside individual. For example, if a wife has an affair with the family physician who had treated both partners and their children for a number of years, the husband might feel violated both by his wife and by the physician, who held a significant role in his life. In essence, the husband must now deal with a sense of double betrayal.

Given that individuals in these trusted positions often represent certain professions or specific institutions, affairs with these persons can lead to disruptions of either partner's relationships with these institutions as well. For example, Leila and Martin both felt overwhelmed after Leila admitted to Martin that she had been having an affair with the pastor of their church. Both Leila and Martin had been quite involved in the church for many years, serving on various committees and assuming positions of leadership. At times, Martin had initiated counseling sessions with the pastor to seek advice about how to address Leila's periodic depression as well as their marital difficulties.

Leila was an active church volunteer, and when the pastor suggested that he and she go together a day ahead to prepare for a weekend church retreat, she felt special and honored. While alone, they had a sexual encounter, which developed into an affair lasting for several months. Finally, Leila disclosed to Martin what had happened, and after further inquiry with other couples, they discovered that the pastor had been involved with other women in the church as well. As soon as they notified church authorities, the pastor was immediately discharged. When the congregation learned what had happened, Martin and Leila were shocked to learn that some members of the congregation concluded that Leila must have seduced the pastor.

Helping this couple deal with the affair was extremely complicated. Martin had to deal not only with his sense of betrayal from Leila but also with violations of other major assumptions and with disruptions of other relationships in his life.

> "I feel like I've lost my whole world. It's horrible enough that my wife cheated and lied to me. But my own pastor and good friend seduced my wife. I can't believe it. I had gone to him and told him about Leila's depression and her problems. He knew her weaknesses and used them to seduce her. I even told him about our marital problems, and he took what I told him and gave her what she wanted from a man, things I couldn't provide. And all the time, he's standing in a pulpit preaching as a man of God. It just disgusts me. Then, to top it off, the whole congregation knows, and unbelievably, many of them are blaming Leila for the affair and us as a couple for dividing the church. We can never set foot in that church, or probably any church, again."

Not only are such affairs complicated for the injured partner, but they can be particularly difficult and confusing for the participating partner as well. The participating partner often recognizes that he or she has greatly disrupted the injured partner's and the couple's life in a multitude of ways. At times, this recognition can lead to an increased sense of guilt, shame, and self-loathing for the participating partner. For example, Leila felt extraordinary guilt for having disrupted Martin's life as well as their broader family life. Her affair was discrepant with her own value system, and in addition, she realized that she had ruined their involvement in their church and perhaps their ability to participate in any church in the future.

> "I really can't believe what I've done. I've always thought I would be one of the least likely people in the world to have an affair, and not only

did I betray Martin, I did this with his trusted friend and our pastor. How much worse can it get? You go to church to try to lead a spiritual life and then defile almost everything you value, right in that church. If there's ever an unforgivable sin, this is it. I've ruined my life, Martin's life, the pastor's life, and our whole spiritual foundation. And there's plenty of blame to spread around. I really messed this up terribly, but it's not like I was the evil temptress who went after this holy man. It seems he had been doing this for years; you literally can't trust anyone. And while the congregation seems to be loving the gossip, it's also destroying the church as the congregation decides who should be hit with the first stone: me, the pastor, or Martin for disclosing the hypocrisy. To be honest, the whole concept of organized religion disgusts me right now."

In dealing with infidelity in such contexts, the general approach to treatment is consistent with what is described throughout this book. The major difference is that a significant emphasis must be placed not only on the violation of trust between the participating and injured partner but also on the violation of trust with the outside person and perhaps with the institution represented by that individual. Moreover, this broader sense of violation of trust often is relevant for the participating partner as well as the injured partner. For example, Leila's self-loathing and guilt were as complicated to address in therapy as were Martin's extreme negative emotions and confusion. It was particularly confusing for the couple to decide how much responsibility should be attributed to Leila and how much to the pastor who had violated his special position of trust. After many months of therapy, Martin and Leila concluded that, while continuing to hold Leila responsible for her personal decision to have an affair, they also needed to accept that they were dealing with an "unhealthy preacher who used his position of trust and authority to prey on women who believed in him and turned to him for support." An important part of the therapy involved helping them to recognize that this experience was not representative of religious leaders or organized religion in general and to resist their initial inclination to overgeneralize from this single, extremely damaging situation with a disturbed individual. This understanding was particularly relevant in this case because the couple's religious and spiritual lives were a central part of their relationship and broader family functioning.

Trusted Personal Relationships

The relationships described previously involve a violation of trust with an outside person who is in a position that has been given special meaning by society, a role that encourages other people to lower typical boundaries when interacting with that person. In addition, a participating partner might have an affair with someone with whom there is a high level of trust because of *personal* relationships that have developed. For example, one partner might have an affair with the other partner's best friend. As in the prior situations, there is a sense of betrayal not only from one's partner but from one's friend as well. Moreover, the very concept of friendship and the trustworthiness of friends in general might be called into question. Even if the couple's relationship survives, the relationship with the trusted friend almost always ends, a casualty of the infidelity.

The injured partner or the couple can almost always decide to end a relationship with a friend; however, the situation becomes increasingly complex if the affair is with a family member. Infidelity with brothers-in-law, sisters-in-law, aunts, uncles, and other family members also occur in real life. When such affairs happen, not only are there multiple betrayals in terms of the participating partner and the other family member, but also the overall security and structure of the extended family can be threatened. Of particular importance is how the couple decides to address the decision of whether to make the affair known to the rest of the family. Many couples report grave concern that making other family members aware of the affair will significantly disrupt or split the broader family as a unit. They note that many family members will likely take sides with one person or the other, depending on the previous quality of the relationships. In addition, having family gatherings or coming together to celebrate holidays or special family events such as birthdays or anniversaries can seem impossible once the affair becomes known. Conversely, if the affair is not made known, finding ways to avoid interacting with the outside person who is a family member can be quite taxing. Being unavailable for holidays and family gatherings on a regular basis can lead to hard feelings or confrontations with members of the extended family.

With such couples, significant attention during therapy will likely need to be focused on the issue of what to tell other family members and how to restructure family interactions in the future. We do not take a given position on this very complex issue, but we do offer cautions consistent with those raised elsewhere in this book. First, the couple must recognize that once this information about the affair is disclosed to other family members, it cannot be retracted. There can, indeed, be significant complications for the broader family as members try to deal with such an extreme violation between family members, and it can be difficult to anticipate how the family might respond. Second, the couple must be clear about the reasons why they would or would not share this information with other family members. Turning to other family members for support in such situations should be done only with great caution because of the likelihood that various family members will choose sides. On the other hand, if the couple has significant concern that the other family member involved in the affair might initiate sexual relationships with additional family members, perhaps even people who are minors, then the couple might decide to share the information judiciously to protect other individuals.

Affairs with Persons in Hierarchical Relationships

The prior relationships are noteworthy because they involve violations with persons who are assumed to be trustworthy, either because of societal norms or personal relationships. Although not totally distinct, other affairs are complicated because the two people involved have unequal authority, power, or influence. Generally, these affairs involve a dual role relationship in which there is some other major basis for interacting in addition to the romantic relationship. Frequently, this kind of relationship occurs in a work setting in which one person has some form of professional authority over the other, such as an immediate supervisor, someone in a higher administrative position, or a teacher. These types of situations are more explicit than those discussed previously, because in this case the individual in the more powerful position often has direct control over the other individual's success in the form of promotions, raises, or job responsibilities.

A complicating factor is whether the less powerful person has free will to make a decision about becoming involved in a romantic relationship or whether implicit or explicit coercion has occurred. For this reason, many businesses and institutions consider it a form of sexual harassment to develop a romantic relationship between two persons within a hierarchy, even if both persons appear to consent to the relationship. The concern is whether the person in the less powerful position really has free will to consent to or reject such a relationship or to terminate it without adverse consequences.

It is important to realize that in such situations neither person might be thinking about the power differential or using it maliciously to develop a romantic relationship. In fact, both persons might be attracted to each other and eager for a relationship to develop. Still, the power differential or influence one person has over the other outside of the romantic relationship can significantly interfere with the less powerful person's ability to make ongoing decisions about the relationship. On the other hand, the person in the less powerful position might actually gain great influence outside of the romantic relationship; having a "fling with the boss" might give one great advantage at work and provide a potential threat to the boss if the relationship goes sour: "I think you might want to give me that raise I've been asking you about."

If the participating partner of a couple in treatment is in the less powerful position, then decisions must be made that are similar to those discussed previously regarding infidelity with a family member or person in a trusted position. First, will the couple make the affair known to the business or institution within which the affair occurred? In some instances, one or both members of the couple may conclude that the participating partner has been abused or treated unfairly by the person in the more powerful position and might want to take either legal or informal action to express the grievance. At times, taking such an action can be difficult for the couple if the participating partner does not want colleagues to know about the affair, but the injured partner wants the outside individual "to pay for what he or she has done." In reaching this decision, the couple must be willing to bear the consequences of making the affair known in the workplace, with an awareness that legal action could result in retaliation against or an attempt to "smear" the participating member of the couple. Equally important, the couple must be cautious that they are not focusing their negative feelings and overall distress on the outside person as a way of avoiding or deflecting a focus on their own relationship and each of them as individuals. In general, we recommend to couples that they not make important, irreversible decisions while they are in a state of extreme distress and confusion, such as during Stage 1. Thus, we typically suggest that the couple proceed slowly before initiating actions such as lawsuits or confrontations in the workplace.

Second, this inequity in power likely influences how the couple attributes responsibility for the affair. If the participating partner was in the less powerful position, then one or both partners may hold the participating partner less responsible. Although this view is understandable, it is important that the couple continue to explore the participating partner's role in the affair so that they do not develop a distorted, overly simplistic conceptualization of how the affair occurred. Totally absolving the less powerful participating partner runs the risk of failing to evaluate changes that one or both partners need to make in the future to minimize the likelihood of another affair.

A different pattern is likely to emerge if the participating partner is in the more powerful position in the affair. In such circumstances, one or both members of the couple are likely to hold the participating partner particularly responsible for the affair. Along with the attributions of increased responsibility, feelings of disgust or disrespect for the participating partner can develop: "I can't believe that as a 40-year-old, well-respected professor, you got involved with a college sophomore. Don't you have any scruples at all? I don't hold her responsible one bit. You should have known better and stopped it before it ever started. You disgust me."

Although the treatment for such couples proceeds in a manner consistent with the steps already discussed, helping the couple develop a well-balanced perspective on the affair can be particularly difficult when the participating partner appears to have abused his or her position of respect or authority in developing the affair. It is also important to remember that the goal of treatment is to help the couple develop a realistic perspective on the affair, and in some instances the picture that evolves will not cast the participating partner in a compassionate light. At the same time, it is critical that, as a therapist, you do not allow your own negative reactions to the participating partner to subtly influence how the affair is conceptualized. Maintaining neutrality can be challenging if the participating partner has behaved in ways that are particularly distasteful to you or are far outside your own value system.

Affairs of Unusual Length or Breadth

Affairs can vary in length from one-night stands to ongoing relationships over many years. Different patterns are likely to lead to differing responses when the affair is first discovered and as the couple explores the context of the infidelity during Stage 2 of treatment. Even when an affair has been ongoing for quite some time, in many instances the relationship with the outside person remains somewhat confined, with an emphasis on emotional or sexual involvement. That is, frequently the participating partner maintains his or her ongoing daily life with the injured partner during the affair, living together, meeting family responsibilities, and perhaps being a good parent to the children. As we have noted previously, the discovery of an affair in this context can be devastating.

The affair tends to be even more upsetting and disorienting when it has become a central part of the life of the participating partner. In some instances, the injured partner concludes that the participating partner has been leading a double life or, even more extremely, that the participating partner's true life was with the outside person and that the committed relationship was a charade or was "staged." For example, the participating partner might have supported the outside person financially, established a secret residence with the outside person, or perhaps had a child with that individual. Such affairs not only disrupt the injured partner's sense of trust of the participating partner and experience of exclusivity, but more broadly they call into question the injured partner's experience of the relationship and perhaps of his or her adult life more generally. Thus, broader assumptions are likely to be challenged as a result of such affairs. Rhonda expressed her devastation after learning about Steve's "double life."

RHONDA: I've been married to this man for 30 years. I helped put him through school, and we both worked hard to raise two children. We decided together that I would give up my career and stay home to raise them, which I was happy to do. It was *our* plan, *our* family, *our* future. And I naively thought that it was working; I thought we both were happy and satisfied. Over the years, I've supported some of my women friends who were having marital problems, and I was always so thankful for Steve's and my relationship. Now I find that Steve's frequent business trips to his company's headquarters on the West Coast for the past 15 years involved being with her, staying in her apartment, and basically living a separate life with her. I literally cannot comprehend it; it seems about as far fetched as saying that martians have been living in our guest room for the past decade, and I just didn't know it. My entire adult life has been a farce; it means nothing.

THERAPIST: Rhonda, I can certainly understand why this feels totally devastating and incomprehensible. And it sounds like it makes you question not only Steve and who he is but also yourself and your own life. Would you clarify what that's like for you?

RHONDA: I wish I could. It's mainly just overwhelming. I think it's that when I married Steve, a big part of my identity became being his wife and mother to our children. I'm not one of these women who are totally self-sacrificing and got lost in the process, but being a wife and mother is a large part of what my life has been about for decades. And over the years, I've looked back on it with a real sense of satisfaction and gratification, and I've looked forward to the future—to retirement, having grandchildren, to traveling with Steve to visit them—and feeling good about what we've accomplished together and how we've given to others. And now it's like I've just awakened to realize that all that good stuff was something I was dreaming, that has nothing to do with reality. (*turning to Steve*) You couldn't just have an affair like most men; you had to set up a whole second life and destroy mine in the process. This isn't just about your involvement with someone else, which would be bad enough; you've robbed me of 30 years of being a wife and mother. Literally, the life that

I thought I had been living all this time doesn't even exist; it was just a fantasy. What's left?

Such affairs can be difficult not only for the injured partner but also for other family members if the affair disrupts their sense of family as well. Tammy was a 23-year-old single woman who worked for her father and thought she was her father's only child and the "apple of his eye" until she discovered a letter to him from an adolescent female calling him "Dad." After looking through his files at work, she found a whole series of letters and cards that made clear to her that her father had a daughter with another woman in a different state. She confronted him, and after an initial denial, he confirmed that he had had a brief affair, which had led to a pregnancy, and that he now had a 17-year-old daughter. Although feeling extremely guilty about what had happened, he had informed his wife years ago and concluded that the only "moral" thing to do was to develop a relationship with this second daughter and support her financially. Although Tammy's mother was aware of the situation, she avoided any discussion of what had occurred. Although the crisis of Stage 1 had long since passed, the couple had never processed the affair, and it had contributed to a gradual withdrawal and distancing in their marital relationship over many years. Tammy's discovery of her half-sister reawakened the issue, which led to couple therapy for her parents to address the affair and their gradually declining relationship. In addition, the three of them entered into family therapy to address Tammy's sense of extreme betrayal by her father and by her mother, who had kept the secret from her as well. In such a situation, the family therapy would proceed generally according to the guidelines presented in this book. However, in Stage 2, there would be less discussion of the details regarding the father's decision to have an affair because this information would be viewed as inappropriate to discuss with their daughter. Instead, a major emphasis would be placed on helping the daughter understand her parents' decision to keep the other child's existence a secret, a major betrayal that she was experiencing. Time would also be spent in helping the daughter define a new sense of family and decide what to do about her half-sister: whether to pursue a relationship with her or not.

Treatment Implications

As we noted earlier, helping couples address these more complicated affairs does not necessarily require special or different intervention techniques beyond those described throughout this text. However, the treatment might require more sessions and certain emphases or points of focus, depending on the complicating nature of the affair. In some ways, the injured partner can be seen as experiencing multiple traumas from these affairs. For example, infidelity involving persons in trusted positions such as clergy or therapists can evoke simultaneous experiences of betrayal from the participating partner, the outside person, and an institution such as a religious organization or the mental health field. Multiple sources of trust have been breached and will need to be addressed in treatment. Similarly, affairs with other family members involve multiple betrayals and require extensive emphasis on real-life decisions, such as whether to tell other family members about the affair and how or whether to interact with the broader family.

When one partner has had an affair in which the outside person has become an integral part of that partner's life, perhaps to the degree that the participating partner seems to be living a double life, then the effects on the injured partner are typically magnified. Although we usually recommend that the couple continue with their couple therapy, at times the injured partner can benefit from individual therapy simultaneously. Such individual intervention should be coordinated with couple therapy and not serve as an alternative forum for the injured partner to avoid addressing difficult issues in couple therapy. Instead, we have found that the amount of time and focus needed to address individual identity issues after such an affair can dominate the couple therapy, leaving inadequate time to address couple issues. In addition, such a broad experience of loss can precipitate a depression or other individual difficulties that might be helped with collateral individual intervention.

Although there are no research findings regarding the impact of these specific types of affairs, our clinical experience suggests that these affairs often lead to notable consequences. Even though many couples stay together after such affairs, injured partners tend to be less trustful of the participating partner and of other people and institutions as well. Thus, they might protect themselves more and maintain tighter boundaries, both with the participating partner and with the outside world. Their experiences have taught them that even supposedly trusted persons and institutions can betray them, as can their partner. Likewise, the participating partner often suffers long-term effects, such as guilt or shame, which can be substantial if that individual concludes that he or she exploited a position of power or influence to encourage an affair with a person in a less powerful position. Similarly, affairs with a family member can create significant shame and guilt as the participating partner recognizes the potential broader disruption to the family and has to face other family members.

Consequently, the treatment of such affairs can be quite challenging for you as a therapist, recognizing the multiple people involved and the effects of the affair that can go beyond the couple themselves. In such complex clinical matters, we have found that having a clear treatment road map can provide important direction, even when the map indicates treacherous, winding, unpaved roads ahead. Although it will likely be quite challenging to create a broad, well-integrated conceptualization of the factors contributing to such affairs, doing so is critical if the couple is to move forward. Chapter 12 provides a discussion of how such conceptualizations can be created and shared to help advance the couple to Stage 3 of treatment.

Summary

Although any affair has the potential to be traumatic with the attendant devastating effects on both partners, certain affairs can be especially complex because of the particular outside partner involved in the affair or the magnitude of the affair. If the affair is with someone who is in a special, trusted position in the participating or injured partner's life, then the affair can have a broader impact. For example, if the affair is with someone who is in a professional role in the couple's life, such as a pastor, physician, or therapist, not only is a betrayal from that person experienced, but also the couple's trust in the institution represented by the outside person can be destroyed as well. Thus, a church is now experienced as a place of hypocrisy rather than a safe refuge. When the affair is with a family member such as an in-law, then not only is there a double betrayal from the outside person as well as the partner, but also the couple must decide how to handle extended family interactions and who, if anyone, in the extended family should be told about the affair.

A somewhat different set of complex dynamics occurs if the affair was with someone who was in a hierarchical relationship with the participating partner, such as a boss or supervisor. Such hierarchical relationships involve greater power in the relationship for one of the two persons and can shift the couple's attributions of responsibility for the affair. If the affair was with the participating partner's boss or superior at work, one or both partners might blame the boss for the affair and excuse the participating partner for his or her role in the affair. Such an approach runs the risk of oversimplifying the context for the affair and can result in failure to examine the changes that need to be made by the participating partner. Likewise, if the participating partner was in the powerful role in the affair, the responsibility given to the participating partner for the affair might be greatly magnified.

Finally, some affairs are particularly complex because of the degree to which the affair is a significant part of the participating partner's life, calling into question the injured partner's experience of the relationship and of life more generally. For example, if the participating partner has been leading a double life with a second residence or children with the outside person, the injured partner might well question the whole meaning of his or her adult life.

In all the prior instances, therapy generally can proceed as outlined throughout this text, with the therapist paying particular attention to these complicating factors and realizing that multiple or extreme betrayals might call for more extensive or longer treatment.

CHAPTER 12

Tying It All Together

Creating a Formulation
of How the Affair Occurred

The therapy sessions and related assignments outside of session described
in Chapters 8–11 provide the couple with an opportunity to examine a
wide range of factors that potentially contributed to the context of the affair.
By this point in therapy, you and the couple will have discussed how their relationship, their social and physical environment, and each individual played a
role in creating the circumstances in which the participating partner decided
to have an affair. With your assistance, the couple will have considered the
immediate, proximal factors that existed close to the time of the affair as well
as the historical, distal factors that might have contributed as well. These
discussions with the couple may have continued for several weeks or months.
Consequently, after sifting through a wide range of possible factors, it is important now to "pull it all together," to develop a thoughtful and comprehensive
formulation of how the affair began, was maintained, and finally ended if it
is over. In essence, although you are not attempting to provide a definitive,
exhaustive explanation for the affair, you and the couple are attempting to
provide a reasoned answer to the questions that preoccupies so many injured
partners as well as participating partners: "Why did you do it?," "What were
you thinking?," "How could this have happened to us?"

By creating this formulation, you and the couple are starting to make a
bridge from Stage 2 to Stage 3 of treatment, which emphasizes moving for-

ward. By gaining an understanding of the affair, the couple can begin to think about their future from an informed point of view. This formulation might include factors that lead one or both partners to a decision to terminate the relationship. Alternatively, it might point out both strengths and weaknesses that need to be taken into account if the couple decides to maintain their committed relationship; it can indicate targets for change in the future as well as domains to maintain or strengthen further.

When offering this formulation, you should continue to emphasize to the couple that developing a broad-based formulation does not justify an affair or excuse the participating partner from responsibility for deciding to have an affair. Otherwise, developing such a formulation might be resisted, particularly by the injured partner, if accepting such a formulation is tantamount to saying, "Of course you had that affair—you couldn't have done anything else—it's not your fault." Similarly, it is important to emphasize that the formulation is not an "equation" for an affair that fully explains its occurrence. Even with all the factors included in the formulation, the circumstances did not necessitate that the participating partner have the affair. Instead, the goal of the formulation is to understand the range of factors that might have increased the likelihood that the participating partner *chose* or *decided* to have the affair.

As a formulation is developed, at least two issues need to be addressed: (1) what factors will be included in the formulation and how they will be organized (i.e., the substance or content that is to be included); and (2) how the formulation will be developed and discussed by the partners and with the therapist (i.e., the process for developing and discussing the formulation).

The Content of the Formulation: What Factors to Include and How to Organize the Material

Each partner's understanding of the affair and how it evolved is likely to flow from the work that has already taken place in therapy up to this point. Given the way that the sessions have been structured during Stage 2 of treatment, formulations often incorporate the four major domains that we have discussed throughout this volume: (1) the couple's relationship, (2) their environment, (3) the participating partner, and (4) the injured partner. The importance or contributions of specific factors within each of these four domains will vary greatly from one couple to the next, and it is important to allow each couple's story and circumstance to speak for itself rather than attempting to fit each story of infidelity into a similar mold. Therefore, in developing a formulation, we do not automatically assume that there are notable factors about the injured partner, for example, that helped to set the context for the affair.

Different approaches can be taken to considering the four domains or breaking them down further, and no single approach is always best. For example, you might find it helpful to consider how factors in each domain contributed to (1) the initiation of the affair, (2) the maintenance of the affair, and (3) the termination of the affair, recognizing that different factors might have been important at various stages of the affair. Concurrently, you would delineate both proximal factors and distal ones. Table 12.1 lists the factors that Pam and Tom viewed as most relevant in understanding the onset of Pam's affair.

An alternative organizational structure might be to consider how certain factors increased the risk for an affair: (1) the presence of negative influences and stressors, such as frequent arguments between the partners; (2) the presence of what might be considered positive qualities in other contexts, such as an emotionally sensitive participating partner; and (3) the absence of protective factors, such as a lack of committed couple friends. Although it is theoretically possible to consider all these factors systematically in developing a formulation—negative, positive, and protective proximal and distal factors in the relationship, environment, and each partner as they apply to the initiation, maintenance, and termination of the affair—such an approach is likely to be far too complex for almost any couple or therapist and runs the risk of becoming too complicated or confusing to be of practical use. Consequently, depending on your personal style as a therapist, the psychological sophistication of the couple, and the ways in which you worked together up to this point in treatment, we recommend that you develop an approach that is not overly complex yet allows for the consideration of all relevant factors. For example, you might work with the couple to consider how their relationship, the environment, and each partner contributed to the context for the initiation of the affair, including both distal and proximal factors as appropriate, and then integrate negative influences, positive qualities, and the lack of protective factors where appropriate.

The Process of Developing and Sharing the Formulation

The prior discussion notes the various categories of contributing factors that might be included in the formulation, but how is such a formulation actually derived after weeks or months of discussion both in the sessions and by the couple outside of the sessions? It is important to decide upon a *process* for bringing these various threads together to weave a meaningful perspective

TABLE 12.1. Major Factors Contributing to the Development of Pam's Affair with Mark: Table Completed by Pam with Input from Tom

Historical or distal factors	Recent or proximal factors

Source: Pam

Family of origin: My dad was confident, assertive, and successful, and I think I came to really like that in males. But he was also pretty thoughtless and not very caring, which I hated. It would be nice to have both.	*Professional*: I continued to move forward in my career, feeling good about myself and the new opportunities I was getting at work. At home, it became awkward discussing my successes with Tom because he wasn't on the same fast track I was. I'll admit I wish I had a partner whom I could relate to about careers and who shared my goals.
Dating history: I always liked to have fun, and I was pretty outgoing. And to be honest, I was physically attractive: Males really liked me and I enjoyed having lots of different boyfriends. I was popular and it felt great.	
Marital history: I was really attracted to Tom because of his sensitivity and caring; I loved that in him. But as our marriage went along, I became really frustrated with his lack of initiative and confidence. He often let me boss him around; it was nice to get my way but in the process I lost respect for him.	

Tom (provided by Pam with Tom's input)

Family of origin: His father was extremely aggressive and abusive. Tom swore never to be this way, and maybe he become unassertive and avoided conflict in the process. But he was successful in making sure he'd never run over other people.	*Professional*: Tom continued to seem comfortable staying in his same position at work, in part because of who he was but also because sometimes he wasn't sure of himself. This seemed okay personally for Tom, but it became more of a problem as I moved ahead at work, sending us in different directions careerwise.
Adolescence: He always felt more comfortable being a follower and team player rather than taking the lead. He seemed to know that I wanted him to lead, but that was never his nature.	

Couple's relationship

Tom said he felt that he was lucky to get me as his wife and wanted to do nothing to rock the boat. I was more assertive than Tom and tended to dominate decisions and Tom went along. In the process, I lost some respect for him, but usually outdebated him when he disagreed. He says he trusted my intelligence, decisions, and values without question; therefore, he didn't question me when he thought my behavior seemed inappropriate or off target.	We both felt we were being good parents, but otherwise we were spending less and less time together with demands of work and children. There were very few conflicts between us, but there wasn't much passion or even fun. We grew more distant both emotionally and sexually. We had lots of casual conversation but not much in depth. Things seemed okay, but our relationship became somewhat boring and mundane more than anything.

(continued)

TABLE 12.1. *(continued)*

Historical or distal factors	Recent or proximal factors
Outside environment	
We both spent long hours at work for many years, Tom being a good team player at work and me working to move ahead. My strong job skills combined with my interpersonal skills meant I was invited to work closely with men in authority on important projects, which put me at some risk for an affair, although I didn't realize it at the time.	I began working more closely with Mark and was impressed by his assertiveness and success, and it was clear that Mark really liked me as well. Mark was a big shot at work, and it felt good to get his attention. Without admitting it, we found reasons to spend more and more time together on projects. Tom ignored signs that he thought my behavior with Mark was inappropriate, and when he did see it, he was uncomfortable raising it with me.

for understanding how the affair took place. Different approaches can be used depending on how the couple works most effectively. Likewise, once the formulation is developed, various strategies for sharing it with the couple can be considered as well.

Developing the Formulation: Individual versus Interactive Strategies

One of the most important decisions to make is whether to have the couple work together as a unit to develop a formulation of the affair or to have the two partners work independently to derive their respective stories. There are several factors to consider in making this decision: (1) the degree to which the partners have developed shared versus differing perspectives on the affair at this point in therapy; (2) the ability of the partners to "work" and talk together as a team in addressing the affair; (3) each person's intellectual, psychological, and verbal abilities to pull the various factors together, develop a reasonable perspective on the affair, and be able to share it with the other partner; and (4) the psychological impact of separate versus shared formulations (e.g., the degree to which one person, usually the injured partner, needs to hear the other partner demonstrate individual understanding for the affair and take personal responsibility).

Shared versus Differing Perspective(s) on the Affair

The focus of Stage 2 of treatment is to help the couple consider various factors that contributed to the context for the affair, with discussion and input from both partners and you as therapist throughout the process. Consequently, in many instances, there is a fair amount of convergence of opinion between the partners regarding the most salient factors, while at the same time the partners might have differing understandings of less central factors. If the two partners have developed a somewhat congruent perspective on how the affair occurred, then it can be helpful to have them work together to create a shared, verbalized formulation. Not only might this approach be efficient, but also it can be useful therapeutically for the couple to experience that they have worked hard and have arrived at a common understanding, even on a topic that is so difficult to confront and understand. Whether this shared understanding leads to the couple staying together and building for the future or deciding to end their relationship, it can be comforting to know that they understand the affair similarly and have discussed and developed an agreed-upon "story" of what happened.

The Couple's Ability to Discuss the Affair in a Constructive Manner

In many instances, this factor is related to whether the partners have derived a common perspective on the affair; when partners have a shared perspective, it often is easier to communicate constructively. Yet these two issues can be disparate. The previous section focuses on whether the partners have a shared perspective of the substantive content of the affair, but the current section focuses on their process of discussing the affair. Even if the two partners understand the affair differently at this point in treatment, some couples are able to discuss these issues in a constructive and respectful manner; if so, then it is easier to have them develop a joint formulation. However, other couples, even after several months in therapy, have a great deal of difficulty discussing the affair without becoming destructive or unproductive and engaging in escalating arguments, a demand → withdraw interaction pattern of blaming and defending, or mutual avoidance or disengagement as the issues become more threatening. When such destructive patterns occur, it is difficult for either person to maintain a thoughtful perspective on the affair when interacting with the partner; instead, they react to each other in the moment and become derailed from the task of developing a thoughtful, reasonable formulation. In such instances, it can be more productive to have each partner work independently. In this way, each person can focus energy and attention on considering the various factors that have been discussed and think of how to discuss or write about the affair unencumbered by the other person's immediate reactions.

Each Partner's Individual Resources

Partners vary considerably in how insightful they are and how well they can verbalize their thoughts, feelings, and overall perspectives, particularly on an emotionally laden topic such as infidelity. If either or both partners struggle on these dimensions, it can be beneficial to have them work together in developing an overall conceptualization, perhaps with assistance from the therapist. Otherwise, not only might the task be frustrating or embarrassing for an individual with limited abilities, but the other partner might inappropriately interpret a seemingly simplistic formulation as a demonstration of lack of involvement or an unwillingness to take responsibility for that person's role in the affair. For example, if a man with limited verbal abilities has had an affair and after months of couple therapy he provides his partner with a short, simplistic interpretation for why he behaved as he did—"We weren't doing well, and she was just there"—she might experience strong disappointment or anger at what she interprets as his disregard for what has been discussed over the previous sessions. Working together, the woman in this example might provide suggestions or guidance that would then assist the man in further elaborating his perspective, in contrast to a short, simple narrative if he were to work alone.

Psychological Impact of Shared versus Individual Formulations

For some couples, it might be more therapeutic to develop a formulation together, but for other couples, individual formulations might be more therapeutic. Previously, we provided an example of the benefits of the two partners deriving a shared formulation together: They have the experience of working together on addressing the affair as a team and concurring on issues that are so important for their relationship. On the other hand, sometimes one partner wants to see evidence that the other individual has grown in his or her understanding of the affair over the course of therapy. For example, the injured partner might view it as important to hear how the participating partner now understands the affair and whether that person has developed more self-insight, takes more responsibility for his or her actions, and so forth. In such circumstances, the injured partner is saying, in essence, "I want to know what you understand after all of these weeks or months of treatment. I don't want to tell you what I think; I want to know what *you* think and feel." Likewise, a participating partner who felt condemned and vilified at the beginning of treatment might now want to know if the injured partner has developed a greater sense of empathy or compassion for the participating partner's behavior. If so, then hearing from the injured partner separately might be important in this case as well.

Sharing the Formulation

If the two partners are working independently in developing formulations, then you must decide whether they are developing their formulations at home between sessions or are doing so during a couple session. If they are developing their formulations independently at home, you can ask them to take one of several approaches that vary in level of formality: (1) Each person is to think about the factors contributing to the affair with plans to discuss these in the next session; (2) each person completes a form, perhaps similar to what is provided in Table 12.1, and brings it to the next session to share; or (3) each person writes a letter or narrative about the factors contributing to the affair, with plans to share the letters before or during the next session. In essence, these three approaches vary in terms of formality and degree to which the contributing factors are written down before the session. In the first two strategies, you still must decide how the information will be shared during a couple session: by having each person provide a full formulation without interruption or by having the couple discuss each factor together.

Sometimes, as noted previously, we have found it very effective when each partner writes a letter sharing that person's understanding of the affair. In composing such a letter, it is important that the writer use tactful, caring language that can be heard by the other partner, while avoiding any distortion or minimization of important factors that contributed to the affair. The participating partner needs to accept responsibility for his or her actions and the injured partner needs to express compassion and understanding for the participating partner's human frailties, to the extent that such expressions by both partners are honest and heartfelt. Furthermore, to the degree that the letter writer is ready to make renewed commitments to the relationship, it can be beneficial to include such commitments in the letter. Although neither person should make premature commitments, if they are ready to make specific changes, these changes can be articulated to provide concrete substance to the letters. In essence, a well-articulated letter includes the following ideas, but only to the extent that they are experienced honestly:

- A thoughtfully worded discussion of the major factors contributing to the context of the affair.
- A statement of responsibility for one's own contributions.

- Compassion and empathy for the other partner and what he or she has been experiencing.

- A recommitment to one's own values, the other person, and the relationship, to the extent appropriate.

- Clarification of specific changes the individual is committed to make.

If these guidelines and principles are reflected in the letter, it can contribute significantly to an experience of healing and moving forward and provide an important transition to Stage 3. Below is a copy of the letter that Bill wrote to Vicki as they finished their sessions in Stage 2 of treatment:

Dear Vicki,

First, I want to thank you from the bottom of my heart for hanging in there with me. I realize that I have put both of us through utter misery, and I don't know if I could do what you have done over the past few months. So thank you for continuing to take care of our marriage, even after I almost ruined it for us. Second, I want you to know that I take full responsibility for what I did. The goal of this letter is for me to try to explain what I understand might have influenced my decision to have an affair, but I still made that decision. No one and no thing forced me to do it; I did it of my own free will.

I am so grateful that we have spent these months together trying to understand how this happened, and I know that I can't do it justice, that I will oversimplify mainly because it is still hard to pull it all together in a way that makes sense. Given that, I also know that all this really begins with me. I was feeling very insecure in our relationship, and I turned to someone else for reassurance that I was still appealing. During our therapy, I've come to realize that this started long before we met. I was indeed a chubby little boy and then a chubby adolescent who never felt attractive or appealing, particularly to females. Luckily, I was bright and willing to work hard, so I always excelled both in school and in almost any activity that I took on. But I always continued to question whether women could really find me to be attractive, and when things would start to go wrong in relationships, I would push for more closeness and reassurance. If that didn't work, I'd try to find someone else to date or find a new girlfriend who would prove that she loved me and wanted to be with me.

Not surprisingly with this history, my first marriage was a failure, and then I found you. I felt that my heaven had finally arrived on earth! It was so wonderful and easy between us, even when James was born. And we had even been great work colleagues, so I thought it would be super when we started our own business together. Sure, we had different work styles and philosophies, but I thought we could overcome that given that we're both very talented and successful. But we couldn't overcome it, and as I tried to move quickly to make business decisions, sometimes unilaterally and sometimes minimizing your input, things really got bad. I know that you have a history of being abused by men, all the way back to your childhood, and have legitimately experienced that your needs or opinions are ignored or devalued by males. I think you learned to protect yourself by withdrawing, closing off, and not being vulnerable when you felt threatened. As we started to have conflicts around the business, I think it led directly into our personal life as well. As we had more frequent arguments and fights, I think you withdrew both emotionally and sexually. And I felt panicky and responded by trying to reach out more to you, which I think led to your withdrawing even further.

After a while, I responded in the typical way that I had learned for decades: I turned to another woman to make me feel better about myself. If I had simply needed someone to talk to about problems we're having, I could have picked one of my male friends, our pastor, or a therapist. Instead, I chose one of our good female church friends; although I didn't admit it to myself, at some level I think I had to be looking for a woman to sympathize with me and make me feel better about myself. From there, you know the rest of the story. And I can't blame her for the affair. It's not as if she continued to pursue me, with me setting limits all the way and finally giving in. I think she and I played this seductive dance, with both of us aware that we were developing an inappropriate relationship under the guise of her supporting me through a difficult time. Once I got so involved with her, I lost all perspective and simply wanted to pursue it. I lied to you and tried to cover it up, but I didn't even do a good job there. Thank goodness you discovered it before I totally wrecked our marriage.

I want you to know that if you're willing to take one more chance with me, I will never, ever do anything like this again. First, having confronted it, I could never repeat this when it is so inconsistent with my own values. More important, I just couldn't do this to you again. I see how it has almost destroyed you. To ask you to take me back and put you through this again would feel like a real crime. You don't deserve to live that way. You're a wonderful person, and my goal is to bring you happiness, not destroy you. Also, I wouldn't do this to our family. I don't want to live that way, and I want us to work together to make sure that it never happens again.

I'm willing to do whatever it takes to make sure that it never happens and do everything possible to make our relationship as strong as it can be. I know that I can't turn to someone else if you and I have difficulties in the future or are distant from each other. Either I have to work it out with you, or I have to tolerate those more difficult times. I know that won't be easy and if I need individual therapy to help, that's fine, or we can continue in couple therapy as long as we need to. I do think that it's important to continue to work on our sexual relationship. I believe a good sex life is important for couples in general, and I know that is one way that I feel close to you. That part of our relationship had been deteriorating long before my affair, and I worry about whether we have now done some permanent damage to it. I won't push you on it, but I hope we can take this at whatever pace we need and to try to make it better. What I will ask from you is that you take a huge risk with me and not shut me out. I promise I will never again take advantage of that trust.

We both entered this marriage as the second chance for each of us. We both had the realization that together our lives could be better than what either of us had ever experienced or perhaps could imagine. Even though I may have shattered that bubble, I still have that fundamental belief that with you I can be better as a person and happier than in any other possible circumstance. Although I haven't been that person for you recently, I commit that if you will continue to give me the opportunity, I will do everything I can to bring you happiness and to live an honorable life together.

I do not know what the future holds, but if we approach it together, I truly embrace it.

With all my love,
Bill

Given the various considerations discussed previously, you might sometimes decide that it is more appropriate to work together with the couple during a therapy session to articulate the formulation that has been developing over the previous sessions. The following is an excerpt of how the therapist might have worked with Vicki and Bill in a session to begin to create the same formulation addressed from Bill's perspective in this letter:

THERAPIST: I see you both brought some notes with you as we had discussed, and I think that will be very helpful tonight. We've spent a number of sessions discussing the various factors that we think might have played a role in Bill's decision to have an affair. And although we've discussed each of those factors as we've gone along and tried to make some sense of things, we haven't really stepped back and tried to pull it all together at one time. So, as we agreed in our last session, let's start to do that tonight, okay?

I thought we might do this in the following way. Let's take one area at a time, for example, what about Bill as an individual made him more likely or vulnerable to having an affair? And let's discuss both more distant, or historical, aspects, such as how he grew up or his earlier relationships as well as what was going on with him individually closer to the time the affair began. Bill, perhaps we could start by asking you to discuss what you think you contributed to this situation, and then we'll have Vicki add her own perspectives. I'll join in, and we'll try to pull that part together before moving on to look at other areas. And let's have you do this by talking directly to each other. Bill, would you begin for us?

BILL: Sure, I'll give it a try. I'm not sure I understand myself all that well, but I think I've started to make some progress based on what we've talked about in here. The most basic thing, I think, is that when things aren't going well for me in a relationship, I first try to reach out to get close, but if that doesn't work, I guess I tend to turn to someone else to feel better about myself. That sounds sort of cliché and immature, but I think that's the crux of it. When you're young and dating, I guess that's okay because people are breaking up and checking out other people all the time. But when you're married, you just can't do that. It's too risky even if you don't plan to get involved.

THERAPIST: You said it sounds sort of cliché; what I couldn't tell is if it seems real to you in your case or whether it is just some sort of nice therapy explanation we created.

BILL: Sort of both, I guess. I mean, I do believe that is what I do or have done, so in that sense it is real. But I don't sit around thinking about it when it is happening. I'm not aware of it at the time; I'm just acting according to what I feel at the moment. I think that's how I do everything; I'm not thinking to myself, "Now I'm doing this or doing that." At least that's how it has been, but now I'm trying to pay attention so I don't mess things up again.

THERAPIST: Right. If you were thinking all the time about what you do, it would get in the way and make it hard to get anything done. But in this area with other women, it sounds like it's important for you to do just that, and it seems like you're making those efforts. And Vicki has said she sees you making those efforts also. So, given this tendency, how do you see that it played out with you and Vicki and your affair?

BILL: Vicki, for a long time I think you and I had a wonderful relationship and I felt great. But when things got tough between us, primarily when we went into business together, I got frightened about what would happen with us. I think I did try to reach out to you more to make things better between us, but maybe I didn't do it very well; I'm not really sure. And I think you pulled back, like you sometimes do when things aren't good. It doesn't justify my affair, but I think I reacted to your pulling back by finding someone else to help me feel better about myself. I felt lonely and unsure of myself, and I went for comfort. It doesn't sound good, but I think that's what happened.

THERAPIST: Bill, thank you. I think you're making an attempt to be honest and open, and you said a lot. Vicki, before we go any further, why don't you let Bill know that you heard what he has said so far? At this point, don't add your own perspective: just let him know that you heard him.

VICKI: Well, I think I do understand what you're saying. It's pretty consistent with what we've discussed in here, and I also agree with it – although it's hard for me to see you as insecure on the outside because I met you when we were working together and you always seem so confident around everyone, were so admired, and so successful. So it's a little hard to imagine you as some insecure person who worries about being accepted or cared about by women. My concern has always been that too many women find you appealing, but I realize that isn't what you experience inside. It sounds like our individual styles really mismatch. When things are tough between us, you first try to reach out in order to feel more secure and I withdraw to protect myself. And for you, if reaching out doesn't work, then you might look elsewhere.

THERAPIST: So, I think we all agree that this is a critical factor in helping us to understand why Bill might have turned to someone else to get reassurance. Vicki, are there other things about Bill from his childhood or his other relationships in the past that you believe might have contributed as well? I realize that you weren't present for most of this, but based on what Bill has told you, things his friends and family members have shared about what he was like, or what we have covered in therapy, are there other things you think we should discuss in that area?

Regardless of the approach that is used to develop and share the formulation, at some point each partner's formulation should be shared in the session, with an opportunity for both people and the therapist to respond, provide input, and perhaps augment or enhance the formulation. Developing and sharing the formulation may take two or more sessions, which prepares the couple for the next phase of treatment—moving forward—when the emphasis shifts from the past to the present and future.

Summary

Stage 2 of treatment is of central importance in helping couples heal from infidelity. Not only does it help them gain understanding for why the affair occurred, but also it sets the stage for where the couple is headed in the future: "If these factors contributed to the affair in the past, then here is what we need to change if we are going to stay together" or "Given my understanding of how this affair came about, this would not be a healthy relationship for me to continue in the future." Given the wide range of factors that have been considered over a number of weeks or months in Stage 2, pulling it all together to develop a formulation for why the affair occurred, was maintained, or finally ended is critical to crystallizing the extensive work that the couple has done to this point in treatment.

In developing the formulation, the couple should consider the extent to which each partner, the relationship, and outside factors contributed to the context of the affair, always holding the participating partner responsible for deciding to have the affair. In developing the formulation, both distal and proximal factors should be taken into account. The process for developing and sharing the formulation can vary, with each partner developing a formulation independently, discussing the formulation together before a session and then bringing it to the session for further discussion, or with the couple working together with the therapist during a session to create and discuss the formulation. Even if each partner works independently outside of the session to develop a formulation, these perspectives are still shared during a session and discussed, with opportunity for both partners and the therapist to respond to each formulation.

Although the formulation at this point is not considered final, it serves as a transition point for shifting to Stage 3 of treatment, which focuses on moving forward. In essence, the couple is soon asked to address the following questions in a more formal way: "Given what you have experienced and now understand about the affair and how it fits into your broader relationship, where do you want to go from here? Do you want to stay together and, if so, let's clarify how we want to proceed and what needs to change and be retained in your relationship. Or do you need to end this relationship and, if so, let's discuss how to do that in a fair and respectful manner." The following chapters discuss how these broad, future-oriented questions are addressed in the next stage.

Resources from *Getting Past the Affair*

Our self-help book for couples, *Getting Past the Affair*, includes information related to the topics discussed in the current chapter. *Chapter 11*, "How Do I Make Sense of It All?," is devoted in its entirety to developing and sharing a formulation of how the affair occurred. Because it is a self-help book, it asks the couple or reader to create this formulation on his or her own, without the possibility of assistance from a therapist or discussions in a therapy session. Thus, you will want to clarify for the couple how to use the material in the chapter while they are in treatment with you. The content of Chapter 11 can serve as a helpful complement to the concepts you will raise in treatment and perhaps describe the goals in different words to help consolidate the ideas. Exercise 11.1 helps the couple construct a summary of the important factors that contributed to the affair, and Exercise 11.2 then asks each person to write a narrative based on the factors identified in the earlier exercise.

PART FOUR

STAGE 3 OF TREATMENT

Introduction to Stage 3 of Treatment

The comprehensive conceptualization of the affair developed in Stage 2 provides a transition to Stage 3, which is intended to help the couple move forward. Now that the partners have a better understanding of the factors that put their relationship at risk for an affair as well as deeper insight into their broader relationship separate from the affair, they are poised to make and implement decisions about their relationship.

Many partners are eager for this next stage, given their desire to put the pain and misery of the affair behind them; however, engaging fully in Stage 3 work can be quite challenging. During this stage, couples are encouraged to reach a critical decision: whether to maintain and strengthen their relationship or to end it. It is often very difficult for couples to make this decision because it requires a firm commitment at a time when their lives have been extremely confusing and disjointed. Moreover, it requires a dichotomous choice—either maintain or terminate the relationship—yet the partners' feelings and thoughts might not be dichotomous because feelings of love and commitment might still be intermixed with hurt, mistrust, and anxiety. Likewise, certain elements of the relationship might appear to be healthy, whereas other factors predict continued difficulties. Making dichotomous decisions when thoughts and feelings are ambivalent is difficult at any time and is particularly complex when the stakes are so high, such as someone's intimate, committed relationship.

To move forward in this difficult context, couples need to take at least three steps to achieve their goals:

- Remove barriers to forgiveness or moving forward.
- Make good decisions about the future of their relationship.
- Implement these decisions and anticipate future issues

REMOVING BARRIERS TO FORGIVENESS

To move forward after an affair, partners need some way to "put it behind" them. For many persons, this process of deemphasizing the hurt from the past and focusing on the present and future is thought of as *forgiveness*. However, some individuals have come to think about forgiveness in ways that create barriers to the process of moving forward as an individual or a couple. For example, in some contexts, forgiveness is equated with weakness and an inability to stand up for oneself or demand appropriate treatment. For other individuals, forgiveness implies that "the slate has been wiped clean" and the participating partner is no longer being held responsible for what happened. Yet other individuals believe, "If I forgive you, you'll betray me again; I have to stay focused on the affair to prevent its recurrence." Although such beliefs are understandable and can potentially serve useful purposes when phrased in less extreme ways, when they are adhered to in an absolute fashion, they typically interfere with the recovery process. Consequently, it can be important to discuss the concept of forgiveness with couples and explore their beliefs about it. In Chapter 13, we provide an extended discussion of a variety of views about forgiveness that may complicate a couple's ability to move forward. When such attitudes are encountered, it is important to help the couple reevaluate their beliefs and seek to adopt less extreme, more adaptive attitudes.

For example, many people believe that forgiveness requires "reconciliation" and remaining in a relationship. In pursuing Stage 3 work, we advocate a different perspective: We encourage couples to distinguish between the decision to forgive versus the decision to stay together or move on separately. We frame forgiveness as a decision to move on emotionally, no longer being dominated by negative thoughts, feelings, or behaviors. In Chapter 13, we discuss strategies that you, as the therapist, can adopt in helping partners pursue this goal.

MAKING GOOD DECISIONS ABOUT THE FUTURE OF THE RELATIONSHIP

After barriers to forgiveness or moving forward have been addressed, the couple is in a position to make important relationship decisions. In order to decide whether to maintain their relationship long term, couples typically need to consider two broad sets of factors: (1) whether another affair is likely to occur in the future and

(2) whether the broader relationship beyond the affair is one that both persons want to maintain. For many couples, the pain after an affair is what brings them to couple therapy. Once the intensity of the pain subsides and some equilibrium has been reestablished, a central question becomes whether another affair is likely to occur in the future. Given that a great deal of therapy has focused on the factors that contributed to the context for the affair, most individuals at this point are able to make thoughtful predictions about the likelihood of future infidelity and what must change to decrease the likelihood. However, even if both individuals are able to reach thoughtful conclusions that the affair is unlikely in the future, they may not necessarily want to continue their relationship. As we discuss in Chapter 14, sometimes the affair has so disrupted or destroyed positive feelings toward the other person, particularly loving and tender feelings from the injured partner toward the participating partner, that the person devoid of positive feelings decides to end the relationship. Helping the couple to understand whether this loss of positive feelings is likely to be a temporary state or a more permanent change is an important discussion elaborated on in Chapter 14.

Furthermore, even if they conclude that another affair is unlikely to occur in the future, some partners might decide to end their relationship based on insights they have gained during Stage 2 work. By contrast, other couples reaffirm the importance of their relationship and the family they have created, committing to continue their relationship. Many couples decide to maintain their relationship while recognizing that significant additional changes are needed.

IMPLEMENTING THE DECISIONS

Even after a couple decides whether to maintain or end their relationship, they still have more work to do. Often a great deal of effort is needed to implement specific elements of these decisions. If a couple decides to stay together, the work from Stage 2 typically provides the direction needed for changes that will help to build an optimal, healthy relationship. Additional couple therapy might be needed, focusing on their broader relationship, individual interventions for one or both partners, or specific changes in how the couple relates to their surroundings, including other people. The range of potential specific changes is almost infinite. In addition, most couples need to address two lingering issues as a result of the affair. First, even if they are successful in generally focusing on the present and the future, for most couples, memories, images, or emotions related to the affair will occasionally reemerge. Helping the couple to anticipate such recurrences and developing a plan for how they will address them is important.

Second, a major theme for couples who decide to stay together involves building or regaining a sense of trust in their relationship. As we discuss in Chapter 14, merely wanting or committing to trust the other person typically is not enough. Couples struggle to understand how they can experience a sense of trust on a broad level within their relationship. Such efforts are difficult, and therapeutic progress is more likely if the couple and therapist can target specific aspects of their relationship in which trust needs to be built. For example, the couple might devise a plan to address questions such as "Can I trust you not to have dinner alone with other women?," or "Can I trust you to come home when you say you will?," or "Can I trust you to listen without judging me if I share how I'm truly feeling in a vulnerable way?" As noted in Chapter 14, building trust in a variety of specific domains can be an effective strategy toward helping the couple develop a broader, more general sense of trust in their relationship overall.

Although many couples stay together after an affair, other couples decide to end their relationship. In many ways, the therapeutic tasks in this situation are similar to helping any couple end a marriage or committed relationship, even when infidelity has not occurred. In addition, issues focal to the infidelity need to be considered in termination with affair couples. Most important, we encourage partners to avoid creating further damage or unnecessary hardship for either partner. Thus, it is important to discourage both partners from using the affair or reactions to the affair as leverage toward a favorable divorce settlement, given that such strategies typically lead to adversarial positions and reciprocal accusations. Also, it is important for both partners to reach an agreement about whether the affair will be disclosed to other individuals, just as they did when the affair was first discovered. Some injured partners might see the merit of keeping the affair confidential while deciding whether to reconcile, but once the decision has been made to terminate the relationship, the injured partner might want to provide justification to other family members or friends for that decision. As discussed during Stage 1, there is no single way to handle such issues, but it is important that both partners be honest about why they might disclose such information and, as much as possible, handle the situation in a way that allows both people to maintain their individual dignity and behave according to their own values. It is easy for partners to become vindictive during a divorce process, particularly those who feel justified by the experience of infidelity. Helping the couple navigate this difficult set of circumstances is an important therapeutic task before ending treatment.

CONCLUDING COMMENTS

In Chapters 13 and 14, we discuss how to help the couple move forward, including a discussion of forgiveness, how to make healthy decisions about the future of their relationship, and how to implement these decisions. Often when couples first begin this difficult process of addressing infidelity, it is impossible to know where the road might take them. Our experience suggests that if the therapist helps them through the process in a manner that we have described in this book, then Stage 3 typically evolves naturally from the earlier stages of therapy. Whether this process results in a joyous reconciliation, a painful termination of their relationship, or something in between, the outcome offers the potential for emotional resolution culminating from the hard work that has transpired over many weeks or months of therapy.

CHAPTER 13

Addressing Issues of Forgiveness and Barriers to Moving Forward

B y the time a couple has completed Stage 2 of treatment, they have spent considerable time and energy reaching an understanding of the major factors that contributed to the development and maintenance of the affair. As a result, much of the therapy has focused on the past, and by this point in treatment many partners are ready to move forward, either together or apart. Often, when there has been a major transgression such as an affair and partners are attempting to move forward, the notion of forgiveness comes to the forefront. Either directly or indirectly, the participating partner often asks, "Can you forgive me?" Likewise, the injured partner grapples with a set of related questions: "Can I forgive you? What does that mean after such a violation of trust? If I forgive you, do I have to stay with you? If I forgive you, will you do it again?" Because the concept of forgiveness is central and often confusing to many people after a major betrayal such as infidelity, we devote the current chapter to helping couples understand and implement forgiveness in a healthy way.

First, we discuss essential characteristics of forgiveness that create a framework for the remainder of this chapter. The model presented here is an elaboration of our stage-process model of recovery from relational traumas, outlined in Chapter 1. Therefore, without labeling it as such, the couple has already been engaging in the forgiveness process through Stages 1 and 2 of treatment. Because forgiving can seem frightening or unsafe to some partners, we discuss the benefits that can result from forgiveness for both individuals and their relationship. Different persons have various views of forgiveness, which can either facilitate or impede their ability to move on from the affair. Therefore, we examine common beliefs that people hold about forgiveness that can be problematic after a deeply hurtful event and ways to help the couple reconsider their beliefs about forgiveness. Even when partners want to let go of their hurt and move forward, often they do not know how to do so; therefore, we discuss intervention strategies that can facilitate the process. Moreover, at times a partner has difficulty forgiving him- or herself. Therefore, we conclude with a brief section addressing forgiveness of self, which often is relevant for both members of the couple.

Defining Aspects of Forgiveness

When introducing the concept of forgiveness with couples, it is important that, as the therapist, you articulate a clear perspective on this important issue in relationships. Although multiple views on forgiveness might be valuable to share with couples, we have found that several core characteristics of forgiveness can serve as the basis for productive discussions and interventions with couples:

- Forgiveness is a process that unfolds over time, typically requiring much energy and effort.
- The process involves an understanding of the individual, relationship, and external factors contributing to the context for the transgression.
- Forgiveness involves no longer being *dominated* by negative emotions and, at times, developing empathy and compassion for the other person.
- Forgiveness does not necessarily imply reconciliation.

First, forgiveness of deep injuries is a *process* that takes time and requires that couples struggle with difficult issues in an effort to regain the ability to move forward. A remorseful partner does not merely ask for forgiveness, which is then granted by a compassionate partner. In Chapter 1, we outlined our model of recovery and discussed the theory that underlies it. As described in that chapter and elsewhere, a primary reason that affairs can be traumatic is that they often shatter individuals' worldviews of their partners, their relationship, and even themselves. Thus, the work required in a healthy recovery process involves reconstructing these worldviews, which takes considerable time and effort. The concern is that for many clients "rapid forgiveness" is likely to involve denial or avoidance that can short-circuit a necessary but painful growth process of learning important information essential to enduring recovery. Research findings indicate that people who say they have forgiven but who have not accomplished the work of forgiveness outlined in this book have less healthy relationships than those who appear to have fully engaged in the forgiveness process (Gordon & Baucom, 1998).

Consequently, even if both members of the couple state that they have already forgiven each other, it can still be valuable to ask them about their understanding or definition of forgiveness and to evaluate the extent to which they have worked through the process outlined in this book. In addition, it is important to emphasize to the couple that, although they can facilitate the forgiveness process through the strategies that we have discussed, forgiveness cannot be forced from a partner. As much as a partner might want to forgive, that person cannot simply will it to happen; patience is critical as the process of letting go of hurts and resentments unfolds.

Second, a central goal of the forgiveness process is to gain a balanced view of each partner and factors that contributed to the affair. By "balanced view," we mean a realistic perspective that considers both positive and negative qualities of each partner and their relationship in terms of a "bigger picture" or "long-term view." Thus, both partners are able to see each other holistically, acknowledging both strengths and weaknesses. One benefit of this broadened perspective is that the partners can make more realistic and accurate predictions about their future together and can understand themselves more clearly. Another benefit is that some individuals might develop or increase their ability to tolerate ambiguity or inconsistencies in themselves and their partners, realizing that relationships and people are not all good or all bad. This perspective might help partners develop greater acceptance and compassion for their own and others' vulnerabilities and weaknesses.

A third aspect of forgiveness involves a release from being dominated by negative emotions, such as anxiety, anger, and hurt. This release does not mean that injured individuals will be entirely free from pain or resentment about what happened; it is unrealistic to expect that forgiveness "wipes the slate clean" or that partners actually "forget" or lose their memory of what has occurred. Instead, the hope is that both partners learn from what has happened. When negative feelings about the affair resurface, couples are encouraged to choose to respond in ways that will be constructive rather than destructive. For example, instead of lashing out in response to past hurts, a couple might choose to strengthen their relationship by spending more quality time together or working together on a task to promote a sense of partnership. Thus, although not ignoring negative emotions, couples can make decisions to behave in ways that will help to create positive emotional experiences rather than ruminating about past negative events.

In some but not all instances, forgiveness implies not only a decrease in negative emotions but also an increase in compassion and warmth toward the partner. For many couples, the work involved in Stage 2 can help effect this change. As one partner becomes aware of the developmental origins and vulnerabilities underlying the other partner's actions, he or she often becomes more empathic and accepting of the partner's shortcomings. For example, Vicki initially struggled to forgive Bill, but she was furious about his affair. In addition, his recent actions reactivated her own long-term fears of abandonment, which made her reluctant to be vulnerable to him. However, as Bill disclosed his history of rejection as a teenager and his struggles in adulthood to prove that he was an attractive and desirable male, Vicki began to feel compassion for him. The therapist helped Vicki to view Bill's strong needs for acceptance and approval as stemming in part from his long-term tendency to feel insecure in relationships. In addition, the therapist helped her see parallels in Bill's experiences and Vicki's own fears about her attractiveness and fears of abandonment. Although Vicki was still distraught that Bill had chosen to have an affair, she could now empathize with his strong underlying needs to be loved and desired. These more empathic feelings eventually helped her to move beyond her anger and toward reengagement with Bill.

A fourth component in this conceptualization is that forgiveness does not necessitate reconciliation. Couples can develop new understanding and emotional release during the forgiveness process, yet still decide to terminate their relationship. Maintaining an unhealthy relationship likely results when people equate forgiveness with reconciliation. Helping individuals to separate these two decisions provides the following important message: "You can forgive and move forward in a healthy manner that at times might include the decision to end your relationship."

For example, as Dennis and Lena struggled with whether he could forgive her for her affair, two of his beliefs about forgiveness became clear: (1) Dennis felt compelled to forgive Lena in order to be a "good" person and (2) he also believed that forgiving Lena required his staying in their relationship if Lena was truly remorseful for her infidelity. Unfortunately, couple therapy also revealed that Lena still had unresolved psychological issues that made her vulnerable to having another affair. She continued to have major substance abuse problems and struggled with emotional insecurity and sexual impulsivity. The therapist helped the couple face this issue and address what it might mean for their future as a couple.

DENNIS: Lena didn't have a chance . . . I know all the horrible stuff that went on in her life, and she just didn't have a chance. I'm not sure she can be in relationships any other way than how she behaved toward me. I don't think she intends to hurt people; I just don't think she knows how to be different. And to be honest, I know she won't change any time soon. But knowing her history, how can I leave her? It would be one more major blow to her.

THERAPIST: So having such compassion for her, it's hard for you to consider ending the relationship. What would it mean about you if you did end it?

DENNIS: It would hurt her. That would be a terrible thing for me to do. I would be abandoning her and going back on my commitment. That's not who I am.

THERAPIST: What do you think your relationship would be like in the future if you stay, knowing her vulnerability to affairs again in the future?

DENNIS: I know it would be hell. We've done this over and over and nothing changes; and I'm so angry at her all the time and so hurt.

THERAPIST: So it seems that it's hard for you to remain compassionate toward her when you're repeatedly being hurt by her actions.

DENNIS: Yes, and we fight all the time. And the kids see it, and I know that's not good.

THERAPIST: So it seems that even though you want to do what is right and honor your commitments to Lena, in many ways your relationship doesn't seem to be healthy, and you don't think it's good for your kids. Do you think it's healthy and rewarding to Lena?

DENNIS: No, I think she hates it. And I hate it too. I hate the way our life is . . .

THERAPIST: Dennis, I can see that you're really struggling. On the one hand, you want to be a compassionate, forgiving person, and on the other hand, it seems you have real questions about whether it's healthy to continue in this relationship. And for you, those two issues seem to be contradictory. Let me suggest how you might think about it in a different way and keep those two issues separate from each other. That is, you can maintain a caring, forgiving stance toward Lena, and it seems that is important to you. But whether to stay in your relationship long term is a different issue. The fact that you care about Lena and forgive her doesn't necessarily mean you need to stay in your relationship long term. What to do about your relationship is a huge and complicated decision for both of you, and you don't have to decide that right now. But I think that tying together forgiveness and whether to stay in your relationship is creating confusion for you in a way that isn't helpful or necessary. What would you think about first allowing yourself to feel compassion for Lena and forgive her for what she has done? Then, separate from that, let's look at all the factors we've discussed over the last several months, and based on that, you can decide whether to continue in your relationship or end it, taking whatever time you need. Do you think you might be able to separate forgiveness from your decision about the relationship?

DENNIS: I don't know . . . I've never thought about it like that. But maybe that would help me get unstuck.

Separating the decision to forgive from the decision about the future of the relationship can be a complex therapeutic task, particularly if both partners are present when the issues are discussed. Sometimes such discussions can occur effectively in conjoint sessions with both partners present, but often these issues are best addressed in individual sessions that allow each partner to explore the issues freely, without concern for how the partner might react. If you do conduct individual sessions, you need to address carefully how pertinent information from those individual sessions will be shared with the partner in subsequent conjoint sessions.

Introducing the Concept of Forgiveness

Once the couple completes Stage 2 work, it is appropriate to introduce the topic of "letting go" or forgiveness to the couple, assuming that it has not already been raised by one of the partners during the course of therapy. Before Stage 3 of treatment, we typically refrain from introducing the word "forgiveness" because of concerns that (1) either partner might be put off by the concept because he or she is still so upset about the affair or (2) the couple might prematurely foreclose on the process of exploring factors that contributed to the affair in order to put the affair behind them more quickly and "move on." However, during Stage 3, couples are likely to be more receptive to discussing forgiveness, particularly if they have successfully addressed the issues focal to Stage 2 and have gained some understanding or compassion for each other and insight into reasons why the affair occurred. Consequently, after the couple has developed a shared narrative of their relationship, we raise the issue of forgiveness and ask the couple to consider how it fits into their recovery.

Often it is helpful to begin the discussion of forgiveness by exploring both partners' perspectives on forgiveness. This exploration can be done directly by asking the couple to share with each other their thoughts about, or definitions of, forgiveness. As they do, you can listen for similarities and differences between their views and the perspective provided earlier in this chapter. At this point, we often give the couple a handout (Table 13.1) that provides them with a way of thinking about forgiveness within the treatment we have already been pursuing. Sometimes the process of hearing both partners' views on forgiveness can highlight potential obstacles, such as when an individual believes that forgiveness necessarily leads to reconciliation but he or she has doubts about continuing the relationship.

Partners might have various beliefs about forgiveness that make it more difficult for them to let go of deep resentments or move on. Therefore, in addition to addressing these problematic beliefs and encouraging partners to continue working through the forgiveness process, it can be useful to discuss positive implications of forgiveness: Why would one person want to forgive another person who has engaged in betrayal and inflicted pain? What good comes from forgiving the partner? Drawing on techniques of motivational interviewing (Miller & Rollnick, 2002), you can initiate this process of contrasting the benefits and potential risks of forgiveness by asking the couple to first list their fears or concerns and validating these concerns when

---

TABLE 13.1. Perspectives on Forgiveness

What forgiveness is:

- A process.
- A release from being dominated by negative thoughts, feelings, and behaviors.
- A chance to learn about and gain more understanding of your partner, your relationship, and yourself.

What forgiveness is *not*:

- Forgetting.
- Reconciliation.
- An immediate event.
- A one-time event.

---

appropriate. Most clients are ambivalent about forgiveness, and both sides of this struggle need to be acknowledged. After validating partners' concerns about forgiveness, you can move the focus toward negative consequences of not forgiving and the benefits of forgiving. If clients do not generate these consequences themselves, it is appropriate for you to point out that chronic, unresolved hurt and anger can have negative emotional and physical consequences for both partners.

For example, such chronic negative emotions can lead to further difficulties, such as depression, irritability toward others and distressed relationships, high blood pressure, headaches or back pain, and chronic fatigue (e.g., Enright, 2001; Fincham, Hall, & Beach, 2006; Younger, Piferi, Jobe, & Lawler, 2004). Likewise, continuing conflict from the affair can have negative consequences for both partners and for their children (e.g., Buehler & Gerard, 2002; Papp, Goeke-Morey, & Cummings, 2007). In contrast, forgiveness has been linked to decreased anxiety and depression, better immune functioning, and cardiac health (e.g., Enright, 2001; Younger et al., 2004). In addition, some research suggests that forgiveness might also be associated with partners' abilities to parent more collaboratively (Gordon, Hughes, Tomcik, & Litzinger, 2006).

The injured partner also should be encouraged to consider the effects that continued anger might have on the participating partner. The participating partner often struggles to let go of his or her own feelings of guilt, shame, and resentment. Although these emotions initially can help the participating partner to take responsibility for his or her behavior, if they persist for too long or at too extreme a level, these self-focused negative feelings can trigger a broad range of additional emotional and physical health problems similar to those we described for the injured partner. A guilt-ridden, depressed participating partner is not in a good position to devote energy and effort toward rebuilding a relationship or make good decisions about how to proceed. In contrast, when injured persons want their relationships to succeed and care for their partners' well-being, letting go of past hurts is likely to promote better emotional and physical health in both partners and may inspire the participating partner to work harder on behalf of the relationship and give more in return.

We encourage all couples to consider issues of forgiveness and how these might contribute to their moving forward; however, for some individuals the concept is so problematic that using the term "forgiveness" hinders rather than helps the process. In such instances, you might help the couple approach moving forward using different terms such as "moving on" or "letting go." For example, you might ask the couple, "What would it mean to you to move on from the affair?" or "What would have to happen for you to be able to let go of your hurt from the affair and put it behind you?"

Problematic Beliefs about Forgiveness

Even when partners are convinced of the value of forgiveness and have worked hard during Stages 1 and 2 of treatment, some persons still have difficulty taking the next steps toward moving forward. Developing understanding about the past is one task, but envisioning the future and taking the necessary steps to reach that future can be frightening. At times, this fear of and resistance to moving forward are compounded because of problematic beliefs that couples hold about the forgiveness process. Nearly everyone has had some experiences with forgiveness, such as having to forgive, being unable to forgive, or wanting to be forgiven. These experiences can shape beliefs about forgiveness and a person's ability to move forward in Stage 3.

Thus, it is important to explore each partner's beliefs about forgiveness that may interfere with letting go of their deep resentments and moving forward. Some of these beliefs might become clear when initially asking the two partners to describe their views about forgiveness. Table 13.2 is designed to help couples identify potentially problematic beliefs that they might have regarding forgiveness. To begin this discussion, you might ask the couple to review the list and identify any statements with which they agree. The partners should then discuss how these beliefs might make the recovery process more difficult for them. For example, if one person believes that forgiveness is synonymous with forgetting, then you can comment that it is unlikely that either person will ever actually forget that the affair occurred. Instead, forgiveness involves a commitment to move beyond negative thoughts and feelings when they do occur. You can guide the couple in discussing the potential consequences of these different beliefs about forgiveness, and help them begin to reconsider their perspectives that could make moving forward more difficult.

During this discussion of beliefs about forgiveness, it is useful to validate any "kernel of truth" that is demonstrated by an individual's beliefs or attitudes. For example, given that many people want to protect themselves after being betrayed, it is understandable that someone might fear being more vulnerable if he or she forgives a partner. Affirming some aspects of partners' current beliefs can help to minimize feelings of invalidation while exploring the benefits and risks of various beliefs with the couple.

TABLE 13.2. Beliefs about Forgiveness

The following statements describe various beliefs about forgiveness that can interfere with moving forward. Consider these statements and how they relate to your own beliefs.

- "If I forgive the affair, then it is unacceptable for me to feel any further negative emotions about what happened."
- "I cannot forgive my partner until my anger has completely gone away."
- "I should not feel angry at my partner if he or she has sincerely apologized."
- "To truly forgive, I have to forget what happened."
- "If I forgive, it means that I am letting my partner get away with doing something hurtful to me."
- "If I understand why my partner behaved in this way, then I have to excuse him or her from taking responsibility for the behavior."
- "Forgiving my partner is the same as saying that what happened does not matter."
- "If I forgive, I will appear weak."
- "If I forgive, I will open myself up to be hurt again."
- "Forgiving my partner means tolerating negative things that he or she has done or continues to do to me."
- "If I forgive my partner, I have to continue the relationship with him or her."
- "I should not forgive my partner if he or she does certain things such as hit me, have an affair, or betray a confidence."
- "I should not forgive my partner until I feel that the score is 'even' between us."

Next, we describe common problematic beliefs about forgiveness, along with examples of how you, as therapist, might explore and evaluate these beliefs with a couple.

Religious and Culturally Based Beliefs

People's beliefs about forgiveness often are closely linked to their religious experiences. Almost all major religions include forgiveness as an important value (e.g., Klassen, 1966; McCullough, Worthington, & Rachal, 1997). However, various religions place different emphases and take different approaches to forgiveness. These differences are useful to consider because they are also likely to impact the partners' views regarding necessary ingredients in the recovery process. For example, in Christianity and Islam, forgiveness often is encouraged regardless of whether or not the offender expresses contrition or engages in acts of restitution; thus, forgiveness is more of an internal process within the forgiver. However, in Judaism, the emphasis regarding forgiveness is dyadic and focuses more on the role of the person requiring forgiveness (Rye et al., 2000). Moreover, some views of Christianity hold that it is a person's religious duty to forgive regardless of the severity of the offense, whereas in Islam forgiveness is viewed more as a matter of choice for the victim (e.g., Rye et al., 2000). Because a couple's beliefs about forgiveness are likely affected by their religious or cultural backgrounds, it is useful to explore how partners' religious or cultural upbringings have helped to shape their views of forgiveness, even among those who do not currently identify themselves as religious.

For example, Peter, who was Christian, had betrayed Ruth, who was Jewish, by having an affair with a female coworker. Ruth had been distant and aloof throughout treatment. Although she participated in Stage 2 work, she showed few signs of softening toward Peter. When the therapist raised the issue of forgiveness in Stage 3, she began by asking the couple about their views on forgiveness. For Peter, forgiveness involved an internal transformation in which one partner sought to understand the other and to work actively to let go of anger toward that person. Ruth, on the other hand, saw forgiveness as requiring significant atonement and restitution by the offending partner before the injured partner could forgive. It became apparent that Ruth had not yet received enough restitution from Peter and thought that his remorse lacked genuineness because it was not accompanied by the appropriate restitution.

Peter and Ruth's therapist encouraged the partners to talk about their early experiences of forgiveness. As the partners discussed their histories with forgiveness, the therapist also directed them to consider each other's approach and to identify elements that they appreciated. Peter was able to see that the idea of atonement might help with the issue of self-forgiveness, an issue that was very difficult for him, and that it would communicate to Ruth his commitment and remorse. Ruth could see that the internal processing that Peter used to achieve forgiveness could help her gain a new and useful perspective on her partner and could promote self-growth. Their therapist helped them to develop a shared perspective on forgiveness, drawing on these positive elements from both partners' views. Forgiveness for them became a process of creating a release from anger through discussions with each other and through symbolic acts of atonement and forgiveness.

Similarly, other cultural backgrounds often affect clients' views about forgiveness. For example, the African concept of "ubuntu" suggests that because members of a community are interconnected, the pain that an offender causes to another individual ultimately causes pain to the offender. In some respects, this communal view helps promote empathy and compassion for the offender and a heightened openness toward reconciliation, because it suggests that the good that results when an injured partner forgives a participating partner will ultimately benefit the injured partner as well.

Other cultural perspectives on forgiveness can also influence moving forward for the couple. For example, the Latino values of "machismo" and "marianismo" might make a woman's affair seem less forgivable than a man's affair; if a man forgives his wife, he might be seen as weak. Even if a partner does not personally hold these views, if family members hold these beliefs, the couple's own forgiveness process can be affected. For example, after much work in therapy, Mario, a Latino who was relatively acculturated into American society, was willing to forgive his wife, Lucia, for her affair. However, he received numerous angry and derogatory comments from his family regarding his decision. Consequently, Mario experienced self-doubt about his decision and struggled with whether he should allow Lucia back into his life. Their therapist intervened by encouraging the couple to consider how they could remain a cohesive team in the face of the family's verbal assaults on Lucia.

Forgiving versus Excusing or Forgetting

In addition to varying cultural and religious beliefs on forgiveness, many individuals differ in the extent to which forgiving is distinguished from "excusing," "pardoning," or even "forgetting." For some people, forgiving an offender means that they no longer hold the offender accountable for the betrayal. In such instances, forgiveness may be seen as tantamount to saying that what happened no longer matters. Not surprisingly, people who equate forgiveness with excusing are often unwilling to forgive their partners for severe offenses. Other partners believe that forgiveness literally implies forgetting that the affair occurred. In fact, some participating partners ask, "Why can't you just forget the past and move on?" If partners believe that they literally must forget what happened, then they often feel incapable of forgiving.

Likewise, for some partners, forgiving an offense implies that negative emotions about what happened are no longer appropriate: "If I forgive you, then I can't be angry with you or feel upset about what happened." Therefore, a partner who still has negative feelings about what happened may believe that he or she is not ready to forgive the other individual. We clarify our own stance that, whereas forgiveness means the person is no longer *consumed* with negative emotions, there is no assumption that *all* negative feelings will disappear. Another problematic belief that some partners hold is that "letting go of the affair" means they should not take what happened in the past to make predictions in the future: "If I forgive you, I should trust you to treat me well from now on." Such a position could mean that the forgiving individual must ignore high-risk behaviors that were related to the affair and behave as if the couple is no longer vulnerable. Such an approach runs contrary to a major tenet of the current treatment in which the couple thoughtfully considers what they have learned in order to plan for the future.

Indeed, what once may have been viewed as innocent and "safe" behaviors may no longer be acceptable or may interfere with moving on because of their association with the affair. In such instances, as therapist, you need to help the couple find realistic ways of altering either person's behavior in order to reduce anxieties created by the affair. For example, the couple might decide to check in regularly by telephone when separated, arrange for other trusted workers to be present when the participating partner is working late, or avoid situations that unnecessarily stir up thoughts and feelings related to the affair. Thus, instead of ignoring risky behaviors as a part of forgiving, the couple must take these behaviors into account as they move forward.

In the following exchange, Tom and Pam's therapist helped Tom to explore his fear that forgiving Pam for her affair would render him more vulnerable in the future.

THERAPIST: Tom, based on some things you've said previously, I wonder if in some ways it seems better for you *not* to forgive Pam, that in some way it protects you or the relationship. Does that fit at all for you?

TOM: I don't know. Given what we've talked about, it sounds odd to suggest it's better not to forgive her, but I think at some level, I do believe that.

THERAPIST: In what ways? Help me understand what you're thinking.

TOM: Well, it seems that by not forgiving, I make sure we don't forget or become complacent about things. I mean, what happened was horrible, and in some ways, I don't want to put that in the past; I want us to remember it so it never happens again. I'm afraid that if we put it in the past, it could happen all over again.

THERAPIST: So it sounds like by not forgiving, you feel you're keeping your relationship on track in some way?

TOM: Yeah, I guess so.

PAM: I don't feel on track. I'm constantly tense and worried that you're going to yell at me, Tom. I can't relax and be myself around you.

THERAPIST: What is that like for you, Pam?

PAM: I hate it. I can't live this way. I want things to be back like they were before.

THERAPIST: Before?

PAM: When we could enjoy ourselves with each other, and things were light and playful. And we weren't walking on eggshells.

TOM: I want that too.

THERAPIST: So, although you think that not forgiving is keeping you on track by making sure you don't forget what happened, it also seems that this approach is creating ongoing bad feelings and keeping you from the really good things that you both want.

TOM: I can see that . . . I'm just so afraid of it all happening again.

THERAPIST: I can understand that, Tom. So, if you were to forgive, it seems that forgiveness would have to mean that something would be different from before the affair, that you wouldn't be at risk for Pam having another affair.

TOM: Yes . . . I can never put myself in that position again to be hurt like that.

THERAPIST: Right, it's certainly understandable that you don't ever want to go through that again. So it sounds like our challenge will be to help you in some way forgive Pam and move forward without increasing the risk of another affair, is that correct?

TOM: Right, if I could do that, I would. But forgiving her feels so risky.

THERAPIST: I wonder if maybe allowing yourself to see both the relationship's vulnerabilities and its strengths might help you here. I don't think forgiveness means turning a blind eye or forgetting what happened: it means knowing what you need to work on and then working on it. Perhaps we could focus your energies on how to make the relationship better as a way of decreasing the risk of an affair rather than continuing to focus on the hurt and anger from the affair. What would you think about taking that approach?

TOM: Yes, I could see that. I wouldn't necessarily be going back to my old rose-colored glasses where I ignored problems, and I wouldn't just be letting Pam off the hook. But I wouldn't be dwelling on the past either, just to keep Pam honest. I mean, this sounds good in theory; I'm just not sure I can do it.

PAM: This sounds good to me, too. I don't want to go back to that old relationship. I need to be aware of the problems and I want to work with you, Tom, to deal with them.

THERAPIST: So let's think about this possibility. How would forgiveness look for the two of you if we started from this perspective . . .

From that point, the therapist and the couple began to generate a picture of what a forgiving but healthy relationship would look like for them.

History Is Destined to Repeat Itself

Another belief held by some injured partners that interferes with forgiveness is "If you hurt me once, you are bound to hurt me again." This attitude can lead to a constant state of vigilance, in which the injured partner mentally rehearses what happened in the past in order to guard against the possibility that it might occur again. However, constantly reliving the affair perpetuates not only the memories but also the deeply hurt feelings. If, as a result of treatment to this point, partners are able to observe real changes in their relationship and understand when and why their relationship gets into trouble, they may be able to relinquish their fear and excessive vigilance.

At other times, the fear of being reinjured might be based on the fact that some issues from the affair have not been addressed or resolved, thus contributing to a lack of safety. For example, Gail wanted to forgive Brad, and they agreed that they had gained much understanding about why he had the affair. They also agreed that his behaviors had changed for the better over the course of treatment. Yet Gail still could not forgive him and continued to rage at him and experience deep pain from the affair. The therapist began to explore Gail's block to forgiving.

THERAPIST: Gail, it seems to me that there's still some "unfinished business" for you about this affair. It seems that you don't feel safe putting this event behind you. Is that right?

GAIL: I don't know; I just can't let it go . . . Some of the things that happened after the affair, I just can't . . . How can I believe the changes I see now, when after I discovered the affair and he said it was over, he still called her and met with her even though she was harassing me? Brad said he was sorry, but I kept finding out new things he hadn't told me! So how can I believe he's different now? I'm so afraid that if I put it behind me . . . How can I know it won't happen again?

THERAPIST: So even though you understand better why Brad had the affair, and you can see that he's really trying to make necessary changes, it's hard to move on when you still don't understand how he continued to misrepresent things after he said it stopped? It makes it hard for you to believe him now when he seemed so sincere before yet continued to see her. Is that right?

GAIL: It's impossible to believe him. I can't make that leap. I want to, but I can't. I just don't trust that he'll be there, that he'll follow through on all this.

THERAPIST: It sounds to me as if there are still several unanswered questions for you, not so much about the affair itself but more about Brad's actions after the affair. Is that right?

GAIL: Yes, I still can't make that fit, and I still can't trust him. Why is he behaving so well now but didn't then? We could be so much farther down the road to recovery if he hadn't behaved the way he did after I found out about the affair.

BRAD: I was so confused at that time; I didn't even know what I was doing.

GAIL: You told me it was over and it *wasn't*!

BRAD: It was, but I couldn't completely let go yet.

THERAPIST: It seems to me that we need to spend some more time exploring that time period after you told Gail the affair was over, Brad, so that she can understand whether there is a difference between then and now.

Additional discussion of the time period after the affair became known was necessary in order to answer Gail's questions and to clarify whether risk factors were still present that the couple needed to address. Over time, Gail began to understand the motivations behind Brad's decisions during the time immediately after the disclosure of his affair, decisions he now deeply regretted.

Thus, in exploring a partner's concern that another affair is likely in the future, it is important to differentiate whether this belief is based on general unresolved fears or on objective remaining risk factors. These two situations call for different interventions: The former involves reappraising the fear, whereas the latter requires further behavior change.

Facilitating the Decision to Forgive

Even when a partner understands the value of forgiveness and is committed to the process, often he or she does not know how to go about forgiving. Or the partner might falter when the couple has a lapse in progress or when new difficulties arise. Therefore, it is useful to help couples recognize that they have begun a process that will take time and sustained effort to complete. Having realistic expectations of the process will aid in preventing hurt feelings and misunderstandings between the partners when they encounter the almost inevitable lapses and difficulties in moving past the affair. Strategies that can help the couple move forward, even after they have committed to forgive each other, are presented next.

Developing Constructive Strategies for Managing Negative Emotions and Thoughts

Couples may find that even though they have committed to move on past hurt feelings, they still struggle with managing negative emotions and reactions to the affair. Although it is important that they are able to share these feelings with each other when appropriate, frequent processing of these emotions can be exhausting for the couple and potentially erode emerging positive emotions. As the therapist, you can teach the couple to avoid escalation of negative feelings by recognizing when they are having particularly "hot thoughts," speaking in a harsh or angry manner, or experiencing other cues of anger. You can then encourage them to use strategies to address these feelings more constructively, such as writing in journals, talking with trusted friends or religious figures, or using outlets such as art or music. Thus, many of the strategies discussed in Chapters 4–6 and recommended during Stage 1 of treatment when emotional intensity is high are also applicable here.

In addition, injured partners often need help managing recurring intrusive memories and negative thoughts regarding the affair. As described in Chapter 6, using strategies for emotion regulation such as those developed in the treatment of anxiety disorders and dialectical behavior therapy can be useful. Partners might find it helpful to redirect their thoughts to a different topic or distract themselves by engaging in a different activity; they also can attempt to disrupt negative thoughts by trying to view the situation from a different, more positive perspective (Linehan, 1993). For example, rather than focusing on their disappointment that they continue to have memories of their partner's affair, they can remind themselves that the memories do not occur nearly as often or that the hurt feelings that accompany the memories are not as devastating or do not last as long as they once did.

Developing Compassion

In some instances, encouraging one person to practice compassion for the partner and the partners' vulnerabilities can help the couple to move forward. Compassion for a partner can involve a deepened understanding of how the partner came to behave in a hurtful way. It also can stem from recognizing the other partner's distress from the affair and wishing to put an end to that pain for the partner. In other cases, developing compassion might be more difficult or even unrealistic. For example, if the participating partner has engaged in numerous affairs or other hurtful behaviors and shows little remorse, it is understandable that the injured partner would be opposed to such strategies or believe that the situation does not merit it.

Drawing on Spiritual Resources

Often when partners feel trapped in ongoing anger and resentment, they can work toward moving on emotionally by considering their own personal or spiritual values. From this perspective, the benefits of forgiveness go beyond personal or relationship consequences and instead involve values regarding the inherent goodness or benefits of forgiving someone who has wronged another person. Drawing on personal or spiritual values can help couples work toward letting go of the past, even when they "don't feel like it." In approaching such issues, it is important to avoid implying a moral prescription that the individual should or must forgive the other individual. Rather, you might inquire about the person's own personal values and beliefs regarding forgiveness and how he or she might try to put those values in place in the current context, even when it is difficult to do so.

Restitution, Remorse, and Reform

Although nothing can "undo" an affair, acts of restitution or seeing that the partner is "going the extra mile" to show caring, concern, and love can serve as concrete expressions of remorse or a commitment to change. As DiBlasio (1998) noted, having a partner perform some real or symbolic act of restitution can be a means of helping couples proceed through the forgiveness process. However, if an injured partner continues to demand large acts of restitution or such demands continue for a long time period, these acts typically no longer serve to strengthen the relationship or promote feelings of closeness but instead appear to be acts of vengeance. If vengeful demands for restitution are becoming problematic, you should address those concerns with the couple. Often it is possible to help the injured partner realize that continued punishment might feel satisfying in the short run, but in the long run it typically prevents the couple from moving forward. More specifically, you might begin by helping the injured partner explore anticipated short-term benefits of these demands for restitution, such as showing the participating partner that he or she cannot get away with such behavior. By starting with benefits, you can validate the injured partner's motives and identify what factors might be maintaining this behavior. Then you can ask the injured partner to think beyond the initial benefits of the vengeful behavior and consider how these efforts negatively affect the relationship and the partner in the long term, such as causing resentment from the participating partner for the "cruel and unusual punishment." Focusing on the long-term effects can help motivate the injured partner to examine how he or she might find other, more constructive methods of meeting the needs that the vengeful behaviors have been serving.

For some couples, it can be helpful to discuss and agree on what acts of restitution will be beneficial. However, for some injured partners, having to ask for expressions of remorse and contrition can render the act meaningless: "I shouldn't have to ask you to say you are sorry or tell you how to make things up to me. You should know what to do, and you should do it because you want to and because it's the right thing to do." Although such a view is understandable, at times the participating partner might want to make things better but does not know what would be helpful or effective. This situation is especially likely if the participating partner attempted to apologize and offer restitution during Stage 1 of treatment but found those efforts to be unsuccessful. Thus, it can be helpful to discuss with the couple at this point what the injured partner would value as sincere demonstrations of remorse and restitution. During these discussions, it is important to emphasize that the meaning of such acts should not be viewed as diminished because they are being requested. Rather such discussions can serve to clarify what acts are valued by the injured partner, with the participating partner responding in his or her own way in a voluntary manner.

Making Forgiveness Explicit

Explicit declarations of forgiveness between the partners can have several advantages as long as both members have a clear understanding about what this declaration means. These statements can demonstrate a commitment to the process of moving forward, even though the process still might be difficult for the partners. As long as both partners recognize that the commitment to moving forward implies a process that is still unfolding, rather than an end that has already been achieved, this commitment can promote greater understanding and patience between the partners when they experience setbacks in letting go. Explicit rituals of seeking and asking for forgiveness can have important resonance and power, which in turn can facilitate a sense of emotional release for the partners (e.g., DiBlasio, 1998). If the process unfolds naturally and is unforced and genuine, it can be a meaningful and salient experience for both partners.

Self-Forgiveness

Participating partners often struggle with issues of forgiveness, particularly in forgiving themselves for the affair. Injured partners also may wrestle with forgiving themselves for their own roles in making the relationship more vulnerable to an affair or for their hurtful or punitive behavior in response to the affair. Partners' difficulties in forgiving themselves can occur for many of the reasons that we have discussed earlier in this chapter. For example, they may fear that forgiving themselves would make it easier to forget what happened or increase the likelihood that they would let down their guard against hurting their partner again. Research has shown that the greater the empathy for the injured partner, the more difficult it is for the participating partner to move beyond guilt and shame and forgive him- or herself (e.g., Zechmeister & Romero, 2002). Furthermore, some partners may believe that further suffering serves as a penance for the pain caused to the injured partner. Thus, it can be important to explore beliefs about self-forgiveness with couples recovering from infidelity. Extreme or prolonged shame and guilt can make it difficult for the participating partner to be engaged in the recovery process when it is most needed. Such feelings can also immobilize the injured partner and prevent constructive changes from occurring.

For example, Peter tended to ruminate excessively on his guilt over hurting Ruth. He could not bear to observe her pain during the sessions and had a tendency to shut down and withdraw at these times. In response, Ruth felt abandoned by him and tried to engage him; when he did not respond to her efforts, she lapsed into angry silence. Their therapist began by encouraging Peter to verbalize to Ruth what he was experiencing. As the depth of Peter's self-contempt became clear, the therapist began to talk with Peter more specifically about self-forgiveness. The therapist helped Ruth understand how Peter's guilt and shame, rather than disinterest, led to his withdrawal and her loneliness. Peter feared that if he forgave himself, Ruth would think he did not care and he might repeat his horrible acts. The therapist helped Peter explore the latter thought by examining all the ways in which he had changed during therapy and evaluate the likelihood that he would, in fact, have another affair. Both Peter and Ruth agreed that the likelihood of another affair was low. Moreover, as a result of the couple's new perspectives on forgiveness, Peter found that symbolic rituals of atonement not only made Ruth feel better but also made Peter feel "freer." Together, the couple came to recognize that Peter was more effective in demonstrating his commitment to the relationship by being engaged and working to improve the relationship instead of retreating into his private shame.

When a couple is addressing self-forgiveness, a careful balance must be preserved. On the one hand, true remorse, guilt, and sadness can serve a constructive role to the degree that such emotional experiences reinforce beliefs that a partner has behaved in hurtful, inappropriate ways and initiate a sincere self-evaluative process. At the same time, extreme and prolonged guilt and shame can stifle the recovery process. Thus, it is important to help both partners experience and express painful emotions that result from the affair and yet move forward.

Summary

In this chapter, we have presented a model of forgiveness as an essential process for partners moving forward emotionally and then reaching and implementing healthy decisions regarding their relationship. Forgiveness can be both a liberating and a frightening experience for couples. It is a concept that has widely varying definitions and perspectives. A variety of strategies discussed in this chapter can facilitate forgiveness of the other person as well as self-forgiveness.

Once a couple has developed a thoughtful conceptualization of how the affair occurred, forgiveness has been addressed, and potential barriers to moving forward have been discussed, the remaining task is for the couple to make a clear decision about whether to stay together and build a meaningful relationship or to end their relationship and move forward separately. The next chapter provides guidelines to help couples take these final steps in the recovery process.

Resources from *Getting Past the Affair*

Our self-help book for couples, *Getting Past the Affair*, includes information related to the topic of forgiveness. *Chapter 12*, "How Do I Get Past the Hurt?," helps couples identify their beliefs about forgiveness and develop a plan for letting go of their pain and anger. Detailed guidelines are designed to help the couple through this process. Tables outline typical beliefs and provide a quick overview of recommended steps, and exercises walk the partners through critical steps. Chapter 12 complements concepts you will raise in treatment and provides descriptions and examples from other couples' experiences that can bring the material alive for couples, possibly helping them identify beliefs they hold about forgiveness that they might not previously have recognized.

CHAPTER 14

Moving Forward

After many weeks or perhaps months of therapy, most couples will have reached a point where they are ready to shift their focus from the past to the present and future. As we discussed in the previous chapter, making this shift does not mean that they have literally forgotten the traumatic events surrounding the affair; nor does it mean they have concluded that the infidelity is acceptable. Instead, it means that the initial crisis and arousal immediately after the affair have likely subsided to some degree, and you and the couple have worked together to develop a fuller, more balanced understanding of the variety of factors that contributed to the development and continuation of the affair. Furthermore, you have discussed issues related to forgiveness in preparing the couple to move forward.

As we have stated repeatedly, forgiveness and moving forward do not require reconciling or continuing the relationship. Instead, they mean that while acknowledging the painful occurrences related to the affair, both persons focus on optimizing their individual and collective lives, either staying together or moving forward separately. We believe that it is important for couples to make an explicit decision about how they will proceed in the relationship, regardless of what that decision might be. Without couple therapy to focus on the infidelity, some partners discuss the affair to some extent and simply continue living together without making a focused, committed decision to move forward in a given manner. An explicit decision is important because it carries with it agreements and responsibilities. If a couple decides to stay together, we discuss with them in detail what changes are needed and what should be maintained in their relationship, along with reaching clear agreements about how to bring about needed changes. Should they decide to end their relationship, likewise we discuss with them how they can move forward in the most respectful and least damaging way possible. Otherwise, couples run the risk of staying together with ongoing resentments and a lack of focus on how to make needed changes. Or, they may end their relationship with angry, resentful feelings that continue to plague them even after their relationship is terminated.

Couples differ in terms of how significant this decision seems to be for them at this point. Some couples have known since they entered therapy that they intend to continue their relationship, but they sought treatment with a goal of gaining understanding and finding some peace with the infidelity. For such couples, at this point in treatment, we still ask them to step back, reevaluate where they are and where they have been, and make an explicit decision to stay together, explaining that such a decision carries with it the types of responsibilities described previously.

Other couples entered therapy without a clear decision about the future of their relationship. For them, this point in therapy can be difficult, confusing, and often anxiety provoking. Some of them may have hoped that, over the course of therapy, life would return to normal as a result of the "healing process," and they may feel confused because their feelings remain somewhat mixed. For others, making a decision with the attendant responsibilities means that they are now giving up their "escape route." That is, before this point, one or both partners might have thought or verbalized, "If I get upset or find it to be too hard, I can always leave." However, deciding to stay in the relationship and recommitting means giving up that option and agreeing to "tough it out" as a couple, even when times are extremely difficult. Likewise, making a firm decision to end the relationship for many partners signals a new phase of life as a single person, with many fears and uncertainties. Therefore, regardless of how couples entered into therapy and the degree to which they might have already reached a decision about the future status of their relationship, we still spend time having them make a clearly articulated formal decision about whether to stay together or separate, and we explore with them the implications of that decision for each partner. Of course, if a couple is not ready to decide at this point, we clarify what factors need further consideration and help them address those issues before proceeding.

Factors to Consider in Deciding Whether to Stay Together or End the Relationship

In deciding whether to continue or terminate their relationship, we recommend that couples consider two broad domains. First, we focus considerable attention on the affair, including all that they have experienced over the course of treatment to this point. The formulation that they have developed, as described in Chapter 12, serves as an excellent starting point for this discussion. In that formulation, you and the couple have discussed how each individual, the relationship, and external factors played a role in the development, maintenance, and termination of the affair. Isolating those factors provides a natural segue for a discussion regarding whether to stay together, and if they choose to do so, what would need to be changed, maintained, or enhanced. Likewise, a careful look at the same factors can serve as the basis for a discussion of why one or both partners believe that their relationship should end.

Second, the couple should assess their relationship more broadly beyond the affair per se; that is, the future of their relationship might involve more than recovery from the affair. In some instances, the affair serves as a major precipitant for both partners to step back and evaluate their lives more broadly. For example, some injured partners might conclude that they can work through the trauma of the infidelity, but the affair has caused them to scrutinize their relationship and realize that in other ways the relationship is unhealthy for them, and they need to terminate it. This happened in Robin and Frank's marriage after Frank's affair. They worked diligently with their therapist, and Robin concluded that in terms of the affair itself, she could forgive Frank and move forward. However, the shake-up caused by the affair resulted in her stepping back and looking at her life and their marriage more broadly. She concluded that over the years their relationship had become imbalanced, with her serving primarily to meet Frank's and the children's needs. As a result, she felt that her own personal growth and development had come to a standstill and that Frank had consistently stifled her attempts to meet her own needs. Although it was a painful process, after careful consideration and much discussion with Frank during therapy, Robin decided to end their 23-year marriage. The couple had successfully addressed the affair itself, but broader relationship issues came into focus for Robin as a result of the affair, which led to her decision to end their relationship.

Issues to Address in Deciding How to Move Forward

Specific Behavior Changes Needed to Decrease the Likelihood of a Future Affair

A major factor for couples to consider regarding the future of their relationship is the likelihood that another affair could occur in the future. In Table 14.1, we have listed a broad set of questions that most couples would benefit from

TABLE 14.1. Factors to Consider in Reaching a Decision about Your Relationship

Evaluating your partner

- Is your partner's affair an isolated event or part of a long-term pattern of betrayals?
- Has your partner been able to make and sustain difficult changes in the past?
- Has your partner made appropriate responses to the affair by
  - Taking responsibility and expressing remorse for his or her actions?
  - Addressing his or her own characteristics that contributed to vulnerability to an affair?

Evaluating your relationship

- Have you and your partner been able to address important relationship factors that contributed to risk of an affair?
- Have you and your partner restored a positive relationship? If not, do you believe you will be able to do so in the future?

Evaluating yourself

- Have you addressed any aspects of yourself or your behavior that might have contributed to a risky situation for you and your partner?
- Have you reached a decision to move on in spite of your hurt?
- Are you able and willing to take gradual, appropriate risks in restoring trust in your partner and your relationship?
- How does your decision take into account your own values and beliefs, including religious beliefs to the degree they are relevant?

Evaluating your relationship with the environment, including other people

- Have you altered the way that you interact with others in the environment in order to promote commitment and safeguard your relationship?
- Is the outside person a threat that needs to be considered or dealt with further?
- Has your relationship created problems or damages in other settings that need to be addressed in order for you to be successful in your intimate relationship?
- How will your decision affect other important people in your life, such as your children?

addressing when deciding how to move forward, either together or separately. Included in this list is a series of questions that fundamentally ask whether both partners are committed to, and are in the process of, making important changes that became apparent in the formulation. For example, as alluded to in Chapter 12, Pam came to recognize that she had a way of relating to men in her work setting that put her at risk for blurring of boundaries, developing inappropriate intimacy, and potential infidelity. She and her coworker, Mark, had set up many long work meetings involving just the two of them, frequently commented on what a great team they were, praised each other's efforts, and hugged when they had successes. During couple therapy, Pam came to recognize this risky pattern and began setting much stronger boundaries with men at work as well as socially. Knowing that Pam was making these changes was critical for Tom before he could decide to continue in the relationship.

However, although both Tom and Pam were committed to making changes and were attempting to do so, they were less successful in another important domain for the future of their relationship. They both agreed that when they interacted with each other, Tom was relatively unassertive and Pam was quite assertive, at times bordering on aggressive. They developed strategies to alter this pattern of interaction, such as having Tom make proposals of what they would do during one evening out a week, in marked contrast to their previous pattern in which Tom would ask Pam what she wanted to do and routinely go along with it. They specified several ways they could create more balance in their day-to-day lives regarding decision making, but they continued to struggle in this area to some degree, even as therapy terminated. Frequently, Tom had difficulty clarifying for himself and articulating to Pam his own preferences and ideas; likewise, Pam had difficulty holding back from expressing her preferences and dominating their decision making. Even though the couple acknowledged their frustration with the difficulty of making these changes, they continued to make efforts in this area, recognizing Pam's tendency to lose respect for Tom when he behaved unassertively. At the end of treatment, both Pam and Tom were committed to their relationship, concluding that their therapeutic work had been highly productive and essential for the future well-being of their relationship, while also recognizing that some of their interaction patterns were difficult to change, even with consistent effort. Thus, for Tom and Pam, their formulation of the factors that increased Pam's risk for infidelity not only clarified a pattern that Pam needed to change at work but also made them aware of a change they needed to make in the way they related to each other.

It is not assumed that a relationship must be completely "affair proofed" as a prerequisite for a couple to decide to stay together. Almost no couples are able to make all the changes they would like to make, and even if they are, there is still no guarantee that an affair could not happen again in the future. Likewise, all desired changes need not have occurred by the end of therapy. Similar to couple therapy to deal with issues other than infidelity, often therapy ends when the partners have acquired the needed skills and motivation to proceed and continue making changes on their own outside of therapy. In addition, some changes are more important than others in the couple's decision regarding their future. For example, it was critical that Pam set firmer boundaries in her interactions with other men; however, her expressing strong feelings about where to eat dinner might be less risky to the relationship, even though it contributes to the maintenance of her dominant position relative to Tom. Therefore, in helping the couple decide about the future of the relationship, you need to help them differentiate between essential changes and changes that are desirable but not prominent in their decision of whether to stay together.

Using the Past to Predict the Future

Whether important behavior changes are already occurring or not, both partners have the somewhat difficult task of predicting what will happen in the future if they stay together. This task can be particularly frightening, given that most couples did not anticipate that they would ever have to confront an affair in their relationship. Will important changes that are occurring now persist long term, or are they short lived and perhaps the result of a threatened divorce or end of a committed relationship? Once the pressure ends, will either individual revert to his or her old ways of behaving? If one individual has committed to make changes but has not been able to do so yet because of a variety of circumstances, can the other partner trust that these will indeed come about, or are they idle promises? One type of information that can be of particular importance in addressing these questions is to turn to the individual's previous behavior. As often stated, unless there is an identifiable way in which the current situation is different from previous circumstances, the best predictor of future behavior is past behavior.

Thus, a participating partner's affair can be viewed within the context of other commitments and value-based behaviors from that partner in the past. For example, Sam and Debbie sought couple therapy when Debbie felt that she was at the "end of her rope." During their 15-year marriage, Sam had at least 11 different affairs, the last 3 with the same woman. Each time when Debbie found out about the affair, Sam seemed extremely remorseful, promised to change, and was very attentive to Debbie, only to initiate another affair in subsequent months. This persistent pattern of infidelity in itself would be sufficient for many partners to conclude that Sam was unlikely to change; in fact, in this domain his past behavior of infidelity had been an excellent predictor of his future behavior for many years. In addition, as they explored their relationship more broadly, Debbie realized that Sam had betrayed her with his dishonesty in multiple areas unrelated to his affairs, such as his frequent promises to be present at the children's events, promises that he rarely kept. Debbie witnessed Sam's dishonesty and betrayals in other areas of his life as well. Much to her discomfort, he underreported his income each year on their tax records, arguing that everyone did it and that he paid more than his fair share of taxes anyway. His financial dishonesty was not confined to an "impersonal government." Debbie was aware that Sam had cheated his business partners on several occasions, always justifying that he had done most of the work and deserved a larger share of the profit. After several months in couple therapy to focus on the affair, Debbie concluded that it was time for her to "face reality." She acknowledged that Sam seemed sincere each time he promised to change, but in large part she had denied what she really believed: that he would never change. She had suffered deep pain when her own parents had divorced, and she had committed to herself that she would never put her own children in a similar position. Also, she had come from a poor family and reveled in the social status that Sam's financial success had provided; therefore, she had denied these strong patterns in Sam's behavior. Once she "took off the blinders," she concluded that, to maintain her self-respect and avoid future bouts of depression resulting from endless disappointment, she needed to end her relationship with Sam, although she would always miss his warmth, fun, and charisma.

Although this example is extreme and somewhat dramatic, many partners in less extreme circumstances are capable of looking at the other individual's broad patterns of behavior over time to assess whether important changes are likely to occur in the future. Consequently, it is appropriate to address the questions in Table 14.1 to evaluate whether the affair is an isolated event or part of a long-term pattern of betrayals and whether the individual has been able, in the past, to make, and to continue making, difficult changes. Almost the opposite of Debbie's conclusions, Vicki felt strongly that Bill would actually accomplish the changes that he needed to make. Although his affair had been very painful for her, she recognized that it was an isolated event that seemed to occur in response to several atypical factors that converged at one time. In fact, other than this one affair, Bill had always been faithful to Vicki and had not shown inappropriate interest in other women. More generally, she had always found him to be an extremely determined person, one of the attributes she most admired about him. When he decided to do something and made a commitment, he almost always followed through. In this context, Vicki was able to give a strong, affirmative answer to the important question of whether Bill had taken responsibility and expressed remorse for his inappropriate behavior. Through the course of their therapy, she concluded that Bill had developed good insight into the bases of his behaviors that contributed to his affair and had made thoughtful and determined commitments to Vicki about what he would change and *how* he would go about making those changes. In addition to avoiding future affairs, Bill also seemed committed to improving the overall quality of their marriage by making more time for Vicki, becoming a better listener when they talked, and including her directly in their joint business decisions. Thus, when she combined her experience of his current willingness to change with his determination and success in making changes in the past, she decided to continue in their marriage with a willingness to make changes herself, while fully expecting Bill to do the same. Combining a person's knowledge of a participating partner's past behavior with the way that he or she has addressed the affair can help the injured partner to make reasonable decisions regarding whether to continue the relationship in the future.

The Role of Emotions in Deciding about the Future

Just as the initial decision to get married or enter into a committed relationship typically is not based exclusively on logic and the prediction of future behavior, partners' decisions about whether to stay in the current relationship after an affair are not based solely on a coherent assessment of contributing factors and future risks. Each partner's emotions are also central in the decision about how to proceed. Even if it seems rather clear that the participating partner is unlikely ever to have another affair, the injured partner might experience a decrease or absence of feelings of love and respect for the participating partner. Some partners believe, "It is simply over, finished. Whatever was there between us in the past is dead." For other partners, the realization may not be this clear, but one partner might recognize that he or she no longer has the intensity of feeling for the other person that would be necessary to maintain their relationship long term. This kind of realization served as a major basis for Gail's decision to end her relationship with Brad after his affair with a female graduate student, Jill. Gail's fury toward Brad and her humiliation while working in the same department with Brad and Jill had subsided, and Gail had made strong efforts in therapy to understand the various factors that contributed to Brad's decision to have the affair. Furthermore, Gail realized that their early relationship was based on Brad's role as a mentor for Gail and that more recently, as she became a professional herself, this style of relating was no longer appropriate. Gail concluded that even though both she and Brad had worked hard to relate as equals, they were not successful. Although this realization was important, the determining factor in her decision to seek a divorce was more emotional in nature. As she told Brad during a therapy session,

GAIL: Brad, this is incredibly difficult to say, given all that we've been through and the efforts we've both made to keep our marriage together. But the reality, at least for me, is that it hasn't worked, and I need to end it. As we've discussed many times, we've needed to find a way to relate as equals, instead of me looking up to you as the successful professor. I don't really think we've been successful at that, but if that was all of it, I would keep trying. But there's something much more important that is hard for me to understand myself or to explain. After we got through the initial emotional roller coaster of your affair, I realized that something had changed within me. It's like something really died in our relationship and my feelings toward you, and I know it's not coming back. I hate saying this because we both have had enough pain recently, but my feelings are gone and I have to move on. And I hope you will too.

BRAD: But . . .

GAIL: Let me finish. You need to understand that this is real. I waited all this time because I wanted to make sure that I wasn't just in shock, or protecting myself, or trying to get back at you for what you had done. And it's not any of that. It's that the joy, the passion, and my desire to be close with you are really gone. Brad, I have already let go and I can't come back.

THERAPIST: Gail, I know that was extremely difficult for you to say, and, Brad, based on what you've said before about desperately wanting to stay married, what you just heard might be your worst nightmare. I know you probably have a lot that you want to say in response, but I think it's critical that you understand why Gail is telling you that your relationship is over. I want to give you all the time that you need to respond, but first let's make sure that you really understand what Gail is telling you. What did you hear?

Just as affairs typically do not end immediately, when one person says "It's over," marriages and committed relationships usually do not end quickly either after such a pronouncement. Brad tried in various ways to persuade Gail to reconsider but without success. As Brad gradually came to accept that their marriage was ending, the remainder of therapy focused on helping the couple terminate their relationship in the least destructive and most respectful way possible. To a degree, this effort was successful although Brad ended their marriage believing that Gail had quit too soon and that he had ruined his best chance at happiness.

In some instances, the emotional response of one partner, usually the injured partner, dictates the future of the relationship but not necessarily in a healthy, adaptive manner. As we have noted previously, some individuals have difficulty regulating emotions, particularly negative feelings. Emotion dysregulation has been discussed in the clinical literature primarily within the context of borderline personality disorders (Linehan, 1993); however, Kirby and Baucom (Kirby & Baucom, 2007a, 2007b) discuss how it cuts across a number of diagnostic and clinical syndromes and affects couples' functioning. We have encountered many situations in which the injured partner has broad difficulties regulating negative emotions, far beyond the trauma of the infidelity per se. For such individuals, the emotional intensity that results from infidelity precipitates ongoing emotional turmoil from which he or she has immense difficulty recovering. Even after many months, any discussion of the affair precipitates extreme distress. Moreover, it appears that the mere presence of the participating partner can serve as a trigger for flashbacks or strong reexperiencing of overwhelming emotions. Such couples are at high risk for divorce when one or both partners conclude that they simply cannot continue in this highly distressing emotional climate; it is as if the crisis of Stage 1 in response to infidelity does not end but continues indefinitely.

Recognitions that the affair has led to important emotional changes or new realizations come not only from the injured partner but from the participating partner as well. For example, Kathy and Mike had what they both described as a "good marriage" for 8 years. At that point, Kathy had an affair with a work colleague, David. She had always wondered whether the quality of her marriage and her feelings for Mike were all that one could expect in life or whether it was possible to have more. Even after doing her best to rule out the intensity that comes with a new relationship such as with David, and recognizing the excitement and intrigue that accompany a secret romantic relationship, she still concluded that the way that she "connected" with David was much more rewarding and gratifying than she had ever experienced with Mike. With David, she was at her best as an individual and experienced what she felt was a healthy, intimate way of relating that she had always envisioned. Although she worked hard in couple therapy to improve her relationship with Mike, she came to recognize that it would never be nearly as good a relationship as she believed she was capable of having, and her limited experience of emotional connection with him would never be fulfilling. After much soul searching, she concluded that, although she was not unhappy with Mike, she wanted more from a marriage and asked for a divorce.

While encouraging both partners to take their emotions into account in making such a large decision, certain cautions are necessary as well. First, as many partners have experienced by this point in therapy, emotions change considerably over time after an affair and often in unpredictable ways. Particularly in the context and trauma of infidelity, what a person feels today might not be what he or she feels tomorrow. These changing feelings account for one reason why couple therapy after infidelity typically requires a number of months; only after extended time can the partners start to experience with some confidence that both their feelings and their thoughts are relatively stable and can serve as the basis for making such a major life decision. As a result, we discourage partners from making quick decisions about the future of their relationship, even if such decisions seem clear and strongly felt. Second, it is important to try to discern whether a lack of feelings toward the partner reflects core feelings about the individual or whether this absence results from a temporary need for an injured partner to protect him- or herself from further pain or to punish the participating partner. All these issues should be addressed during the course of therapy so that current feelings or lack of emotion can be understood and acted on appropriately.

Therefore, just as with other individual and couple-related decisions, we encourage partners who are deciding about the future of their relationship to take into account both (1) their logic, reasoning, and best predictions about their future behaviors and (2) their emotions and desires related to their partner and the relationship. At times, both logic and emotions lead to the same conclusions; however, in other circumstances, the two might be quite contrary. For example, as noted in the prior discussion of Debbie and Sam, Debbie had been captivated by Sam's charisma for many years and also was extremely frightened by the possibility of divorce. Therefore, she had ignored her own logical conclusion that, after multiple affairs, Sam was unlikely to remain faithful in the future. When she finally allowed herself to experience the reality that he was unlikely to change, she gave primary emphasis to his pattern of consistent infidelity as a prominent factor in her decision to seek a divorce. She came to realize that, in her circumstance, her logic needed to take precedence over her feelings for Sam and her fears of being alone and subjecting her children to divorce.

There is no clear rule of thumb to use in guiding couples as they combine their reason and emotions in reaching such important decisions. Our major recommendation is that both sets of factors should be taken into account, and each factor should be noted for what it is without one factor contaminating the other. For example, just because an individual still has strong positive feelings for a partner, these feelings should not be used to distort the individual's logic about the likelihood of infidelity again in the future. Instead, it is much more valuable to acknowledge the strong feelings, along with the recognition that the couple is still at risk for infidelity in the future. A good decision must take both of these factors into account.

Making a decision about the future of a relationship becomes increasingly complex as each person takes into account not only what is best for him- or herself but also for other persons who are affected by the decision. What is best for one person is not necessarily best for other individuals significantly affected by the couple's decision to stay together or separate. That is, one person's continued growth and well-being might best be served within the context of the relationship, but the other partner might be happier if the relationship ends. Also quite appropriately, almost all couples want to take into account the impact that a divorce or staying together will have on their children. If the couple concludes that both partners and the children are best served by a given decision, then the resolution is straightforward. However, if a given decision is in the best interest of some members of the immediate family but not others, then deciding how to proceed is much more complex. For example, Jasmine experienced conflicting feelings when she concluded that she would be happier if her marriage with Norm ended after his affair, but she felt reluctant to put her children, ages 6 and 9, through a divorce. The children's biological father—her first husband—had been killed in an automobile accident, and it had been difficult for the children to develop a trusting, loving relationship with Norm. Over time, they had bonded deeply with him, and she could not envision putting them through another loss because of her own unhappiness. There are no easy decisions in such circumstances, and declarations from friends, such as "You have to put your own needs first" or "The needs of your children have to take precedence," often are oversimplifications of very complex family situations. There is no algorithm or clear formula for how to combine the needs of the various people who are central in such situations to arrive at a decision regarding the future of the relationship, and we make that clear to couples as they grapple with these complexities. What we believe to be important is that the various factors are articulated, both people have a clear understanding of how each person perceives the situation, and they push themselves to make a thoughtful decision that takes into account the emotional and practical needs of the people who are centrally affected by the couple's relationship.

The Role of the Therapist in Helping the Couple Make a Decision about the Future of the Relationship

As with all decisions that the couple makes, the ultimate conclusion they reach regarding the future of their relationship rests with them. As a therapist, your primary role is to ensure that the process proceeds appropriately. You need to be certain that all the factors discussed previously are articulated, that both partners' perspectives are fully heard and respected, and that both partners and the couple as a unit are making reasonable decisions. At the same time, you should not adopt the attitude that "whatever the couple decides is fine; it's up to them." It is true that the couple will decide what to do, but it is not true that any decision is fine. If one or both partners seem to be ignoring important factors or if their reasoning in putting these factors together is grossly distorted, then, as a therapist, you need to point out the distortions and help the couple consider all important information appropriately, even if they eventually reach a decision that is different from what you consider optimal. For example, if Debbie had decided to continue in her relationship with Sam after his 11 affairs and concluded, in spite of evidence to the contrary, that he would change, the therapist might address this decision as follows:

DEBBIE: This is really hard, and I know I'm taking a risk that can sound silly. But I love Sam, and this time I think that he means it. I think he's really going to change, and I believe that, even after so many affairs, he won't hurt me again. I don't think I'll ever stop believing in him, so I want to stay in the marriage and give it another try.

THERAPIST: That is a huge decision, and I imagine a lot of people might think it *is* silly. However, as we've discussed, your ultimate responsibility is to the people most centrally involved here: you, Sam, and your children. And, Debbie, your love for Sam is apparent. I think it also is admirable that you believe people can change, even after a long-term pattern of unacceptable behavior. But, I want to push you further. In addition to just believing in Sam in some general way, let's see if we can help you articulate what you have learned during our work together and outside of our sessions that would lead you to conclude that this time it will be different. You've told me that you said the same thing each time you found out about a previous affair, and then the pattern repeated itself. I want to hold both you and Sam accountable. Why would it be different this time? What has changed, and what else would need to change? All those questions that we have been addressing all along. I'd like to hear from you first, Debbie. And, Sam, it is critical to hear from you as well. Are you really likely to change, and how will that occur? I think we need to consider more than your current motivation and commitment to change since relying on that hasn't worked well for the two of you in the past; we need to be specific about what is different this time.

Couples make many decisions that are different from what a therapist might conclude is optimal, and most therapists understand that couples need to reach their own conclusions because they are the ones who will live with the implications of those decisions. Our experience suggests that instead of being too forceful and directive with couples regarding decisions about the future of their relationship, some therapists have a tendency to hold back when the couple is discussing their future, even when the therapist sees the couple ignoring important issues or overemphasizing certain factors in a way that is likely to lead to unexpected consequences. In such circumstances, we view it as part of the therapist's role to note this distorted or misguided process and help the couple continue to explore and discuss the issues further until they can reach a decision that is based on a thoughtful integration of the many complex factors involved.

Implementing the Decision

How to Proceed If the Couple Decides to End the Relationship

At this point in therapy, some couples will decide to end their relationship. Such a decision might be based on the hurt and pain surrounding the affair or the belief that an affair is likely to happen again in the future. Likewise, the infidelity can serve as an impetus to explore the couple's relationship more fully, and such broader examination can lead one or both partners to decide that the relationship needs to end. When a partner reaches such a decision, the therapist's role is similar to situations in which any couple in therapy decides to terminate their relationship. A broad discussion of how to help couples bring their relationship to a close is beyond the scope of the current discussion, but helpful presentations of this topic are available in other sources. For example, Epstein and Baucom (2002) provide a discussion of this important topic from a cognitive–behavioral perspective, and our self-help book for couples addresses this issue as well (Snyder et al., 2007). Overall, we try to help couples end their relationship in a manner in which both people are able to maintain a sense of personal dignity, and each partner not only respects the way that the other person has handled the situation but also concludes, "I liked the way that I handled the situation. I acted within my own value system. And although it was tempting at times to get dirty, I didn't do that."

In addition to the guidelines that we would use with any couple divorcing or ending a relationship, certain issues need to be emphasized within the context of infidelity. First, we explicitly recommend that the injured partner avoid using the infidelity and potentially damaging related information as a way to manipulate or intimidate the participating partner, either in terms of reaching a particular legal settlement or in achieving other desired ends. For example, the injured partner may have copies of e-mail exchanges between the participating partner and the outside person that would be damaging if shared with other people, such as children or colleagues. This was the case for June, whose husband, Al, had an affair with his coworker, Marty. Not only did their e-mail exchanges contain sexually explicit information, but they also made fun of their boss and joked about how company funds had supported their "business trips" together. June recognized the explosive nature of these e-mails, which she had printed, but in spite of her wish to retaliate, she assured Al that she would not share these messages with his company or threaten to use them to obtain a better divorce settlement. She realized that, although she might derive momentary pleasure in watching him lose his job, treating anyone that way was not consistent with her own value system. In essence, June was behaving according to a recommendation that the therapist offered early in treatment: "Do not let the other person's hurtful actions provoke you to behave in ways that you yourself do not respect."

Although both partners might begin the termination of their relationship with a constructive mind-set, when one person behaves in a destructive or self-serving manner during the termination of the relationship, there can be a strong pull for the other partner to respond accordingly. In particular, if the participating partner behaves in a hurtful or destructive way once the couple has decided to end the relationship, it can be very difficult for the injured partner to resist the urge to "even the score." Your role as a therapist is to help the couple get through these difficult times and maintain an atmosphere of civility. It can be difficult to accomplish these goals when the two partners have decided to move on separately and, therefore, the well-being of the relationship is no longer a priority. In most cases, we continue working with couples through this phase of terminating their relationship.

Furthermore, during termination it often is necessary to revisit an issue discussed in Chapter 4: what to say to other people about the infidelity. Early in treatment when the partners are still deciding about the future of their relationship, they might agree to keep the affair private in case they decide to maintain their relationship. They understand that telling other people such as their parents and friends might create difficulties if they decide to stay together. However, that motivation is no longer relevant if they are terminating their relationship. Often the injured partner wants to tell other people about the affair at this point, both to receive support for the agonizing experience he or she has been through and to provide justification for ending a marriage or committed relationship. We do not attempt to impose any particular resolution regarding what to tell and to whom, but we do provide several guidelines to couples as they make these decisions as discussed next.

Be Honest about Your Motivations

As mentioned previously, at times one partner—most likely the injured partner—wants to hurt the other individual by disclosing highly personal and compromising information about the affair to other people. As in almost all contexts in working with couples, we caution partners against using vengeance or punishment as a way to meet their individual needs. Consequently, it is important to have both partners understand the true bases for their behavior and avoid rationalizing hurtful behavior. Hopefully, both partners will be discreet and share information with other individuals only when doing so serves a valuable purpose, such as to receive support, and the individual is an appropriate person to turn to for that reason.

Whenever Possible, Inform the Other Partner about Your Plans to Talk to Others

If both partners are willing to do so, it can be valuable for them to have discussions during this latter phase of therapy—as well as in the future—regarding whom they plan to tell about the affair, what level of detail they plan to include, and their reasons for sharing information with this person. Given that the two partners have common family members and mutual friends and associates, awkwardness and unpredictability can be minimized if both partners are honest and forthcoming about what they are telling to whom. Otherwise, the other partner might experience anxiety and embarrassment around mutual friends, not knowing who knows what. Of course, these conversations between the two partners will not always take place ahead of time, given that some of these disclosure conversations with other people evolve unexpectedly. In such instances, it is preferable if both partners agree that they will inform the other partner as soon as possible after the conversations have occurred. Some couples handle these situations productively, whereas others, particularly injured partners, insist, "I'll say what I want to say. It's none of your business what I tell anyone. You did it, and if I decide to tell someone the truth about what happened, that's your problem, not mine." Such a position suggests a willingness, or perhaps a motivation, to hurt the other person, and we encourage that individual to exercise caution before behaving in a vindictive manner. We remind such persons that they might be compromising their own values and that vengeful behavior often results in similar behavior from the other person.

Not only does the couple need to decide who will be informed, but it is preferable if they can agree on which of them will communicate the information and what level of detail will be shared. In some instances, one or both individuals might have strong relationships with the other partner's family. For example, Gail had close relationships with Brad's parents and wanted them to understand her painful decision to divorce Brad. Although Brad did not want his parents to be aware of his affair, Gail insisted that they know. When Brad realized that she would not negotiate on this point, he convinced Gail to let him talk to them initially and acknowledge what he had done. Then Gail would talk with them about her decision, focusing on her own feelings and her desired ongoing relationship with Brad's parents.

Give High Priority to Children's Needs in Deciding What to Say

A special case of who should know what information and how it should be communicated involves the couple's children. In making decisions about the children's knowledge of an affair when a couple is terminating their relationship, the principles discussed previously apply. Thus, telling the children about a parent's affair should not be done as a way to punish that parent. Moreover, when partners need to turn to other people for support, we strongly recommend that they turn to people other than their children, particularly if the children are minors. Many injured partners express that it is very difficult to resist telling the children, particularly if the children are opposed to the divorce and continue asking why it is happening. In these situations, injured partners might say, "I shouldn't have to take the blame for ruining the family. I can't stand it when the children are crying and begging me not to get a divorce, and it appears that I am the one tearing their world apart." To counterbalance these strong feelings, we encourage both partners to think about what is best for the children long term. Many individuals who have had an affair are otherwise good, loving parents. In most instances, it is preferable for children to maintain strong, caring relationships with both parents, particularly during such frightening times. Therefore, it can be unwise to say things to children that will damage their relationship with one parent. Consequently, we suggest to parents that they be quite cautious in what they tell their children about the affair. Parents need to remember that they will continue to have this option in the future as the children get older, but once the information has been revealed to the children, it cannot become confidential again. If one parent insists that the children know about the affair and refuses to compromise on this position, then it is still valuable for the couple to discuss exactly what information will be shared and how they will share it. We have seen couples handle this type of situation in a variety of ways: the two parents together telling the children, the participating partner telling them, or the injured partner telling the children while the participating partner refuses to be part of such a conversation.

Helping any couple end a long-term, committed relationship or marriage can be very difficult, particularly when the relationship is further complicated by infidelity. In some instances, even with concerted efforts by the therapist, the relationship ends with anger, hostility, and legal efforts by both partners to get as much as possible for themselves. On the other hand, following the guidelines described previously, we have often been successful in helping couples treat each other respectfully and maintain their dignity as they bring their relationship to a close.

How to Proceed If the Couple Decides to Stay Together

Many couples make a decision to stay together in their relationship after an affair. In such instances, we communicate two important messages to them: (1) Although this decision is critically important, reaching the decision in and of itself does not imply that the couple's work is done and (2) making a commitment to stay together involves pledging to do whatever is necessary to make the relationship as strong and gratifying as possible for now and for the future. With regard to the decision to continue in their relationship, we ask both partners to make this statement in a clear, definitive way that both partners can understand. In most instances, the partners both state their decision in a brief and caring manner and then move forward to focus on building their relationship. The following dialogue is an example of how Bill and Vicki declared their commitment during a therapy session:

THERAPIST: Both of you have suggested and maybe even have been explicit about wanting to stay together, but given all the hard work you've done, I think it might be valuable if each of you tells the other in very clear terms the decision you have made about whether to stay together.

BILL: Sure, I'm delighted to do that. I absolutely want to continue in our marriage. I can't believe that I almost destroyed it, and I am so thankful that you are willing to give me another chance. I want this to work more than anything I have ever wanted, and I will not mess it up again, no matter what happens. Vicki, I love you so much, and although I realize that we can never make this pain disappear, I'm going to do everything possible to make you happy and treat you like the amazing person that you are.

VICKI: Thank you, Bill. I know that you feel that way, but I really needed to hear you say it. It's been awful, and I don't want to be a Pollyanna about it. But at the same time, I do think we've learned from all of this, and we have the potential to have a better relationship than we did before. So, I really do forgive you, and I also commit to doing everything I can to make our marriage great. And in case that wasn't clear, I have decided that I do want to stay married to you.

Vicki and Bill found this pronouncement to be very meaningful, and it was all they needed to say. At times, some couples want to do something more symbolic to demonstrate their recommitment to each other. For example, they might write a letter to each other in which they express their feelings and recommitment. Other couples might have a more extensive recommitment ceremony, either just between the two of them or with close people in their lives present, sometimes including clergy. Of course, in these more public ceremonies, the reasons for the recommitment are not explicitly addressed. Other couples might write down their resentments and the hurts they have been "holding onto" on pieces of paper and tear them up or burn them. Yet other couples might do something together that they really enjoy to celebrate a new phase of their relationship, ranging from having dinner at their favorite restaurant to taking a trip together. We find that couples vary greatly in terms of their desire for some symbolic act, and we think it is most important that each couple proceed in a way that is most meaningful for them. What we find to be critical is that, if couples have some such act, ceremony, or celebration, it not be viewed as a final act and not detract from the focus of the second issue: identifying concrete actions that the partners need to take in order to build the strongest relationship possible.

The next steps for couples vary, depending on the work and conceptualization that have occurred to this point in therapy. They might have recognized that one or both partners need individual therapy to address long-standing personal issues that affect the relationship and put them at risk for an affair. They might conclude that they need to interact with the environment in different ways, such as joining a couple's group that will support them as a unit. Many couples will have pinpointed areas in their relationship that need to be addressed, and these issues now become the focus of couple therapy in much the same way that couple therapy might have progressed in the absence of infidelity. That is, the emphasis in treatment shifts from a major focus on the past to a focus on how the couple can best move forward. Even so, as the couple knows by now, the impact of the infidelity does not disappear. Thus, in addition to addressing a wide range of relationship difficulties typical of many couples, partners who have decided to stay together after an affair also need to address several issues that we now discuss.

Addressing Flashback-Type Phenomena

Although the frequency, duration, and intensity of flashbacks likely have decreased over the months since the affair has ended, couples need to be aware that they may still recur in spite of the couple's recommitment and focus on the future. The same triggers or stimuli that evoked flashbacks previously might continue to have this effect. In addition, it can be helpful for couples to know that they might experience distress or flashbacks on the anniversary of important events related to the affair. These flashbacks can be handled in much the same way as discussed in Chapter 5. For example, Vicki and Bill envisioned that they both might experience distress on the 1-year anniversary of the day Vicki confronted Bill about his affair. They decided that they would not necessarily bring up the affair on that day, although either person was free to do so if it seemed important. Instead, they decided that they would go out that evening to a movie, something they both enjoyed. They were not attempting to deny or avoid the reality of the past. Instead, they believed that planning to go to a movie could help them focus their attention elsewhere, while at the same time serving as an indirect acknowledgment that they wanted to be together on such a difficult evening. Most important, we believe that couples need to have realistic expectations about the future and not become discouraged when feelings, thoughts, or images of the affair resurface. They should understand that such experiences are typical of many couples and do not signify that the couple has dealt with the infidelity inappropriately or that their relationship is doomed. Having these conversations with the couple soon after they make the decision to stay together can help to prepare them and give them the proper mind-set to be able to handle flashbacks if they do recur.

Building/Rebuilding Trust

By definition, infidelity implies that a betrayal has occurred and that a major basis of trust has been violated. Given that betrayals such as infidelity disrupt basic assumptions about the participating partner and the relationship, there often is a "spreading effect," in which violated trust in this one important area leads to a broader, more fundamental experience that the participating partner is not trustworthy. Therefore, in most instances, even when both partners recommit to the relationship, they still have to make efforts to develop a new sense of trust in each other and the relationship. Partners' act of deciding to stay in the relationship does not mean that trust suddenly reappears. In fact, the events surrounding the affair along with the deception that typically accompanies it provide strong evidence that the participating partner at times has not been honest and forthcoming. To ignore these experiences would seem to be an expression of denial that is unhealthy in most couples' relationships. Consequently, couples should not equate commitment and love with trust, particularly in these circumstances. Partners struggle with how to approach this issue, and it is not uncommon for injured partners to make statements such as, "I love you, and I am committed to our relationship. And I want to trust you, but given what has happened, I don't. I wish I did, but I honestly don't know how to make that happen."

After a major betrayal, trust cannot simply be willed as a result of caring or desire. Thus, exhortations to "just trust me" are ineffective, even if the injured partner would like to do so. Likewise, intervening to increase trust on a broad, global level is difficult, if not impossible. Instead, a global sense of trust is likely to evolve based on multiple experiences that a partner is dependable and honest in *specific*, important domains. Therefore, we help couples clarify which areas of their relationship already involve a good sense of trust at present and which areas need attention. Couples can approach this issue by completing the following sentences:

- "I trust you to . . . "
- "I trust you with . . . "

- "I don't trust you to . . ."
- "I don't trust you with . . ."
- "I have some but not full trust regarding . . ."

For example, Tom answered some of these questions in the following way when thinking about Pam:

TOM: I know I can trust you in many ways. Obviously, I know I can trust you with the children to be a good mother; I never worry about that. And I know I can trust you with money; you've always been very responsible, and it's not like I worry that you're going to steal the money and set up a secret bank account. Plus, I generally trust that you're a responsible person; you meet all of your professional responsibilities, and you do all your chores and tasks at home in a top-notch way.

THERAPIST: And how about Pam's interaction with you? Will you tell Pam in what ways can you trust her and not trust her?

TOM: Well, in terms of our interactions, I'm still not sure that I can trust you to let me be myself with my own opinions, feelings, and preferences. It's hard for me to express them in the first place, and if I try, I still feel like you overwhelm me. You seem to have such strong opinions, and if I disagree with you, I feel like you tell me why you're right and I'm wrong, and you make me feel stupid. So even though you say you want to know what I think and feel, I'm not sure I believe you or trust you; it's as if you want to hear me as long as I agree with you. Those are some of the things that are important to me.

THERAPIST: Exactly, Tom, that *is* important. You both have talked about trying to change how you interact, and you both have said you want Tom to be more assertive with his feelings and opinions. It sounds like one reason that you don't do that, Tom, is because you don't trust that Pam will respect your opinions and feelings; is that right?

TOM: Yes, that's right.

THERAPIST: So that might be an important area where we try to build a greater sense of trust by setting it up so that the two of you have different experiences when you, Tom, try to open up with Pam. That is, you'll come to trust her if you both behave differently; does that make sense?

In discussing these areas of trust and mistrust, partners raise a wide variety of issues, from very concrete domains such as trusting the other person to remember to bring home groceries, to psychological issues such as the one just mentioned regarding trusting the partner with one's own feelings, to areas focusing on issues such as how the partner interacts with attractive, appealing people. All these domains are appropriate for discussion, and cumulative positive experiences across these domains can contribute to a more general sense of trust as well. Although issues certainly can arise in both directions, in most instances, struggles regarding trust focus on the extent to which the injured partner can trust the participating partner. For the couple to have successful trust-building experiences, both partners must fulfill their relative roles. Injured partners must take gradual steps to put themselves in a somewhat vulnerable position to experience whether the participating partner can be relied on in some specific domain. That is, developing trust in another person involves placing oneself in a position of uncertainty and seeing what happens. Participating partners must be reliable and follow through on a consistent basis. In helping the couple create experiences that can lead to the development of trust, you should encourage them to frame it in a way that is not viewed as a "test" of the participating partner to see if that individual succeeds or fails. Instead, the couple should work together to maximize the likelihood that they will be successful in promoting a broader sense of trust over time. In many instances, the couple will need to have a decision-making conversation in which they discuss how they will interact and what will contribute to the greatest likelihood of a successful experience.

The therapeutic principle of graduated exposure is important as the couple structures these experiences. That is, the injured partner is placing him- or herself in a vulnerable position that is likely to create some anxiety as a result of the uncertainty about what will happen. We talk to couples about taking small steps, thinking of ways they can place themselves at some small degree of risk without creating a situation that feels highly dangerous. Thus, the injured partner should take a small chance in an area, such that if the interaction is not successful, the person is not overwhelmed or distraught. Likewise, the interactions should not tax the abilities or resources of the participating partner, so that he or she can be successful and build trust with the injured partner. The following is an example of how the therapist helped Tom and Pam begin making efforts to develop trust regarding Tom's ability to disclose his thoughts and feelings.

THERAPIST: Good, let's think about how we can set up situations where Tom can start to trust that if he expresses his thoughts and feelings, Pam will respect them and not overwhelm him. To a large extent, this will likely happen if you simply follow the guidelines for couple conversations that we've discussed and practiced many times before. But this is about more than just using good communication skills; it is about developing a sense of trust that if one of you opens up and shares your inner thoughts and feelings with the other, the person who is listening will honor those thoughts and feelings and not "trample" on them in some way. So, Pam, in part it requires having a certain mind-set. We're going to start by asking Tom to choose some area in which he wants to share some of his thoughts and feelings with you, but not some topic that is so intense and vulnerable that it would make him highly uncomfortable to share it. Pam, what is crucial is that you get across the message to Tom that "when you open up and share what you are feeling and thinking, you can be assured that I will listen and respect what you tell me, regardless of whether I have the same thoughts and feelings or not. I won't take over; I won't tell you why you're wrong; I'll just try to listen and understand." If you can get that message across, Tom will start to trust that it is safe to open up to you. And that is your goal: to make it safe so that he can trust that you will be there for him if he takes the chance to share with you. Does that make sense to you?

PAM: Yes. I know this is still a problem for us, and I've been uncertain how to change it.

THERAPIST: Good. We've already talked about some of the mechanics of how you can do that, such as making good eye contact, using body language to show that you're interested, and reflecting his most important thoughts and feelings when he finishes speaking, without evaluating what he has said. But those are just tools, and you mainly need to get across in a sincere fashion that you are accepting and nonjudgmental. Of course, that doesn't mean that you're always going to agree with Tom. When you share your own perspective, it might be quite different from his. And, Tom, when Pam does share her own point of view, it will be important for you to accept that as well, without necessarily agreeing. Do you both understand what I am asking you to do? (*The therapist has a brief dialogue with each partner clarifying their roles and how this fits into the concept of building trust.*) Let's begin then. Tom, let's choose an area that has relevance and importance where you'd like to share some thoughts and feelings with Pam. But don't select something that would be extremely uncomfortable for you to talk about or an area where she might have real difficulty listening and accepting your thoughts and feelings. We'll work our way up to more difficult topics and discussions over time. What are some areas that we might consider?

In the prior example, to a large degree the actual conversation that results from this exercise might look like many couple conversations in which one partner shares thoughts and feelings. However, the conversations are being framed from the perspective of trust building and would be discussed from that perspective, both in setting up the conversation and evaluating the inter-action after it occurred. For Tom and Pam, this area was important because they had identified assertiveness as a key factor in what Pam found attractive in men.

Other domains of trust building might focus less on how the partners communicate with each other and more on other types of interactions. For example, a couple might discuss how they can develop trust that each partner will come home on time or be at other locations at prearranged times. In this instance, trust almost equates with dependability in doing what one person says he or she will do. Couples may also have extensive discussions about how the participating partner will interact and set boundaries with other individuals who could be a threat to the relationship. In Chapter 4, we discussed how Gail and Brad developed an agreement stipulating that he would notify her if he received any correspondence from Jill, the woman with whom he had a recent affair. In ending the affair, he had told Jill not to contact him again. Brad and Gail agreed that if Jill did contact him, he would not respond to Jill but would tell Gail immediately. Although Gail could never be certain that he was following through and it was painful to learn that Jill had e-mailed Brad, she came to trust that he was not communicating with Jill after he twice told her of Jill's recent e-mails to him, which he deleted without a response.

Our experience suggests that, for many couples, over time there is a grad-ual evolution not only with regard to trust in specific domains but also in terms of a more general sense of trust, to the degree that it is appropriate. At the same time, some partners express that once the affair has occurred, they can no longer have absolute trust that it will never happen again, no matter how much time has passed since the affair or how the participating partner is now behaving. In spite of this recognition of trust with some limitation, many couples can move forward to build stronger relationships with a basis of trust that serves them well.

Summary

After a couple has come through the initial crisis of confronting an affair, has spent considerable time understanding the variety of factors that contributed to the participating partner's decision to have the affair, and has addressed issues of forgiveness and how to move forward either together or apart, the partners are in a position to make a decision about the future of their relationship. Making that decision and implementing it have been the focus of the current chapter. In making this decision, each individual needs to take into account both (1) his or her reasoned perspective about whether the affair is likely to recur and whether the overall relationship can be strong and gratifying and (2) his or her emotions about staying in the relationship. A good decision will be based on both of these broad sets of factors as well as an understanding of how the decision will affect the other partner as well as other individuals central to the relationship, such as children. Most important, the decision should include a consideration of specific changes that are needed if the couple is to stay together or separate.

Some couples decide to end their relationship after one partner has had an affair. When the couple makes this decision, we do not consider our work with them to be complete. Instead, we believe it is important to help them bring their relationship to a close in a way that is as respectful of each person as possible, attempting to avoid hurtful and destructive actions that would harm either partner or other people they care about deeply, such as their children. Of great importance, if couples have children, they must address what the children will know about the affair and how this information will be communicated. Our general recommendation is to be extremely cautious in discussing such matters with children in order to preserve appropriate parent–child roles and to maximize the possibility that both partners can continue to have loving relationships with their children in the future.

When a couple decides to stay together, a wide variety of factors might need to be addressed, but in all such cases, two specific factors resulting from the affair should be discussed during this phase of therapy. First, the couple needs to be aware that occasional flashbacks are likely to occur in the future, and the couple must decide how they will address such flashbacks if they do occur. Second, infidelity by definition involves a breach of trust, and the couple needs to develop a strategy of how to rebuild trust within their new, evolving relationship. Rather than leaving them to attempt to establish trust on a broad, general level, we intervene with couples and help them pinpoint specific aspects of their relationship in which they need to build a sense of trust. We then work with them to design interactions in those specific areas that proceed in a gradual manner in order to enhance their experience of interacting in predictable, reliable ways that lead to reestablishing trust.

Resources from *Getting Past the Affair*

Our self-help book for couples, *Getting Past the Affair*, includes information related to the topics discussed in the current chapter. *Chapter 13*, "Can This Marriage Be Saved?," is devoted to helping the couple decide whether to stay together in their relationship or move forward separately, along with a discussion of what factors to take into account. Thus, it can serve as a useful adjunct to your therapeutic work with the couple. Exercise 13.1 guides the reader through a consideration of various factors relevant to this decision. The chapter also includes a discussion (pp. 303–307) regarding building trust if the couple stays together and how to attend to the needs of children if the relationship ends. Exercise 13.2 focuses on ways to implement the decision once it is made.

Chapter 14, "What Lies Ahead?"—the final chapter in the self-help book—can serve as a helpful resource for the partners as they move forward. It includes a discussion of anticipating setbacks, avoiding unnecessary risks, and continuing to communicate. It could be used in the final stage of treatment or at the very end as the partners terminate therapy, serving as a tool to help them maintain their perspective and more effectively navigate the challenges ahead.

CHAPTER 15

Concluding Comments

Addressing infidelity is complex, demanding, and often emotionally draining both for the couple and for their therapist. Many couples in this situation feel that they are living a nightmare from which they cannot awaken. Life seems confusing and out of control. An important source of support from the past—the partner—is no longer available for comfort during this turmoil. In such circumstances, a knowledgeable, confident, comforting professional can help the couple traverse the difficult landscape before them. Unfortunately, many couple therapists report that they lack perspective on how to proceed and find the issues raised by infidelity to be overwhelming. In this book, we have provided a broad outline of therapeutic stages that apply to working with couples recovering from infidelity, along with general principles to guide the therapist. Simply stated, the treatment proceeds through three major stages: (1) progressing through the initial crisis, (2) understanding how the affair came about, and (3) moving forward.

Stage 1 occurs immediately after discovery of the affair when the couple is in crisis and negative emotions typically are at their peak. During this stage, the therapist's goal is to guide the couple through the crisis by helping them reestablish some sense of equilibrium and minimize further damage. Stage 2 involves helping the couple gain understanding by reexamining the affair and the factors that contributed to it. Before the couple can move forward in their relationship, they need to understand why these painful events occurred. Stage 2 is where the bulk of the work occurs. Finally, in Stage 3—moving forward—the partners decide whether to stay together or end their relationship, and they identify and begin implementing the specifics involved in these decisions.

Although these stages are easy to conceptualize, guiding the couple through the process is challenging at each stage. During Stage 1, many couples are in emotional crisis and require considerable support. The therapist often receives unanticipated telephone calls at times outside of office hours, and the therapy sessions are frequent and prolonged. The therapist must be comfortable addressing strong, negative emotions and potentially destructive behaviors and must be prepared to offer guidance and direction when partners are overwhelmed and dysregulated.

Stage 2 presents its own unique challenges. Revisiting a trauma is painful for almost anyone, even if it resulted from a natural disaster or was inflicted by strangers. However, when the trauma was inflicted by a committed partner, revisiting the trauma and experiencing the related emotions can be overwhelming. Helping both partners be as open and nondefensive as possible requires extensive therapeutic skill, given that the couple often uncovers painful realities with incumbent tendencies to blame and defend. In our research investigating partners' mood after each treatment session, we found that both partners often expressed increased depressed mood and anxiety during Stage 2 as they confronted these difficult issues. Likewise, almost any therapist who has compassion for clients also will experience distress during this stage of therapy. Listening as both partners describe and, in a way, relive these hurtful experiences can be emotionally draining for the therapist. It is essential that, in addition to demonstrating compassion for the couple, the therapist also maintains enough perspective to help the couple engage in these difficult conversations and glean from them important information to facilitate their understanding of the context for the affair. Gaining this insight allows both partners to construct at least a partial answer to the question "How could this happen?" and also prepares them to move forward with their relationship.

In Stage 3, the partners face a different set of complex challenges as they are asked to decide whether to stay together or end their relationship. Although the turmoil of Stage 1 has subsided and they may have gained considerable understanding during Stage 2, the critical decisions required in Stage 3 can seem daunting. As a result, some partners would prefer to avoid making a decision. If the partners decide to terminate the relationship, they are giving up a way of life and becoming single again, perhaps after many years of marriage or a committed relationship. If the couple decides to stay together, they often must engage in significant work to build or rebuild a healthy relationship, at times when one or both partners still feel depleted by the trauma of the affair. Thus, helping the couple take this next step and implement important yet difficult life decisions is extremely challenging.

Thus, we recognize that working with couples recovering from infidelity is hard work. Our hope is that the guidelines, suggestions, and therapeutic techniques discussed in this volume will be of assistance as you help couples through this difficult process. At present, treatment outcome research for infidelity is still in its early stages, and we do not yet know which interventions within the approach described here contribute directly to overall effectiveness. We believe that it is crucial to help couples achieve the major goals in each of the three stages and that a wide range of specific therapeutic interventions from diverse theoretical perspectives might be helpful during each stage. We have suggested numerous specific strategies that we have used with success but have no strong conviction that these are the only effective interventions for achieving these important goals. This perspective is consistent with a broad body of empirical findings on couple therapy for distressed couples in which several different theoretical orientations have demonstrated efficacy, yet no single theoretical approach has demonstrated consistent superiority over the others (Baucom, Shoham, Mueser, & Daiuto, 1998; Snyder et al., 2006).

As a result, while keeping in mind the major goals and challenges of each stage, we strongly encourage therapists from various theoretical orientations to proceed creatively in adapting techniques from their respective theoretical orientation as well as integrating strategies outlined in the current volume toward addressing infidelity. In recent years, the field has gained a great deal from basic research on infidelity (cf. Allen et al., 2005), and treatment outcome research on infidelity is beginning to evolve (Atkins, Eldridge, Baucom, & Christensen, 2005; Baucom et al., 2006; Gordon et al., 2004) . Therefore, we anticipate that our clinical interventions will continue to be refined to develop maximally effective treatments for couples dealing with the aftermath of infidelity.

Although demanding, we have also found it extremely rewarding to work with couples as they garner the courage to face the complex circumstances surrounding infidelity. We agree with the long-standing belief that a time of crisis is also an opportunity for change and growth. In almost every instance in our clinical work with these couples, the partners have been presented with both a challenge and an opportunity for living their lives in a new way. At times, they must let go of the past and venture forward alone, whereas on other occasions, they must work to create a new chapter of their life together. In either case, as a knowledgeable, well-informed clinician, you have an opportunity to help both partners at a time of deep distress as they work to make a healthy passage into the next chapter of their lives.

References

Abrahms Spring, J., & Spring, M. (1996). *After the affair: Healing the pain and rebuilding trust when a partner has been unfaithful.* New York: HarperCollins .

Allen, E. S., Atkins, D. C., Baucom, D. H., Snyder, D. S., Gordon, K. C., & Glass, S. P. (2005). Intrapersonal, interpersonal, and contextual factors in engaging in and responding to extramarital involvement. *Clinical Psychology: Science and Practice, 12*(2), 101–130.

Amato, P. R., & Previti, D. (2003). People's reasons for divorcing: Gender, social class, the life course, and adjustment. *Journal of Family Issues, 24,* 602–626.

Amato, P. R., & Rogers, S. J. (1997). A longitudinal study of marital problems and subsequent divorce. *Journal of Marriage and the Family, 59,* 612–624.

American Psychiatric Association. (2000). *Diagnostic and statistical manual of mental disorders* (4th ed.). Washington, DC: Author.

Atkins, D. C. (2003). *Infidelity and marital therapy: Initial findings from a randomized clinical trial.* Unpublished doctoral dissertation, University of Washington.

Atkins, D. C., Eldridge, K. A., Baucom, D. H., & Christensen, A. (2005). Infidelity and behavioral couple therapy: Optimism in the face of betrayal. *Journal of Consulting and Clinical Psychology, 73,* 144–150.

Atkins, D. C., Yi, J., Baucom, D. H., & Christensen, A. (2005). Infidelity in couples seeking marital therapy. *Journal of Family Psychology, 19*(3), 470–473.

Atwood, J. D., & Seifer, M. (1997). Extramarital affairs and constructed meanings: A social constructionist therapeutic approach. *American Journal of Family Therapy, 25,* 55–74.

Baucom, D. H., Gordon, K. C., Snyder, D. K., Atkins, D. C., & Christensen, A. (2006). Treating affair couples: Clinical considerations and initial findings. *Journal of Cognitive Psychotherapy, 20,* 375–392.

331

Baucom, D. H., Shoham, V., Mueser, K. T., & Daiuto, A. D. (1998). Empirically supported couple and family interventions for marital distress and adult mental health problems. *Journal of Consulting and Clinical Psychology, 66*, 53–88.

Beach, S. R. H., Jouriles, E. N., & O'Leary, K. D. (1985). Extramarital sex: Impact on depression and commitment in couples seeking marital therapy. *Journal of Sex and Marital Therapy, 11*(2), 99–108.

Beck, A. T., Steer, R. A., & Brown, G. K. (1996). *Manual for the Beck Depression Inventory–II*. San Antonio, TX: Psychological Corporation.

Betzig, L. (1989). Causes of conjugal dissolution: A cross-cultural study. *Current Anthropology, 30*, 654–676.

Brown, E. M. (1991). *Patterns of infidelity and their treatment*. New York: Brunner/Mazel.

Buehler, C., & Gerard, J. M. (2002). Marital conflict, ineffective parenting, and children's and adolescents' maladjustment. *Journal of Marriage and Family, 64*, 78–92.

Buunk, B. P., & Bakker, A. B. (1995). Extradyadic sex: The role of descriptive and injunctive norms. *Journal of Sex Research, 32*, 313–318.

Cano, A., Christian-Herman, J., O'Leary, K. D., & Avery-Leaf, S. (2002). Antecedents and consequences of negative marital stressors. *Journal of Marital and Family Therapy, 28*, 145–151.

Cano, A., & O'Leary, K. D. (2000). Infidelity and separations precipitate major depressive episodes and symptoms of nonspecific depression and anxiety. *Journal of Consulting and Clinical Psychology, 68*, 774–781.

Charny, I. W., & Parnass, S. (1995). The impact of extramarital relationships on the continuation of marriages. *Journal of Sex and Marital Therapy, 21*, 100–115.

Daly, M., & Wilson, M. (1988). *Homicide*. New York: Aldine de Gruyter.

Derogatis, L. R., & Savitz, K. L. (1999). The SCL-90–R, Brief Symptom Inventory, and matching clinical rating scales. In M. E. Maruish (Ed.), *The use of psychological testing for treatment planning and outcomes assessment* (2nd ed., pp. 679–724). Mahwah, NJ: Erlbaum.

DiBlasio, F. A. (1998). The use of decision-based forgiveness intervention within intergenerational family therapy. *Journal of Family Therapy, 20*, 77–94.

Edwards, J. N., & Booth, A. (1976). Sexual behavior in and out of marriage: An assessment of correlates. *Journal of Marriage and Family, 38*, 73–81.

Ehrensaft, M. K., & Vivian, D. (1996). Spouses' reasons for not reporting existing marital aggression as a marital problem. *Journal of Family Psychology, 10*, 443–453.

Ellis, A. (1969). Healthy and disturbed reasons for having extramarital relations. In G. Neubeck (Ed.), *Extramarital relations* (pp. 153–161). Englewood Cliffs, NJ: Prentice Hall.

Enright, R. D. (2001). Forgiveness is a choice: A step-by-step process for resolving anger and restoring hope. In R. D. Enright (Ed.), *Reconciling* (pp. 263–276). Washington, DC: American Psychological Association.

Epstein, N., & Baucom, D. H. (2002). *Enhanced cognitive-behavioral therapy for couples: A contextual approach.* Washington, DC: American Psychological Association.

Fals-Stewart, W., Birchler, G. R., & O'Farrell, T. J. (2003). Alcohol and other substance abuse. In D. K. Snyder & M. A. Whisman (Eds.), *Treating difficult couples: Helping clients with coexisting mental and relationship disorders* (pp. 159–180). New York: Guilford Press.

Fincham, F. D., Hall, J., & Beach, S. R. H. (2006). Forgiveness in marriage: Current status and future directions. *Family Relations, 55,* 415–427.

Fruzzetti, A. E., & Fruzzetti, A. R. (2003). Borderline personality disorder. In D. K. Snyder & M. A. Whisman (Eds.), *Treating difficult couples: Helping clients with coexisting mental and relationship disorders* (pp. 235–260). New York: Guilford Press.

Glass, S. P. (2003). *Not "just friends": Protect your relationship from infidelity and heal the trauma of betrayal.* New York: Free Press.

Glass, S. P., & Wright, T. L. (1985). Sex differences in type of extramarital involvement and marital dissatisfaction. *Sex Roles, 12*(9/10), 1101–1119.

Glass, S. P., & Wright, T. L. (1992). Justifications for extramarital relationships: The association between attitudes, behaviors, and gender. *Journal of Sex Research, 29*(3), 361–399.

Glass, S. P., & Wright, T. L. (1997). Reconstructing marriages after the trauma of infidelity. In W. K. Halford & H. J. Markman (Eds.), *Clinical handbook of marriage and couples interventions* (pp. 471–507). Chichester, UK: Wiley.

Gordon, K. C., & Baucom, D. H. (1998). Understanding betrayals in marriage: A synthesized model of forgiveness. *Family Process, 37,* 425–449.

Gordon, K. C., & Baucom, D. H. (1999). A multitheoretical intervention for promoting recovery from extramarital affairs. *Clinical Psychology: Science and Practice, 6,* 382–399.

Gordon, K. C., & Baucom, D. H. (2003). Forgiveness and marriage: Preliminary support for a measure based on a model of recovery from a marital betrayal. *American Journal of Family Therapy, 31,* 179–199.

Gordon, K. C., Baucom, D. H., & Floyd, F. J. (2008). *Forgive or just move on?: Preliminary evidence for different strategies and their implications for marital relationships.* Unpublished manuscript.

Gordon, K. C., Baucom, D. H., & Snyder, D. K. (2000). The use of forgiveness in marital therapy. In M. E. McCullough, K. I. Pargament, & C. E. Thoresen (Eds.), *Forgiveness: Theory, research, and practice* (pp. 203–227). New York: Guilford Press.

Gordon, K. C., Baucom, D. H., & Snyder, D. K. (2004). An integrative intervention for promoting recovery from extramarital affairs. *Journal of Marital and Family Therapy, 30,* 213–231.

Gordon, K. C., Baucom, D. H., & Snyder, D. K. (2005). Treating couples recovering from infidelity: An integrative approach. *Journal of Clinical Psychology: In-Session, 61*(11), 1393–1406.

Gordon, K. C., Dixon, L. J., Baucom, D. H., & Snyder, D. K. (2007, November). *It pulled the rug out from under me.* . . . Paper presented at the 41st annual meeting of the Association for Behavioral and Cognitive Therapies, Philadelphia.

Gordon, K. C., Hughes, F. M., Tomcik, N. D., & Litzinger, S. (2006, November). *Widening circles of impact: The role of forgiveness in individual, marital, and family functioning.* Paper presented at the 40th annual meeting of the Association for Behavioral and Cognitive Therapies, Chicago.

Gottlieb, B. H. (1996). Theories and practices of mobilizing support in stressful circumstances. In C. L. Cooper (Ed.), *Handbook of stress, medicine and health* (pp. 339–356). Boca Raton, FL: CRC Press.

Gottman, J. M. (1979). Detecting cyclicity in social interaction. *Psychological Bulletin, 86,* 338–348.

Gottman, J. M. (1994). *Why marriages succeed or fail and how to make yours last.* New York: Simon & Schuster.

Gottman, J. M. (1999). *The marriage clinic: A scientifically-based marital therapy.* New York: Norton.

Greeley, A. (1994). Marital infidelity. *Society, 31,* 9–13.

Greene, B. L., Lee, R. R., & Lustig, N. (1974). Conscious and unconscious factors in marital infidelity. *Medical Aspects of Human Sexuality, 8,* 97–105.

Heyman, R. E. (2001). Observation of couple conflicts: Clinical assessment applications, stubborn truths, and shaky foundations. *Psychological Assessment, 13,* 5–35.

Holzworth-Munroe, A., Marshall, A. D., Meehan, J. C., & Rehman, U. (2003). Physical aggression. In D. K. Snyder & M. A. Whisman (Eds.), *Treating difficult couples: Helping clients with coexisting mental and relationship disorders* (pp. 201–230). New York: Guilford Press.

Horowitz, M. J. (1985). Disasters and psychological responses to stress. *Psychiatric Annals, 15*(3), 161–167.

Horowitz, M. J., Stinson, C., & Field, N. (1991). Natural disasters and stress response syndromes. *Psychiatric Annals, 21*(9), 556–562.

Howell, A., & Conway, M. (1992). Mood and suppression of positive and negative self-referent thoughts. *Cognitive Therapy and Research, 16,* 535–555.

Jacobson, N. S., & Christensen, A. (1996a). *Acceptance and change in couple therapy: A therapist's guide for transforming relationships.* New York: Norton.

Jacobson, N. S., & Christensen, A. (1996b). *Integrative couple therapy: Promoting acceptance and change.* New York: Norton.

Janoff-Bulman, R. (1989). Assumptive worlds and the stress of traumatic events: Applications of the schema construct. *Social Cognition, 7,* 113–136.

Janus, S. S., & Janus, C. L. (1993). *The Janus report on sexual behavior.* New York: Wiley.

Johnson, S. M. (1996). *The practice of emotionally focused marital therapy.* New York: Brunner/Mazel.

Johnson, S. M., & Denton, W. (2002). Emotionally focused couple therapy: Creating secure connections. In A. S. Gurman & N. S. Jacobson (Eds.), *Clinical handbook of couple therapy* (3rd ed., pp. 221–250). New York: Guilford Press.

Johnson, S. M., & Greenberg, L. S. (1985). Emotionally focused couples therapy: An outcome study. *Journal of Marital and Family Therapy, 11*(3), 313–317.

Johnson, S. M., & Greenberg, L. S. (1995). The emotionally focused approach to problems in adult attachment. In N. S. Jacobson & A. S. Gurman (Eds.), *Clinical handbook of couple therapy* (pp. 121–141). New York: Guilford Press.

Joseph, S., Yule, W., & Williams, R. (1993). Post-traumatic stress: Attributional aspects. *Journal of Traumatic Stress, 6*(4), 501–513.

Karney, B. R., Bradbury, T. N., Fincham, F. D., & Sullivan, K. T. (1994). The role of negative affectivity in the association between attributions and marital satisfaction. *Journal of Personality and Social Psychology, 66*, 413–424.

Kirby, J. S., & Baucom, D. H. (2007a). Integrating dialectical behavior therapy and cognitive-behavioral couple therapy: A couples skills group for emotion dysregulation. *Cognitive and Behavioral Practice, 14*, 394–405.

Kirby, J. S., & Baucom, D. H. (2007b). Treating emotional dysregulation in a couples context: A pilot study of a couples skills group intervention. *Journal of Marital and Family Therapy, 33*(3), 1–17.

Klassen, W. (1966). *The forgiving community*. Philadelphia: Westminster Press.

Lauman, E. O., Gagnon, J. H., Michael, R. T., & Michaels, S. (1994). *The social organization of sexuality*. Chicago: University of Chicago Press.

Lawson, A. (1988). *Adultery: An analysis of love and betrayal*. New York: Basic Books.

Linehan, M. M. (1993). *Cognitive-behavioral treatment of borderline personality disorder*. New York: Guilford Press.

Lusterman, D. (1997). Repetitive infidelity, womanizing and Don Juanism. In R. F. Levant & G. R. Brooks (Eds.), *Men and sex: New psychological perspectives* (pp. 84–99). New York: Wiley.

Marshall, A. G. (2005, June 11). Ringing changes on illicit affairs. *TimesOnline*. Available at *www.timesonline.co.uk/tol/life_and_style/health/features/article531753.ece*.

McCann, I. L., Sakheim, D. K., & Abrahamson, D. J. (1988). Trauma and victimization: A model of psychological adaptation. *The Counseling Psychologist, 16*, 531–594.

McCullough, M. E., Worthington, E. L., Jr., & Rachal, K. C. (1997). Interpersonal forgiving in close relationships. *Journal of Personality and Social Psychology, 73*, 321–336.

Miller, W. R., & Rollnick, S. (2002). *Motivational interviewing: Preparing people for change* (2nd ed.). New York: Guilford Press.

Murphy, J. G. (2005). Forgiveness, self-respect, and the value of resentment. In E. L. Worthington (Ed.), *Handbook of forgiveness* (pp. 33–40). New York: Routledge.

Papp, L. M., Goeke-Morey, M. C., & Cummings, E. M. (2007). Linkages between spouses' psychological distress and marital conflict in the home. *Journal of Family Psychology, 21*, 533–537.

Prins, K. S., Buunk, B. P., & Van Yperen, N. W. (1993). Equity, normative disapproval, and extramarital relationships. *Journal of Social and Personal Relationships, 10,* 39–53.

Rathus, J. H., & Feindler, E. L. (2004). *Assessment of partner violence: A handbook for researchers and practitioners.* Washington, DC: American Psychological Association.

Resick, P. A., & Calhoun, K. S. (2001). Posttraumatic stress disorder. In D. H. Barlow (Ed.), *Clinical handbook of psychological disorders* (3rd ed., pp. 60–113). New York: Guilford Press.

Rye, M. S., Pargament, K. I., Ali, M. A., Beck, G. L., Dorff, E. N., Hallisey, C., et al. (2000). Religious perspectives on forgiveness. In M. E. McCullough, K. I. Pargament, & C. E. Thoresen (Eds.), *Forgiveness: Theories, research and practice* (pp. 17–40). New York: Guilford Press.

Sexton, T. L., Gordon, K. C., Gurman, A. S., Lebow, J. L., Holtzworth-Monroe, A., & Johnson, S. M. (2008). *Recommendations from the Division 43: Family Psychology Task Force on Evaluating Evidence-Based Treatments in Couple and Family Psychology.* Unpublished manuscript.

Singer, J. A., & Salovey, P. (1988). Mood and memory: Evaluation of the network theory of affect. *Clinical Psychology Review, 8,* 211–251.

Smith, T. W. (1994). Attitudes toward sexual permissiveness: Trends, correlates, and behavioral connections. In A. S. Rossi (Ed.), *Sexuality across the life course* (pp. 63–97). Chicago: University of Chicago Press.

Snyder, D. K. (1997). *Manual for the Marital Satisfaction Inventory.* Los Angeles: Western Psychological Services.

Snyder, D. K. (1999). Affective reconstruction in the context of a pluralistic approach to couple therapy. *Clinical Psychology Science and Practice, 6,* 348–365.

Snyder, D. K., & Abbott, B. V. (2002). Couple distress. In M. M. Antony & D. H. Barlow (Eds.), *Handbook of assessment and treatment planning for psychological disorders* (pp. 341–374). New York: Guilford Press.

Snyder, D. K., Baucom, D. H., & Gordon, K. C. (2007). *Getting past the affair: A program to help you cope, heal, and move on—together or apart.* New York: Guilford Press.

Snyder, D. K., Castellani, A. M., & Whisman, M. A. (2006). Current status and future directions in couple therapy. *Annual Review of Psychology, 57,* 317–344.

Snyder, D. K., & Doss, B. D. (2005). Treating infidelity: Clinical and ethical directions. *Journal of Clinical Psychology: In-Session, 61,* 1453–1465.

Snyder, D. K., Heyman, R., & Haynes, S. N. (2005). Evidence-based approaches to assessing couple distress. *Psychological Assessment, 17,* 288–307.

Snyder, D. K., & Wills, R. M. (1989). Behavioral versus insight-oriented marital therapy: Effects on individual and interspousal functioning. *Journal of Consulting and Clinical Psychology, 57,* 39–46.

Spanier, G. B., & Margolis, R. L. (1983). Marital separation and extramarital sexual behavior. *Journal of Sex Research, 19,* 23–48.

Straus, M. A., Hamby, S. L., Boney-McCoy, S., & Sugarman, D. B. (1996). The

Revised Conflict Tactics Scales (CTS2): Development and preliminary psychometric data. *Journal of Family Issues, 17*(3), 283–316.

Sullivan, M. J. L., & Conway, M. (1991). Dysphoria and valence attributions for others' behavior. *Cognitive Therapy and Research, 15,* 273–282.

Taft, C. T., Watkins, L. E., Stafford, J., Street, A. E., & Monson, C. (2007, November). *PTSD and relationship functioning: A meta-analysis.* Paper presented at the 41st annual meeting of the Association for Behavioral and Cognitive Therapies, Philadelphia.

Treas, J., & Giesen, D. (2000). Sexual infidelity among married and cohabiting Americans. *Journal of Marriage and Family, 62,* 48–60.

Vaughn, P. (1998). *The monogamy myth.* New York: Newmarket Press.

Veroff, J., Douvan, E., & Hatchett, S. J. (1995). *Marital instability: A social and behavioral study of the early years.* Westport, CT: Praeger.

Whisman, M. A., Dixon, A. E., & Johnson, B. (1997). Therapists' perspectives of couple problems and treatment issues in couple therapy. *Journal of Family Psychology, 11,* 361–366.

Whisman, M. A., Gordon, K. C., & Chatav, Y. (2007). Predicting sexual infidelity in a nationally representative sample: The relative contributions of vulnerability, stressors, and opportunity. *Journal of Family Psychology, 21,* 320–324.

Whisman, M. A., & Snyder, D. K. (2007). Sexual infidelity in a national survey of American women: Differences in prevalence and correlates as a function of method of assessment. *Journal of Family Psychology, 21,* 147–154.

Wiggins, J. D., & Lederer, D. A. (1984). Differential antecedents of infidelity in marriage. *American Mental Health Counselors Association Journal, 6,* 152–161.

Worthington, E. L., Jr. (Ed.). (2005). *Handbook of forgiveness.* New York: Brunner-Routledge.

Younger, J. W., Piferi, R. L., Jobe, R. L., & Lawler, K. A. (2004). Dimensions of forgiveness: The views of laypersons. *Journal of Social and Personal Relationships, 21*(6), 837–855.

Zechmeister, J. S., & Romero, C. (2002). Victim and offender accounts of interpersonal conflict: Autobiographical narratives of forgiveness and unforgiveness. *Journal of Personality and Social Psychology, 82,* 675–686.

Index

Page numbers followed by a *t* indicate tables.

Abandonment, associated feelings of, 5
Accountability, partners' roles and, 59–60
Acknowledgment of contributions, as
    contributing factor, 233t
Acknowledgment of feelings, 80t
Activities, as outside factor, 197–198
Advocate, therapist as, 58–59
Affairs. *see* Complex affairs; Infidelity
Affective-reconstructive therapy, 18
African culture, 289–290
Aggression
    assessment of, 29–30, 36
    expressions of, 76
Alcohol. *see* Substance use
Alliance, therapeutic. *see* Therapeutic
    environment
Ambivalence, infidelity and, 8t
American Psychological Association,
    research and, 21
Anger
    as contributing factor, 233t
    denial of, 127
    forgiveness and, 19, 286
    infidelity and, 8t
    meaning stage and, 148
    regulation of, 44

Anxiety
    assessment of, 33, 34
    associated feelings of, 12
    as contributing factor, 233t, 236
APA. *see* American Psychological
    Association
Approach factors, infidelity and, 8t
Arguing, as contributing factor, 150t
Arousal, PTSD and, 113
Assessment
    addressing long-term dysregulation and,
        141
    Beck Depression Inventory-II, 34
    of couple's relationship, 26–31
    domains, strategies, and treatment
        implications regarding, 27–28t
    of expectations, 37–38
    of individual strengths/vulnerabilities,
        33–36
    initial considerations regarding, 25–26
    introduction to, 24–25
    of outside stressors/resources, 36–37
    of outside-affair relationship, 31–33
    provision of initial formulation and,
        38–41
    of readiness for Stage 2, 163–164

G

Getting Past the Affair: A Program to Help You Cope, Heal, and Move On–Together or Apart (Snyder et. al.), 22–23, 42, 97, 119, 143, 170, 190, 209, 240, 269, 300, 327
Goals, treatment
  forgiveness as, 281
  during impact stage, 66–67
Grief, as contributing factor, 198–199, 233t
Guided discovery, 105
Guilt
  assessment of, 33, 34
  infidelity and, 8t
  as recovery-interfering quality, 230

H

Health care. *see* Self-care
Hierarchical relationships, complex affairs and, 247–249
Honesty
  motivations and, 316
  partners' roles and, 60
Hope, partners' roles and, 61
Hopelessness, assessment of, 36
Household chores. *see* Routines

I

Ignoring
  as contributing factor, 233t
  as therapeutic strategy, 214
Images, emotionally focused couple therapy and, 140
Impact stage
  challenges/risks during, 67–70
  complex affairs and, 251
  goals for, 66–67
  introduction to, 65
  overview of, 15–16
  summary of issues surrounding, 70–71, 328–329

Implementation of decisions, moving-on stage and, 275–276, 314–325
Impulsivity, as contributing factor, 225
Individual functioning, disruption of, 110–112
Individual partner factors. *see* Partner considerations
Individual strategies, formulation and, 259
Infidelity
  case examples of, 3–4
  complex affairs and. *see* Complex affairs
  consequences of, 10–11
  continuation of, 93–95
  framework for, 8t
  frequency of, 7
  previous incidents of, 26
  reasons for, 7–10
  talking about instances of, 88–89t
  three-stage approach to treatment of, 11–20
Influence
  as contributing factor, 233t
  by therapist, 69–70
Initiation, formulation and, 257
Insecurity, infidelity and, 8t, 9
Integrative behavioral couple therapy, 18
Interactive strategies, formulation and, 259
Interpreter, therapist as, 58
Interventions. *see also* Treatment
  assessment and, 24
  complex affairs and, 251–252
  efficacy of standard, 4–5
  flashbacks and, 114–118
  moving-on stage and, 19–20
  substance use and, 226
  by third parties, 6
Intimacy. *see also* Emotional intimacy; Sexual intimacy
  as contributing factor, 150t, 173, 174–175t, 233t, 234
  deficits in, 181–183, 183–184
  disruption of, 100, 102–104
  infidelity and, 7, 8t
  restoration of, 157
Intrusions, 193–198, 194t
Islam, forgiveness and, 288–289